Workbook for

Introductory Medical-Surgical Nursing

ELEVENTH EDITION

BARBARA K. TIMBY, RN, BC, BSN, MA
Professor Emeritus
Medical-Surgical Nursing
Glen Oaks Community College
Centreville, Michigan

NANCY E. SMITH, RN, MS
Professor and Chair
Department of Nursing
Southern Maine Community College
South Portland, Maine

Wolters Kluwer | Lippincott Williams & Wilkins
Health
Philadelphia • Baltimore • New York • London
Buenos Aires • Hong Kong • Sydney • Tokyo

Executive Editor: Chris Richardson
Product Development Editor: Helen Kogut
Editorial Assistant: Zachary Shapiro
Production Project Manager: Marian Bellus
Design Coordinator: Joan Wendt
Illustration Coordinator: Doug Smock
Manufacturing Coordinator: Karin Duffield
Prepress Vendor: Absolute Service, Inc.

11th Edition

9 8 7 6 5 4 3 2 1

Printed in the United States of America

ISBN: 978-1-4511-8722-9

Care has been taken to confirm the accuracy of the information presented and to describe generally accepted practices. However, the authors, editors, and publisher are not responsible for errors or omissions or for any consequences from application of the information in this book and make no warranty, expressed or implied, with respect to the currency, completeness, or accuracy of the contents of the publication. Application of this information in a particular situation remains the professional responsibility of the practitioner; the clinical treatments described and recommended may not be considered absolute and universal recommendations.

The authors, editors, and publisher have exerted every effort to ensure that drug selection and dosage set forth in this text are in accordance with the current recommendations and prac- tice at the time of publication. However, in view of ongoing research, changes in government regulations, and the constant flow of information relating to drug therapy and drug reactions, the reader is urged to check the package insert for each drug for any change in indications and dosage and for added warnings and precautions. This is particularly important when the recom- mended agent is a new or infrequently employed drug.

Some drugs and medical devices presented in this publication have Food and Drug Administra- tion (FDA) clearance for limited use in restricted research settings. It is the responsibility of the health care provider to ascertain the FDA status of each drug or device planned for use in his or her clinical practice.

LWW.COM

DRC1013

Contributors

David Payne, MA, BA
Freelance Development Editor
Signal Mountain, Tennessee

Judy L. Slone, RN, MSN
Professor
Department of Nursing
Glen Oaks Community College
Centreville, Michigan

Preface

This Workbook accompanies the 11th edition of *Introductory Medical-Surgical Nursing* by Barbara K. Timby and Nancy E. Smith. It is designed to help you practice and retain the knowledge you have gained from the textbook and provide a basis for applying that knowledge in your nursing practice. Each chapter of this Workbook is divided into three sections: "Assessing Your Understanding," "Applying Your Knowledge," and "Getting Ready for NCLEX."

ASSESSING YOUR UNDERSTANDING

The first section of each Workbook chapter concentrates on the basic information of the textbook chapter and helps you to remember key concepts, vocabulary, and principles. Types of exercises include the following:

- **Fill in the Blanks**. Fill in the blank exercises test important chapter information, encouraging you to recall key points.
- **Labeling**. Labeling exercises are used where you need to remember certain visual representations of the concepts presented in the textbook.
- **Matching**. Matching questions test your knowledge of the definition of key terms.
- **Sequencing**. Sequencing exercises ask you to remember particular sequences or orders, for instance, testing processes and prioritizing nursing actions.
- **Short Answers**. Short answer questions cover the facts, concepts, procedures, and principles of the chapter. These questions ask you to recall information as well as demonstrate your comprehension of the information.

APPLYING YOUR KNOWLEDGE

The second section of each Workbook chapter consists of exercises that ask you to apply the knowledge you've gained from the textbook chapter. Activities include **short answer questions** and **critical thinking exercises**. Each unit also includes a **case study activity** in which you will read a case study and then answer related questions. This activity helps you to think like a nurse and apply the knowledge that you have gained through your reading and studying to a particular client situation.

GETTING READY FOR NCLEX

The third and final section helps you practice answering NCLEX-PN questions to help reinforce the knowledge you have been gaining. In keeping with the NCLEX style, the questions presented are multiple-choice, multiple-multiple choice, and fill in the blank dosage calculation items, asking you to reflect, consider, and apply what you know and to choose the best answer out of those offered.

RESOURCES ON thePoint

The answers for all of the exercises in this Workbook are provided to your instructor on thePoint website that accompanies the textbook. Your instructor may share answers with you to allow you to check your own work, or he or she may assign Workbook chapters as assignments. You will find other helpful student resources including additional NCLEX-style chapter review questions on thePoint website.

We hope you will find this Workbook to be helpful and enjoyable, and we wish you every success in your studies toward becoming a nurse.

—*The Publishers*

Contents

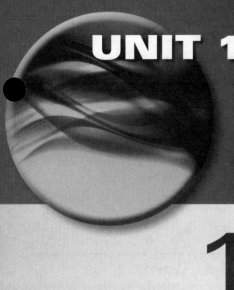

UNIT 1

NURSING ROLES AND RESPONSIBILITIES

1 Concepts and Trends in Healthcare

LEARNING OBJECTIVES

1. Explain the concepts of health, holism, wellness, illness, disease, and the health-illness continuum.
2. Describe how clients with chronic illness may still be considered healthy.
3. Differentiate health maintenance and health promotion.
4. Identify members of the healthcare team.
5. Describe three levels of care that the healthcare delivery system provides.
6. Describe problems related to access to healthcare.
7. Describe Medicare, Medicaid, and Medigap insurance.
8. Explain how a prospective payment system (PPS) works.
9. Explain how the different types of managed care organizations work.
10. Discuss the difference between capitation and fee-for-service insurance.
11. Discuss the effects of cost-driven changes on healthcare.
12. Discuss methods for monitoring quality of care.
13. Describe national and worldwide healthcare campaigns designed to improve healthcare and healthcare outcomes.
14. Identify trends that influence future healthcare policy.

SECTION 1:   ASSESSING YOUR UNDERSTANDING

Activity A   *Fill in the blanks by choosing the correct word from the options given in parentheses.*

1. _____ is a state of being sick. *(Sickness, Illness, Disease)*

2. The _____ is an active partner in nursing care. *(HMO, PPO, client)*

3. _____ refers to the full range of services available to people seeking prevention, identification, treatment, or rehabilitation of health problems. *(Home care delivery system, Healthcare delivery system, Fitness programs)*

4. _____ is a state of complete physical, mental, and social well-being and not merely the absence of disease and infirmity. *(Holism, Wellness, Health)*

5. _____ is a federally funded, state-run program that provides medical assistance for individuals and families with limited incomes and resources. *(Medicare, Medicaid, Medigap)*

Activity B *Write the correct term for each description.*

1. A perspective of viewing a person's health as a balance of body, mind, and spirit. _____

2. A group of people that consists of specially trained personnel who work together to help clients meet their healthcare needs. _____

3. A federally run program financed primarily through employee payroll taxes. _____

4. An inpatient hospital classification system used to group services for clients with similar diagnoses. _____

5. A constant and intentional effort to stay healthy and achieve the highest potential for total well-being. _____

Activity C *Match the types of care given in Column A with the descriptions given in Column B.*

Column A

_____ 1. Tertiary care

_____ 2. Home hospice care

_____ 3. Primary care

_____ 4. Skilled nursing care

_____ 5. Secondary care

Column B

a. Occurs in facilities or units that offer prolonged health maintenance or rehabilitative services, such as long-term care or extended care facilities.

b. Includes referrals to facilities for additional testing such as cardiac catheterization, consultation, and diagnosis.

c. Care is provided in hospitals where specialists and complex technology are available.

d. Resources for terminally ill clients and their families.

e. The first resource person or agency that clients contact about a health need. This initial contact is often with a family practitioner, internist, or nurse practitioner.

Activity D *Briefly answer the following questions.*

1. What is the difference between illness and disease?

_____

_____

_____

2. Which individuals are covered by Medicare?

_____

_____

_____

3. Differentiate health maintenance and health promotion.

_____

_____

_____

4. Identify the members of the healthcare team.

_____

_____

_____

5. Which groups of people are most likely to be underserved by the healthcare system?

_____

_____

_____

Activity E *Briefly answer the following questions about this client situation.*

A client's healthcare coverage is through a point-of-service (POS) plan. The client has decided to seek a second opinion about treatment options for a current healthcare issue from a physician outside the POS group. The client failed to get preapproval from her primary physician.

1. What problem does this create for the client?

_____

_____

_____

2. How does this type of POS control cost?

_____

_____

_____

3. What advantages are there to belonging to a POS plan?

_____

_____

_____

4. How does a POS plan differ from a preferred provider organization (PPO) or physician hospital organization (PHO)?

_____

_____

_____

SECTION 2:   APPLYING YOUR KNOWLEDGE

Activity F *Give rationale for the following questions.*

1. Why must members of a health maintenance organization receive authorization for secondary care?

_____

_____

_____

2. Why do some individuals delay seeking early treatment for their health problems?

_____

_____

_____

3. Why is there much criticism of the prospective payment system?

_____

_____

_____

Activity G *Answer the following questions related to concepts and trends in healthcare.*

1. What are the various methods used to ensure the quality of care?

_____

_____

_____

2. What is managed care? What are the goals of managed care?

_____

_____

_____

3. What is an integrated delivery system? What are the services provided by a fully integrated delivery system?

_____

_____

_____

4. What is the role of the nurse in illness prevention and early detection?

_____

_____

_____

Activity H *Think over the following questions. Discuss them with your instructor or peers.*

1. What are the concerns related to cost-driven changes in healthcare? What are the benefits of cost-driven healthcare?

_____

_____

_____

2. What are the advantages of using a clinical pathway to provide client care?

_____

_____

_____

3. Discuss issues with access to care and health disparities in your communities.

_____

_____

_____

4. Discuss the role of the nurse in national and worldwide healthcare campaigns.

_____

_____

_____

Activity I *Read the following case study. Use critical thinking skills to discuss and answer the questions that follow it.*

On a routine visit to her primary care office, a 45-year-old female was seen by the nurse practitioner. The client reported that she was experiencing fatigue, frequent thirst, and increased need to use the bathroom. She also said that her appetite had increased and she seemed to get hungry again soon after eating. The nurse practitioner also noted that, according to her chart, the client was overweight at 196 lb and had experienced gestational diabetes with her last pregnancy 10 years earlier. The nurse talked with the client about what she was experiencing, answered her questions, encouraged her, and discussed a course of action to achieve a diagnosis.

The nurse practitioner ordered laboratory tests, which confirmed that the client had type 2 diabetes.

The client belonged to a preferred provider organization (PPO) that encouraged her to attend diabetes education classes and a support group. The PPO also paid for the client's diabetic testing supplies, such as a glucometer, lancets, and test strips. The nurse practitioner scheduled follow-up appointments over the next few months to monitor the client's blood sugar levels and support her coping efforts. The client is following her diet and diabetes regimen closely. She is determined to stay as active and healthy as possible to reduce the chance of any future complications.

1. What were the signs and symptoms that brought the client's concerns to the attention of the nurse?

_____

_____

_____

2. Where does the client see herself along the health-illness continuum?

_____

_____

_____

3. Did the nurse address the client from a holistic perspective?

_____

_____

_____

4. How does providing the client with the tools she needs to manage her disease benefit her and her PPO?

_____

_____

_____

SECTION 3: GETTING READY FOR NCLEX

Activity J *Answer the following questions.*

1. When using a holistic approach to nursing care, the nurse must address which of the client's needs?
   1. Physical, emotional, developmental, psychological, and basic needs
   2. Spiritual, psychological, developmental, individual, and emotional needs
   3. Sociocultural, developmental, spiritual, physical, and psychological needs
   4. Individual, spiritual, basic, developmental, and physical needs

2. The nurse is on a busy medical-surgical unit on the 3 to 11 PM shift. The role of the nurse in caring for clients on this floor includes which of the following activities?
   1. Diagnosing illness and communicating the diagnosis to the client
   2. Prescribing medication and communicating with the pharmacy about the dosage
   3. Advocating for the physician and carrying out orders
   4. Collecting data and diagnosing human responses to health problems

3. A 50-year-old female client is instructed by the nurse to take all medications just ordered by the physician, to get screened in 6 months for a mammogram, and to obtain a colonoscopy. These activities by the client represent which of the following?
   1. Health promotion
   2. Health maintenance
   3. Health prevention
   4. Health detection

4. For which of the following clients should the nurse recommend Medicare?
   1. 75-year-old client with high blood pressure
   2. 35-year-old client with urinary tract infection
   3. 55-year-old client with signs of hepatic disease
   4. 15-year-old client with asthma and breathlessness

5. A client is set up for a cardiac catheterization to determine if he has a blockage in his coronary arteries. What type of care does this represent in the healthcare system?
   1. Tertiary care
   2. Secondary care
   3. Primary care
   4. Hospice care

6. Three clients come to the hospital for different surgeries. One has a total hip replacement, the second has a total knee replacement, and the third has a shoulder replacement. All of these inpatient hospital surgeries are classified the same way and are reimbursed at the same rate under DRG 209. This is an example of what type of financial payment system?
   1. Managed care organization (MCO)
   2. Preferred provider organization (PPO)
   3. Prospective payment system (PPS)
   4. Health maintenance organization (HMO)

7. A nurse is assigned to the outcomes measurement committee for the hospital. Which of the following is the goal of this committee?
   1. To identify clients of interest to the hospital
   2. To measure quality through the use of surveys
   3. To determine which cases are risk management issues
   4. To use standardized indicators to measure healthcare quality

8. A nurse is providing care to a client using a standard set of guidelines that determine aspects of care appropriate for a specific type of client. This set of guidelines is called which of the following?
   1. Case management trend report
   2. Guideline for client safety
   3. Clinical pathway
   4. Diagnosis-related report

9. Which agency helps increase quality and years of healthy life and eliminates health disparities through the Healthy People 2020 initiative?
   1. Centers for Disease Control
   2. U.S. Department of Health and Human Services
   3. U.S. Surgeon General
   4. Institute for Healthcare Improvement

10. The LPN identifies from the client's interaction that a 25-year-old African American client does not have the ability to pay for healthcare for herself and her family. This represents what kind of issue?
    1. Access to financial help issue
    2. Access to charity care issue
    3. Access to quality issue
    4. Access to care issue

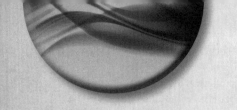

2 Settings and Models for Nursing Care

LEARNING OBJECTIVES

1. Define nursing.
2. Describe the different roles of the LPN/LVN and RN.
3. List three ways to classify healthcare agencies in which nurses practice.
4. Describe settings in which nurses practice and nurses' roles in each setting.
5. Compare nursing care delivery models.
6. Define case management and explain the nurse case manager's role.

SECTION 1: ASSESSING YOUR UNDERSTANDING

Activity A   *Fill in the blanks by choosing the correct word from the options given in parentheses.*

1. _____ have been the traditional sites for much of the nursing workforce. *(Inpatient units, Dialysis units, Same-day surgery units)*

2. _____ emerged in the 1950s to accommodate staff with varying levels of education and skill. *(Patient-focused care, Total care, Team nursing)*

3. _____ maximizes fiscal outcomes without sacrificing quality through careful oversight of a client's healthcare. *(Case management, Patient-focused care, Primary nursing)*

Activity B   *Write the correct term for each model of nursing care delivery description.*

1. The method by which one nurse provides all the services that a particular client requires. _____

2. The method of nursing where distinct duties are assigned to specific personnel. _____

3. The updated version of primary care and team nursing that uses an RN partnered with an LVN/LPN, respiratory therapist, and/or unlicensed personnel. _____

Activity C

Match the facilities or settings given in Column A with the clients who would receive the type of care provided in Column B.

Column A

_____ 1. Acute care

_____ 2. Long-term acute care

_____ 3. Subacute care

_____ 4. Skilled nursing care

_____ 5. Intermediate care facilities

_____ 6. Rehabilitation care

_____ 7. Hospice care

_____ 8. Ambulatory care

_____ 9. Home care

_____ 10. Community health centers

_____ 11. Alternative healthcare settings

Column B

a. Nursing homes that provide custodial care for clients who cannot care for themselves because of mental or physical disabilities.

b. Clients are relatively healthy and do not need extended care but may need some assistance with ADLs.

c. Service clients with complicated or high-risk surgeries, massive trauma, or critical illness.

d. Clients who receive outpatient surgeries or treatments such as diagnostic tests or dialysis.

e. Clients who require care that is more intense than traditional long-term care but less intense than acute inpatient care.

f. Clients receive care in the home setting; care addresses long-term and short-term needs and can provide comprehensive services.

g. Clients who require long-term wound care, ventilator support, or have other conditions that are potentially unstable but do not have rapid changes.

h. Provides care for clients diagnosed with a terminal illness whose life expectancy is fewer than 6 months.

i. Clients who have the potential to regain function but need skilled observation and care during an acute illness.

j. Provide a range of services to clients within the districts, counties, or communities they serve.

k. Clients receive physical and occupational therapy to help them regain as much independence with ADLs as possible.

Activity D

Briefly answer the following questions about this client's situation.

An 82-year-old female has been living alone in her home for the past year, depending on assistance from her neighbors. The neighbors have been helping with transportation, medications, laundry, and light housekeeping. The client realizes she can no longer depend on the goodwill of her neighbors and decides to move to an assisted living center. She feels this would best meet her needs.

1. What concerns/problems should the client be aware of when considering an assisted living healthcare setting?

_____

_____

_____

2. What advantages are there to choosing this type of healthcare setting?

_____

_____

_____

3. How does this care setting differ from a boarding home?

_____

_____

_____

_____

_____

_____

_____

_____

SECTION 2: APPLYING YOUR KNOWLEDGE

Activity E *Give rationale for the following questions.*

1. Why is functional nursing confusing for the client?

_____

_____

_____

2. How did the concept of team nursing emerge?

_____

_____

_____

3. Why is the approach of primary nursing expensive? Can this model be used effectively in contemporary nursing?

_____

_____

_____

4. Why doesn't Medicare reimburse intermediate care facilities (ICFs)?

_____

_____

_____

Activity F *Answer the following questions related to settings and models for nursing care.*

1. Describe the LPN/LVN's role in providing nursing care.

_____

_____

_____

2. Why did the case method become impractical? What is the contemporary model of the case method?

_____

_____

_____

3. Who are the team members involved in team nursing? What is the unique feature of team nursing?

_____

_____

_____

4. What type of care is provided by hospice? What type of special training does hospice staff receive?

_____

_____

_____

Activity G *Think over the following questions. Discuss them with your instructor or peers.*

1. What is your definition of nursing? How does your definition align with the American Nurses Association (ANA) description of the six essential features of contemporary nursing practice?

_____

_____

_____

2. What type of nursing model would you prefer to practice? Why?

_____

_____

_____

Activity H *Read the following case study. Use critical thinking skills to discuss and answer the questions that follow it.*

A small local hospital employs a nurse case manager to oversee clients from admission to discharge. She has been following the progression of a 56-year-old male who is 3 days postoperative from a total knee replacement. This client had problems with postoperative complications last year for the same procedure on the opposite knee. The case manager notes that the client is not progressing according to his clinical pathway. She speaks with the RN who is caring for this client along with an LPN and a physical therapist and asks to be updated on how the client is doing. The RN states that the client has not yet achieved the appropriate degree of range of motion in his knee for this phase of his recovery, as reported by the physical therapist. The RN also reports that the client sometimes refuses to ambulate with his walker when requested to do so, secondary to pain. The LPN has documented in the chart that the client requests pain medication frequently and, according to his medication sheet, has been receiving it as ordered by the physician. The LPN has also documented that the client still requires assistance with some ADLs.

The client lives alone, and the plan is to discharge the client to live independently at home. The case manager talks with the client about an alternative discharge care setting to allow the client to recover at a slower pace over the next few weeks before returning to independent living at home.

1. What were the indicators to the case manager that the client wasn't ready for a home discharge yet?

_____

_____

_____

2. What alternative care setting(s) would be appropriate for this client and why?

_____

_____

_____

3. What current model of nursing is reflected in the care of this client?

_____

_____

_____

4. Do you feel the case manager's actions were based on appropriate allocation of resources for the hospital, or did she provide for the client's safety and quality of care?

_____

_____

_____

SECTION 3: GETTING READY FOR NCLEX

Activity I *Answer the following questions.*

1. Which of the following statements represents one of the essential features of the American Nurses Association 2012 definition of nursing?
   1. Coordinating care, in collaboration with a wide array of healthcare professionals
   2. Putting the patient in the best condition for nature to act upon him
   3. Carrying out those activities contributing to health, recovery, or a peaceful death
   4. Regaining independence through the use of knowledge and self-care

2. An LPN delivers care to a client in a nursing home and encounters a problem with the client's care that cannot be independently managed. In this situation, what action by the LPN is appropriate?
   1. Call the director of the facility for instructions.
   2. Ask for assistance from the client's family member.
   3. Obtain advice from another LPN.
   4. Obtain further direction from the RN supervisor.

3. The nurse works in a subacute setting. Which of the following distinguishes the subacute setting?
   1. RNs manage this setting, and LPNs do not participate in this level of care.
   2. Clients are in these facilities for 120 days or longer.
   3. Frequent assessment and periodic review of the client's progress is necessary.
   4. The client's condition changes rapidly and requires highly skilled care.

4. Which of the following describes hospices?
   1. They provide custodial care for people who cannot care for themselves.
   2. They provide physical and occupational therapy to clients and their families.
   3. They provide care for clients diagnosed with a terminal illness.
   4. They provide skilled nursing and rehabilitative care.

5. What types of clients require more intensive case management?
   1. Clients who experience complications
   2. Clients who do not have chronic illnesses
   3. Clients who undergo unnecessary diagnostic testing
   4. Clients for whom expensive resources are overused

6. How do insurance companies assess the case manager's effectiveness?
   1. By evaluating the case manager's use of tools, such as clinical pathways
   2. By assessing whether the case manager's priority is "bottom line"
   3. By determining the volume of outcome data collected by the case manager
   4. By measuring the cost of services provided to the case manager's clients

7. Which of the following describes the service provided by home health nurses?
   1. Assumes 24-hour accountability for the client's care
   2. Plans care in the primary nurse's absence
   3. Provides care for a small group of clients
   4. Manages both long-term and short-term health needs

8. Which of the following describes the total care model of hospital-based nursing care?
   1. One private duty nurse provides all the services that a particular client requires.
   2. One nurse carrys out all the care for one or a small group of clients.
   3. Distinct duties are divided among specific nursing personnel.
   4. Each nurse partners with one or more assistive personnel to care for a group of clients.

9. Which of the following statements is the definition of nursing given by Virginia Henderson?
   1. Helping people carry out those activities contributing to health or a peaceful death
   2. Applying scientific knowledge to the processes of diagnosis and treatment
   3. Promoting a caring relationship that facilitates health and healing
   4. Integrating objective data with the client's subjective experience

10. Which of the following describes the case method of nursing?
    1. A nurse assumes all the care for a small group of clients.
    2. Distinct duties are assigned to specific personnel.
    3. Accommodates staff with varying levels of education.
    4. One nurse provides all the services that a particular client requires.

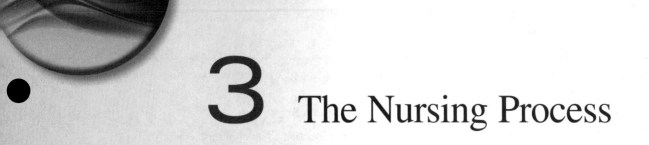

3 The Nursing Process

LEARNING OBJECTIVES

1. State the purpose of the nursing process.
2. Describe the five steps of the nursing process.
3. Define assessment.
4. Discuss the parts of a nursing diagnostic statement.
5. Differentiate types of nursing diagnoses.
6. Explain the five levels of human needs as identified by Maslow.
7. Explain how nurses use the hierarchy of needs to establish nursing priorities.
8. Define expected outcomes.
9. Explain the implementation phase of the nursing process and its relationship with documentation.
10. Explain the purpose of evaluation.
11. Give reasons why expected outcomes may not be accomplished.
12. Define critical thinking and its relevance to the nursing process.
13. List characteristics of critical thinkers.
14. Describe concept care mapping as a method to think critically about client care needs.
15. Relate concept care maps to the nursing process.

SECTION 1:   ASSESSING YOUR UNDERSTANDING

Activity A   *Fill in the blanks by choosing the correct word from the options given in parentheses.*

1. _____ serves as a comparison for future signs and symptoms and provides a reference for determining whether a client's health is improving. *(Baseline data, Client database, Ongoing assessment)*

2. _____ identifies and defines a health problem that independent or physician-prescribed nursing actions can prevent or solve. *(Assessment, Nursing diagnosis, Evaluation)*

3. The plan of care identifies _____ for achieving the outcomes. *(interventions, diagnoses, assessments)*

Activity B   *Write the correct term for each description.*

1. Specific nursing directions so that all healthcare team members understand what to do for the client. _____

2. The process that provides a systematic method for nurses to plan and implement client care to achieve desired outcomes. _____

3. The step of the nursing process that carries out the written plan of care; performs the interventions; monitors the client's status; and assesses and reassesses the client before, during, and after treatments. _____

Activity C

Match the type of nursing diagnoses given in Column A with the corresponding explanation given in Column B.

Column A

_____ **1.** Actual nursing diagnosis

_____ **2.** Health promotion nursing diagnosis

_____ **3.** Risk nursing diagnosis

_____ **4.** Syndrome diagnosis

Column B

a. Identifies a potential problem.

b. Identifies a diagnosis associated with a cluster of other diagnoses.

c. Identifies an existing problem.

d. Reflects clinical judgment of a client's motivation to increase well-being and advance health behaviors.

Activity D

Given are the human needs developed by Abraham Maslow in a jumbled order. Put the needs in order from highest priority to lowest by writing the corresponding numbers in the boxes below.

1. Esteem and self-esteem needs

2. Safety and security needs

3. Physiologic needs

4. Self-actualization needs

5. Love and belonging needs

☐→☐→☐→☐→☐

Activity E

Briefly answer the following questions.

1. How does a collaborative problem differ from a nursing diagnosis? What is the goal of a collaborative problem?

_____

_____

_____

2. What are the parts of a diagnostic statement?

_____

_____

_____

3. A client's lack of progress may result from which deficits in the nursing care plan?

_____

_____

_____

4. How does the nursing process assist nurses to acquire critical thinking and problem-solving skills?

_____

_____

_____

SECTION 2: APPLYING YOUR KNOWLEDGE

Activity F

Give rationale for the following questions.

1. Why should the nurse actively involve the client and family in care planning?

_____

_____

_____

2. Why should expected outcomes be specific, realistic, measurable, and client-centered?

_____

_____

_____

Activity G *Answer the following questions related to the nursing process.*

1. What are the responsibilities of the nurse during the assessment of a client?

_____

_____

_____

2. What are the functions served by accurate and thorough documentation in the medical record? What information should a nurse document?

_____

_____

_____

Activity H *Think over the following questions. Discuss them with your instructor or peers.*

1. You are assessing a client with postoperative right hip pain following a total hip arthroplasty. What information will you need to gather?

_____

_____

_____

2. What nursing diagnoses will you consider? What are the types of nursing diagnoses you will list?

_____

_____

_____

3. What level of priority will you give the diagnoses?

_____

_____

_____

4. How can you actively involve the client in planning and achieving positive outcomes?

_____

_____

_____

5. What would be specific, realistic, measurable, and client-centered outcomes? What would be appropriate time frames to measure the client's responses?

_____

_____

_____

6. How would you evaluate the client's responses and compare the actual outcomes to the expected outcomes?

_____

_____

_____

7. What information will be included in your documentation?

_____

_____

_____

Activity I *Read the following case study. Use critical thinking skills to discuss and answer the questions that follow it.*

A 74-year-old male is admitted with a diagnosis of chronic heart failure (CHF). The client states upon admission that he had slept the past two nights in his recliner due to shortness of breath, a moist cough, and swelling in his ankles and feet. He said that he had gained 5 lb in the last week with no changes in his diet and that activity made him very short of breath and fatigued. Upon admission, he was placed on a pulse oximeter and oxygen at 2 L per nasal cannula. The pulse oximeter showed an oxygen saturation of 91%. Vital signs were slightly elevated with an apical pulse of 94 beats/minute, but stable, with a respiratory status of 24 to 26 breaths/minute at rest. The client is accompanied by his wife who states she has been helping him dress and bathe for the last week because he becomes so short of breath.

The nurse for the oncoming shift receives report and enters the room to introduce herself to the client and his wife, complete her assessment, and obtain the client's weight. The client states he's too *fatigued* to get up and be weighed. The nurse notes that the client's respiratory effort has increased and his *respirations are now 34 to 36 breaths/minute* and *labored*. His lung sounds have *moist crackles*, and his *apical pulse is 108 beats/minute*. The client's *pulse oximeter* has dropped to *89%*. His *oxygen remains at 2 L/NC*. The wife asks the nurse if she can speak to the dietitian to learn what dietary changes will need to be made when her husband returns home.

1. Which situation in the case study should the nurse address first: weighing the client, addressing the respiratory issues, calling the dietitian, or getting the client up? Use Maslow's hierarchy of human needs in your decision making.

_____

_____

_____

2. One of the nursing diagnoses formulated for the client in the given case study is Excess Fluid Volume. What would be an appropriate goal or outcome for this nursing diagnosis?

_____

_____

_____

3. Using the given case study, what focus assessment data, gathered by the nurse, should be added to the following concept care map? (Italicized words are possible answers.)

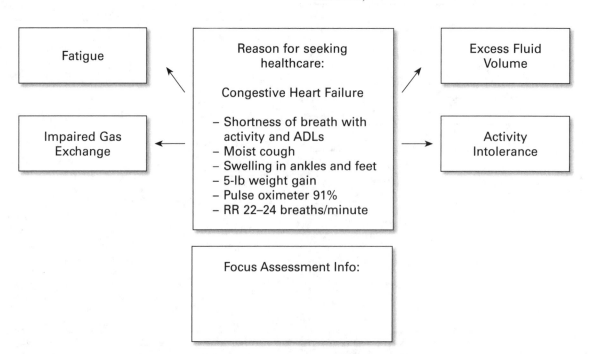

Fatigue

Reason for seeking healthcare:

Congestive Heart Failure

– Shortness of breath with activity and ADLs
– Moist cough
– Swelling in ankles and feet
– 5-lb weight gain
– Pulse oximeter 91%
– RR 22–24 breaths/minute

Excess Fluid Volume

Impaired Gas Exchange

Activity Intolerance

Focus Assessment Info:

SECTION 3: GETTING READY FOR NCLEX

Activity J *Answer the following questions marking the best response.*

1. As the nurse educator teaches a group of new students about the nursing process, which of the following is the best explanation for its purpose?
   1. It helps to systematically plan and implement care to meet a client's desired outcomes.
   2. It allows the nurse to follow steps to ensure consistency of care among professionals.
   3. It provides a language that only nurses can understand that facilitates client safety.
   4. It represents a step-by-step process that anyone can follow regardless of education.

2. There are five steps to the nursing process. When Nurse A begins with setting priorities, defining expected outcomes, and determining interventions, which step is being peformed?
   1. Assessment
   2. Diagnosis
   3. Planning
   4. Implementation

3. The nurse has developed a nursing diagnosis with a client who has determined that she wants to learn more about diet and exercise. What type of nursing diagnosis reflects the motivation by a client to increase well-being?
   1. Actual nursing diagnoses
   2. Risk nursing diagnoses
   3. Syndrome diagnoses
   4. Health promotion nursing diagnoses

4. Client A has been admitted to the hospital with severe internal bleeding following a motor vehicle accident and the loss of two of his family members. According to Maslow, which of the following needs (level) is the highest priority for the nurse when caring for a client?
   1. Love and belonging needs
   2. Self-actualization needs
   3. Esteem and self-esteem needs
   4. Physiologic needs

5. Due to prior demonstration of critical thinking skills, the nurse manager puts a veteran nurse in charge. Critical thinking is outlined in the text as which of the following?
   1. Structured, biased, and logical thinking
   2. Intentional, contemplative, and outcome-directed thinking
   3. Broad, scientific, and one-directional thinking
   4. Outcome-directed, broad, and biased thinking

6. The nurse arrives on the unit, gets report, and enters the client's room. What is the first step in the nursing process that the nurse will use?
   1. Planning
   2. Implementation
   3. Assessment
   4. Evaluation

7. A nurse educator is teaching a group of students about the steps in concept care mapping. What is the first step in this process?
   1. Diagnosis
   2. Planning
   3. Assessment
   4. Evaluation

8. A nurse, implements the nursing care plan for a client but fails to document in the medical record the interventions and the response to these interventions. The functions of documentation in (Alfaro-LeFevre, 2006) that come from accurate and thorough documentation include which of the following? Select all that apply.
   1. Creates a legal document
   2. Communicates care
   3. Supplies validation for reimbursement
   4. Substantiates the care provided by ancillary staff

9. A nurse's expected outcome for a client who is post-partum includes a goal of minimal pain of 3 on a scale of 1 to 10 by the end of the 7 AM to 3 PM shift. The client has taken Motrin every 4 hours as ordered: at 8 AM (pain level of 6 and 30 minutes later pain level of 2) as well as at 12 noon (pain level of 5 and 30 minutes later pain level of 2). Which part of the nursing process is the nurse using when analyzing the data?
   1. Assessment
   2. Evaluation
   3. Implementation
   4. Diagnosis

10. The following is a nursing diagnostic statement: Acute Pain related to tissue trauma secondary to total knee replacement as evidenced by verbalization of pain of 8 on scale of 1 to 10, restlessness, and inability to concentrate. What part of this nursing diagnosis is the name or label?
    1. Related to tissue trauma secondary to total knee replacement
    2. As evidenced by verbalization of pain of 8 on scale of 1 to 10
    3. Acute Pain
    4. Inability to concentrate

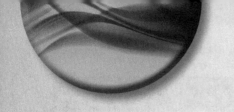

4 Interviewing and Physical Assessment

LEARNING OBJECTIVES

1. Explain the purpose of the interview and physical assessment.
2. Define subjective and objective data, symptoms, and signs.
3. Summarize the three phases of the interview process.
4. Explain the components of an interview.
5. Differentiate a systems method of assessment from a head-to-toe method of assessment.
6. Identify four assessment techniques.
7. Describe general assessment measures that all nurses can perform.

SECTION 1:   ASSESSING YOUR UNDERSTANDING

Activity A   *Fill in the blanks by choosing the correct word from the options given in parentheses.*

1. _____ are statements the client makes about what he or she feels. *(Subjective data, Objective data, Baseline data)*

2. When objective data are abnormal, they are called _____. *(symptoms, signs, chief complaints)*

3. The nurse should ask _____ questions when interviewing a client. *(exhaustive, open-ended, closed)*

4. The _____ method of physical assessment begins at the top of the body and progresses downward. *(systems, chief complaint, head-to-toe)*

Activity B   *Write the correct term for each description.*

1. A client's feelings of discomfort. _____

2. An assessment that determines how well a client can manage activities of daily living (ADLs). _____

3. Asking for detailed information about one body system or problem. _____

4. The approach used during the physical examination, which assesses each body system separately.
_____

5. The current reason the client is seeking care.
_____

Activity C   *Match the assessment techniques given in Column A with the corresponding assessments given in Column B.*

Column A	Column B
_____ 1. Inspection	a. Detects tenderness in the body.
_____ 2. Palpation	b. Detects changes in skin color.
_____ 3. Percussion	c. Detects abnormal lung sounds.
_____ 4. Auscultation	d. Detects changes in skin texture.

Activity D *Describe the following assessment techniques.*

1. Describe the procedure used for inspection.

_____

_____

_____

2. Describe the procedure used for palpation.

_____

_____

_____

3. Describe the procedure used for percussion.

_____

_____

_____

4. Describe the procedure used for auscultation.

_____

_____

_____

Activity E *Briefly answer the following questions.*

1. What is the importance of the initial assessment performed by a nurse?

_____

_____

_____

2. What information regarding psychosocial and cultural history should a nurse collect when conducting an interview with a client?

_____

_____

_____

3. What does the nurse examine and observe during the physical assessment of a client?

_____

_____

_____

4. The technique of inspection should include what measures?

_____

_____

_____

SECTION 2: APPLYING YOUR KNOWLEDGE

Activity F *Give rationale for the following questions.*

1. Why does the nurse establish a rapport and ensure that the client is comfortable during an interview process?

_____

_____

_____

2. Why does the nurse inquire about the client's use of alcohol and tobacco when collecting the health history?

_____

_____

_____

3. Why does the nurse obtain a family history when collecting the health history?

_____

_____

_____

4. When assessing a client, why should a nurse ask general questions about each body system?

_____

_____

_____

Activity G *Answer the following questions related to interviewing and physical assessment.*

1. What does the nurse identify through the systematic assessment of a client?

2. What practices should the nurse follow during the preinterview period?

3. What information should the nurse obtain when discussing the client's past medical problems?

Activity H *Think over the following questions. Discuss them with your instructor or peers.*

1. What necessary modifications will the nurse need to make when interviewing and performing an assessment on an older adult with Alzheimer's disease?

Activity I *Read the following case study. Use critical thinking skills to discuss and answer the questions that follow it.*

The nurse receives a new admission. The client is an 18-year-old male diagnosed with appendicitis. During the interview process, the nurse completes a focused assessment when collecting data about the history of his illness. When reviewing the systems of the body, once again, the nurse performs a focused assessment about the gastrointestinal system. When the interview is complete, the nurse prepares the client for a physical assessment. The nurse asks permission to touch the client and explains the overall process to the client, continuing to explain as she works. The nurse begins at the client's head and works her way down the body. She observes the client's guarded posture and color of skin and assesses the warmth of the client's skin with the back of her hand. The nurse uses her stethoscope to listen for heart, lung, and bowel sounds. She continues until she has completed her full assessment. She then uses her fingertips to palpate for any tenderness of the abdominal muscles. The client complains of *pain* with rebound tenderness in the RLQ. He states that he has been vomiting and has had no appetite for the past 24 hours. The nurse then completes a focused assessment of the client's pain, ending with vital signs that indicate a low-grade temperature of 100° F.

1. What focused assessment data do you think the nurse collected about the client's history of present illness, gastrointestinal system, and pain?

2. How would the nurse provide for the privacy of this client?

3. What assessment techniques and method of physical assessment did the nurse use?

_____

_____

_____

4. Relate the information from the given case study with the following concept care map. What nursing diagnosis in the concept care map should have the highest priority? (Italicized words are clues to the answer). Why?

_____

_____

_____

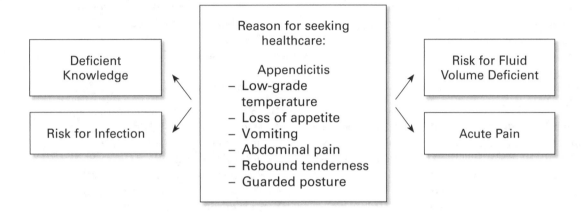

Deficient Knowledge

Risk for Infection

Reason for seeking healthcare:

Appendicitis
– Low-grade temperature
– Loss of appetite
– Vomiting
– Abdominal pain
– Rebound tenderness
– Guarded posture

Risk for Fluid Volume Deficient

Acute Pain

SECTION 3: GETTING READY FOR NCLEX

Activity J *Answer the following questions by marking the best response.*

1. Which of the following nursing assessment components is important when assessing older adults or physically challenged clients?
1. Chief complaint
2. Psychosocial history
3. Functional assessment
4. Past health history

2. What should a nurse do if a client or family member is unable to remember the name of a drug that caused a previous allergic reaction?
1. Identify the drug from another source such as the prescribing physician.
2. Ask the client or family member to describe the allergic reaction.
3. Inquire about the purpose of the drug.
4. Inquire about the family history of drug allergies.

3. Which of the following nursing interventions should the nurse perform when interviewing and performing physical assessments on older adults? Select all that apply.
1. Keep the room cool and ventilated.
2. Allow rest periods during the physical examination.
3. Observe the client performing ADLs.
4. Encourage the client to change positions frequently.
5. Ensure that the client's family member is present.

4. A nurse enters the room and determines that a client is ashen gray in color. What assessment skill has the nurse used?
1. Palpation
2. Percussion
3. Auscultation
4. Inspection

5. A nurse enters the room of a client and begins the interview. The client responds to a question regarding his respiratory system by stating the following: "I had pneumonia in 1995 and was hospitalized for 2 weeks. It was frightening because I almost died." What kind of data has the nurse collected?
   1. Objective data
   2. Subjective data
   3. Symptomatic data
   4. Chief complaint data

6. An LPN/LVN takes the blood pressure of a client and documents the finding as 130/80 mm Hg. The LVN/LPN has collected which type of data?
   1. Objective data
   2. Subjective data
   3. Symptomatic data
   4. Psychological data

7. The nurse is conducting an interview and asks the client an open-ended question. Which of the following questions are considered open-ended? Select all that apply.
   1. "What brought you to the hospital?"
   2. "Are you feeling pain right now?"
   3. "Does your abdomen hurt in this location?"
   4. "In what ways do you feel alone?"
   5. "Do you have family members who live near you?"

8. A nurse enters a client's room and detects pulsations in the client's carotid area. The actual use of the fingertips to detect pulsations is identified as what assessment technique?
   1. Palpation
   2. Percussion
   3. Inspection
   4. Auscultation

9. A nurse identifies that a client is having difficulty breathing and listens with the stethoscope to identify normal and abnormal breath sounds. The nurse is using which of the following assessment techniques?
   1. Percussion
   2. Palpation
   3. Auscultation
   4. Inspection

10. When performing an initial assessment on an older client, the nurse can best determine what the client is able to manage by himself or herself by asking which of the following questions?
    1. "Are there stairs in your house?"
    2. "Can you describe what you do everyday?"
    3. "Do you live by yourself?"
    4. "Do you wear glasses all of the time?"

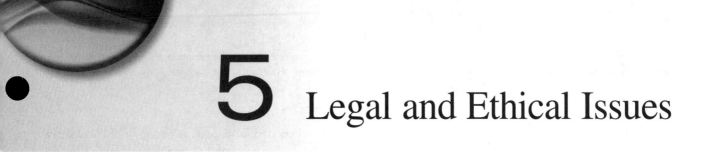

5 Legal and Ethical Issues

LEARNING OBJECTIVES

1. Explain the difference between laws and ethics.
2. Categorize sources of U.S. law.
3. Differentiate intentional and unintentional torts.
4. Summarize negligence, malpractice, and liability.
5. Describe measures such as risk management that help limit nurses' liability in malpractice suits.
6. Describe procedures and regulations to protect client information.
7. Discuss informed consent, advance directives, and do-not-resuscitate (DNR) orders.
8. Explain utilitarianism, deontology, duties, and rights.
9. Summarize the characteristics of ethical values.
10. Define six professional values.
11. Describe factors that affect healthcare ethics.
12. Explain an ethical decision-making model.

SECTION 1: ASSESSING YOUR UNDERSTANDING

Activity A *Fill in the blanks by choosing the correct word from the options given in parentheses.*

1. One of the two systems or theories that predominate in nursing ethics is _____. *(autonomy, deontology, beneficence)*

2. _____ is the duty to maintain commitments of professional obligations and responsibilities. *(Fidelity, Veracity, Justice)*

3. _____ guarantees fundamental freedom to all people in the United States. *(Statutory law, Constitutional law, Administrative law)*

4. Negligence involving licensed healthcare workers is referred to as _____. *(malpractice, intentional tort, limiting liability)*

5. _____ is the duty to be fair to all people regardless of age, sex, race, sexual orientation, or other factors. *(Justice, Veracity, Beneficence)*

6. _____ means that the person is legally responsible. *(Liability, Malpractice, Negligence)*

7. _____ is safeguarding the clients' rights and supporting their interests. *(Beneficence, Nonmaleficence, Advocacy)*

8. _____ is the duty to tell the truth, providing factual information so the client can exercise autonomy. *(Advocacy, Beneficence, Veracity)*

Activity B *Write the correct term for the descriptions about the legal and ethical issues.*

1. The outcome-oriented approach for decision making. _____

2. The rules or principles a person uses to make a decision about what is right and wrong. _____

3. The law which applies to disputes that arise between individual citizens. _____

4. The duty to do no harm to the client. _____

5. The client's right to self-determination or the freedom to make choices without any opposition. _____

6. An unofficial, handwritten, personal account of an incident made at the time of occurrence and updated as needed. _____

7. The duty to do good for the clients assigned to the nurse's care. _____

8. Law that is based on precedent, or the court will make new rules if the precedent is outdated. _____

Activity C
Match the terms associated with the legal and ethical issues given in Column A with their related explanations or definitions given in Column B.

Column A

_____ 1. Informed consent

_____ 2. Living will

_____ 3. Medical durable power of attorney

_____ 4. Do-not-resuscitate orders

Column B

a. The client designates another person to be the healthcare proxy.

b. A written medical order for end-of-life instructions.

c. A document that states a client's wishes regarding healthcare if he or she is terminally ill.

d. Voluntary permission granted by a client for medical staff to perform an invasive procedure on the client.

Activity D
Briefly answer the following questions.

1. What is tort law?

_____

_____

_____

2. What are intentional torts? Provide examples.

_____

_____

_____

3. What are unintentional torts? Provide examples.

_____

_____

_____

4. What is risk management?

_____

_____

_____

5. What are the advantages of deontology?

_____

_____

_____

6. What are the different types of assault?

_____

_____

_____

SECTION 2: APPLYING YOUR KNOWLEDGE

Activity E
Give rationale for the following questions.

1. Why is it essential for the nurse to document forewarning a client about a potential hazard to his or her safety and the client choosing to ignore the warning?

_____

_____

_____

2. Why is it difficult to reconcile nonmaleficence with medical care?

_____

_____

_____

3. Why does the state board of nursing have the authority to implement disciplinary procedures?

_____

_____

_____

4. Developments in science and technology now pose serious ethical issues. Explain this concept using examples.

_____

_____

_____

Activity F   *Answer the following questions related to legal and ethical issues.*

1. Give examples of felonies involving healthcare.

_____

_____

_____

2. What are the nursing interventions required if the nurse must apply restraints and no current medical order exists?

_____

_____

_____

3. What measures should be taken by health professionals to protect the privacy of the clients?

_____

_____

_____

4. What are the principles of the Good Samaritan law?

_____

_____

_____

5. What is the difference between negligence and malpractice? How is malpractice determined?

_____

_____

_____

_____

_____

_____

Activity G   *Answer the following questions related to the statement given.*

A nursing student has just graduated from a nursing program and is about to take her licensure exam.

1. Which agency is involved in approving her nursing program, overseeing procedures for her licensure examination, and hopefully issuing her license to practice?

_____

_____

_____

2. What defines the scope of her nursing practice and identifies her legal title as a nurse?

_____

_____

3. What guides the ethical practices of her profession?

_____

_____

_____

_____

_____

_____

Activity H   *Think over the following questions. Discuss them with your instructor or peers.*

1. Use an ethical decision-making process to evaluate the following situation:
   - A 24-year-old client is in a motor vehicle accident and deemed "brain dead." The client's parents are deceased; he has no siblings and is unmarried.
   - The client has no living will and no instructions on his driver's license indicating a preference for or against organ donation.
   - Two maternal aunts are present, and both indicate that they are opposed to organ donation and have no reason to believe that their nephew would have wished that his organs be donated. They believe the client would want life support immediately withdrawn.
   - His girlfriend is also present; she and the client have been dating for 18 months. She states that she and the client have had conversations about organ donation and his wishes were to donate if possible. She states that the client would want to remain on life support until his organs could be harvested.

2. Does your decision reflect the utilitarian or deontology view of ethics?

   _____

   _____

   _____

   _____

   _____

   _____

   _____

   _____

   _____

Activity I   *Read the following case study. Use critical thinking skills to discuss and answer the questions that follow it.*

A 42-year-old male is involved in a high-speed chase with the police and crashes his vehicle, causing deep lacerations to his forehead and arm. The police bring the client to the local emergency room to be treated prior to taking him to jail. The client is intoxicated, bleeding, yelling loudly, and threatening to harm staff and other clients in the ER. His blood alcohol level is twice the legal limit. He yells that he wants to leave and can't be held against his will. His wounds are bleeding, but he won't allow anyone to attend to them. He is assured by staff that they want to help him, but he continues to yell threats. The police warn the client to behave himself. The client is moved into a room by himself to keep him away from other clients in the ER. The nurse approaches the client to clean the lacerations before the physician sutures the wounds. The client shoves the nurse, kicks over the tray of equipment, and continues threatening anyone who comes near him. Staff members once again explain the procedure for suturing, but the client continues to yell and threaten everyone. The police officer remains at the bedside to help control the client's behavior. The nurse informs the client that if he agrees to hold still, does not hit anyone, and allows his wounds to be sutured, he can leave. She informs the client that if he doesn't cooperate, they may need to restrain him further for his own safety. The client momentarily agrees, but when the physician begins to set up the suture tray, the client knocks it over, yells, and tries to hit a passing lab technician. The client wrestles with police and is put back in bed. The physician orders the client to be restrained × 4 just long enough to sew him up and discharge him.

1. Would the nurse's statement about possibly restraining the client further if he didn't cooperate be considered informative or assault? Why?

   _____

   _____

   _____

2. Is the staff guilty of battery by attending to the client's wounds without his consent?

   _____

   _____

   _____

3. Would placing the client in restraints × 4 long enough to attend to his wounds be considered false imprisonment? Why?

_____

_____

_____

4. What should be included in the nurse's documentation about this client situation?

_____

_____

_____

SECTION 3: GETTING READY FOR NCLEX

Activity J *Answer the following questions.*

1. Which of the following actions places a nurse at risk for being accused of invading a client's privacy?
  1. The nurse verbally attacks a client's character in front of other clients.
  2. The nurse writes a damaging statement that is read by others.
  3. The nurse allows unauthorized persons to observe the client during care.
  4. The nurse offers exaggerated negative opinions about the clients.

2. A client tells the unlicensed assistive personnel (UAP) that it seemed like the surgical wound "gave way" when turned in bed. The UAP reports this to the RN, who says, "When you get a minute take a look at the wound for me." A half-hour later the client yells out that the wound has come apart and is bleeding. Which of the following poses potential liability for the nurse?
  1. The nurse failed to call the doctor after the UAP's report.
  2. The nurse failed to document what the UAP said.
  3. The nurse failed to monitor changes in the client's status.
  4. The nurse failed to treat the client with respect.

3. A pre-op client needs to sign the consent form for surgery. When the RN signs as a witness to the client's signature, it validates which of the following things? Select all that apply.
  1. The client is competent to sign.
  2. The client's consent is voluntary.
  3. The client has all questions answered.
  4. The client' signature is authentic.
  5. The client understands what he or she is signing.

4. A family requests that a client with terminal cancer not be told about the diagnosis or prognosis. The client says to the RN, "I know something is seriously wrong with me, but the doctor says everything is fine. Do you know what is wrong with me?" Which of the following statements by the RN supports the ethical principle of veracity?
  1. "I think you should speak with the M.D. about your concerns."
  2. "The M.D. would never tell you incorrect information."
  3. "What makes you think that something is really wrong?"
  4. "Your family requested that you not be told your diagnosis."

5. A nurse is faced with an ethical dilemma re: the client's care. If the nurse uses a deontological argument, which of the following would apply?
  1. Consequences are the only important consideration.
  2. Consequences are good if they bring pleasure.
  3. Duty is equally important.
  4. The greatest good for the greatest number.

6. An order is written to discontinue the tube feeding on a client who has been comatose for two years. How will a nurse who embraces utilitarian philosophy most likely react?
  1. The nurse will oppose the decision as immoral.
  2. The nurse will support the decision as a necessity.
  3. The nurse will think that an ethics committee should decide.
  4. The nurse will want more information before carrying out the order.

7. A nurse enters the client's room and discovers the client has fallen. Which of the following is the most accurate documentation?
1. "Client collapsed when getting out of bed."
2. "Client found on floor next to the bed."
3. "Client got out of bed after being told to stay in bed."
4. "Client tried to get the urinal and fell out of bed."

8. An elderly client is admitted for persistent incontinence and burning on urination. The client has difficulty communicating because of a heavy accent. Who should make the decisions regarding the client's care?
1. The client.
2. The client's son.
3. The physician.
4. The primary care giver.

9. The nurse is administering a scheduled medication to a mildly confused client. The client states, "This pill looks different than any I take". What should the nurse do?
1. Ask what the other pills look like.
2. Check the original medication order.
3. Encourage the client to take the medication.
4. Explain the purpose of the medication.

10. A client with terminally ill with cancer has three treatment options for managing the pain. The nurse determines that one option will be of most benefit and does not confer with the client about the client's preferred choice. Which ethical principle has this nurse violated?
1. Autonomy
2. Beneficence
3. Justice
4. Nonmalificence

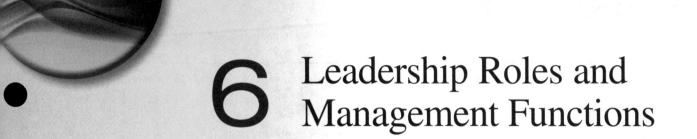

6 Leadership Roles and Management Functions

LEARNING OBJECTIVES

1. Differentiate leadership and management.
2. Define three styles of leadership.
3. Outline the purpose of power in the leadership role.
4. Describe the role of the LPN/LVN in managing client care.
5. Distinguish delegation and supervision.
6. Compare responsibility and accountability.
7. Discuss problems that may occur with delegation and supervision.
8. Describe the role of the LPN/LVN in collaboration and advocacy.
9. Explain the role of the LPN/LVN in resource management.
10. Discuss methods of managing time effectively.

SECTION 1:   ASSESSING YOUR UNDERSTANDING

Activity A   *Fill in the blanks by choosing the correct word from the options given in parentheses.*

1. _____ involves qualities related to a person's character and behavior as well as roles within a group or organization. *(Leadership, Management, Supervision)*

2. _____ means promoting the cause of another person or an organization. *(Collaboration, Advocacy, Acuity)*

3. A team effort to achieve client care outcomes is called _____. *(collaboration, advocacy, resource management)*

Activity B   *Write the correct term for each description.*

1. The ability to control, influence, or hold authority over an individual or a group. _____

2. Procrastination, inefficient use of time, inability to delegate, and socializing. _____

3. Transferring to a competent individual the authority to perform a selected nursing task in a selected situation. _____

4. The term used to measure the degree of a client's illness and identify the care required to meet the client's needs. _____

Activity C *Match the types of power given in Column A with related examples given in Column B.*

Column A

_____ **1.** Reward power

_____ **2.** Coercive power

_____ **3.** Legitimate power

_____ **4.** Expert power

_____ **5.** Referent power

_____ **6.** Informational power

Column B

a. Power due to knowledge one has that others need to accomplish certain goals.

b. Power attained through the ability to grant favors or rewards.

c. Power that results from knowledge, expertise, or experience.

d. Power exerted through threat of punishment.

e. Power exercised through a designated position.

f. Power due to association with others who are powerful.

Activity D *Briefly answer the following questions.*

1. What qualities must effective leaders and managers possess?

_____

_____

_____

2. What are the overall goals of the manager?

_____

_____

_____

3. What are the five rights of delegation?

_____

_____

_____

4. What are the three basic steps for managing time?

_____

_____

_____

SECTION 2: APPLYING YOUR KNOWLEDGE

Activity E *Answer the following questions related to leadership roles and management functions.*

1. Explain the role of LPN/LVN as a leader/manager in various healthcare settings.

_____

_____

_____

2. What steps are required by an LPN/LVN to carry out the five rights of delegation?

_____

_____

_____

3. Describe the role of supervision as it relates to delegation.

_____

_____

_____

4. What are the cost-conscious measures the nurse should follow?

_____

_____

_____

5. What are the traits that distinguish the integrated leader/manager from those who are just leaders or managers?

_____

_____

_____

_____

_____

_____

Activity F   *Think over the following questions. Discuss them with your instructor or peers.*

1. Prioritize the given tasks, indicating which tasks the LPN should attend to and which tasks the LPN should delegate.
   (i)   A client who does not experience adequate pain relief from a prescribed analgesic
   (ii) A client with diabetes mellitus who requires an insulin injection
   (iii) A client who is very scared about a surgery scheduled for later in the week
   (iv) A client who is stable and requests assistance to the bathroom
   (v)   A client who requires a dressing change

2. An LPN is assigned as the team leader in a long-term care facility. Which type of leadership style would be ideal in this care facility? What issues with delegation and supervision may occur for the LPN as a result of his or her position as the team leader?

_____

_____

_____

Activity G   *Read the following case study. Use critical thinking skills to discuss and answer the questions that follow it.*

The nurse receives her assigned group of clients and takes report. Today, she is working with an unlicensed assistive person (UAP). The nurse delegates the tasks of vital signs and morning care to the UAP. She instructs the UAP that a specific client needs his walker when transferring and asks the UAP to let her know the blood pressure for the client in room 345. The nurse then quickly reviews the morning labs and begins the task of completing physical assessments on all her clients before passing morning medications.

As the nurse enters the room of her second client, she recognizes the client's visitors. The nurse becomes involved in a lengthy conversation with them about their recent vacation. The nurse is late getting to her next client but continues to socialize with other colleagues and visitors along the way. As the nurse finally approaches the last client's room, a visitor recognizes her from his prior hospitalization and they stop to chat about the local football team. Later, when her assessments are complete, the nurse heads to the medication room only to be sidelined by a fellow nurse. Her colleague asks her to help move a client who just returned from recovery. Even though the nurse is quite late in passing her meds, she agrees to help because she doesn't want to say no. Throughout the shift, the nurse checks on the UAP to see how she is doing with her assignment and provides positive feedback but fails to make notes about the information given her from the UAP.

When passing medications, a client complains to the nurse that one of her medications makes her extremely nauseated and asks if she can take something else instead. After making a few inquiries of the client, the nurse states that she will contact the physician and let him know the situation. The nurse contacts the physician, who orders another medication. The nurse informs the client of the change.

By the end of the shift, the nurse is still lagging behind schedule and doesn't complete her documentation until 30 minutes after her shift ends.

1. If you were supervising the nurse in the case study, how would you evaluate her time management skills?

_____

_____

_____

2. Was the nurse in the case study appropriate in her delegation and supervision of client care?

_____

_____

_____

3. How did the nurse demonstrate advocacy and collaboration?

_____   _____

_____   _____

_____   _____

SECTION 3:   GETTING READY FOR NCLEX

Activity H   _Answer the following questions._

1. Student nurses are discussing the advantage of a democratic leadership style. Which of the following statements is correct?
1. Staff members acknowledge the manager's role.
2. Staff members share the process of making decisions for the group.
3. Subordinates contribute to decision making and policy making.
4. Subordinates perform at high levels because of their independence.

2. Which of the nurses described in the following situations is engaged in the following situations is engaged in coercive power?
1. The charge nurse teaches the new nursing assistant how to use a blood pressure device.
2. The nurse, spouse of the medical director, persuades others to join a professional organization.
3. The nurse in charge of scheduling controls how the vacation and holiday requests are granted.
4. The team leader is passionate about heart health and gets other staff involved with a heart walk.

3. Which of the following techniques is useful in learning to manage time?
1. Assess expectations for 24 hours at a time.
2. Do one thing at a time and avoid multitasking.
3. Use a worksheet to identify specific tasks.
4. Avoid delegating tasks.

4. The LPN/LVN may experience some problems with delegation and supervision of tasks. Which of the following is the solution when confronting problems?
1. Focus primarily on client care needs.
2. Have the UAP perform tasks alone.
3. Be friendly with coworkers.
4. Ask the UAP to evaluate the client's response.

5. Which of the following is the power a nurse has because of his or her association with others who are powerful?
1. Coercive power
2. Referent power
3. Legitimate power
4. Reward power

6. An LPN/LVN supervisor is working as a charge nurse in a long term care facility. When is the LPN/LVN responsible for supervising tasks delegated to the UAP?
1. Immediately upon receiving the direction until the task is done
2. Upon implementation of the task, throughout procedure, including evaluation
3. When the procedure is completed
4. For as long as the client is on the unit

7. An LPN/LVN is taking care of a client and changes a dressing that should not have been changed. The LPN/LVN seeks out the RN and lets the RN know what transpired. The LPN/LVN demonstrated what trait?
1. Responsibility
2. Advocacy
3. Collaboration
4. Accountability

8. A leader communicates an organizational change through an email to the nurse managers and asks them to convey the change to the staff. This is an example of what type of leadership?
1. Laissez-faire
2. Democratic
3. Autocratic
4. Multicratic

9. A nurse often focuses on group process, information gathering, feedback, and empowerment when involved with nursing unit decisions. What role is this nurse involved in?
1. Leadership
2. Management
3. Supervision
4. Delegation

10. An LPN/LVN is involved with maintaining client dignity by being well-informed about the client's care, supporting the client's decisions, and communicating the client's wishes. This is an example of what role for the LPN/LVN?
1. Collaboration
2. Advocacy
3. Responsibility
4. Accountability

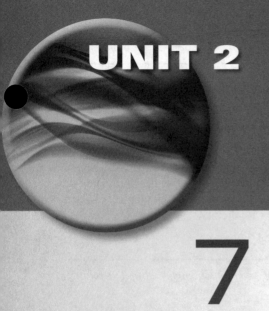

7 Nurse–Client Relationships

LEARNING OBJECTIVES

1. List four roles that nurses perform within the nurse–client relationship.
2. Describe three phases in a nurse–client relationship.
3. Differentiate between verbal, nonverbal, and therapeutic communication.
4. Give examples of therapeutic and nontherapeutic communication techniques.
5. List and explain five components of nonverbal communication.
6. Name and explain the four proxemic zones.
7. Explain what is meant by a client's "comfort zone."
8. Differentiate between task-oriented and affective touch.
9. Name three groups of clients for whom alternative communication modalities are required.
10. List six factors to consider before teaching clients.
11. Explain the learning styles of cognitive, affective, and psychomotor learners.
12. Compare informal with formal learning.
13. Discuss three techniques for evaluating learning comprehension.

SECTION 1: ASSESSING YOUR UNDERSTANDING

Activity A   *Fill in the blanks by choosing the correct word from the options given in parentheses.*

1. A(n) _____ is one who performs health-related activities that a sick person is unable to perform independently. *(caregiver, educator, collaborator)*

2. _____ is an exchange of information. *(Hearing, Communication, Listening)*

3. The _____ processes information best by listening to or reading facts and descriptions. *(cognitive learner, affective learner, psychomotor learner)*

4. An organized arrangement of content in a specific time frame is known as _____. *(formal teaching, a teaching plan, a learning style)*

5. _____ refers to using verbal and nonverbal communication to promote a person's physical and emotional well-being. *(Therapeutic communication, Touch, Proxemics)*

6. _____ refers to a person's intellectual ability to understand, remember, and apply new information. *(Motivation, Learning capacity, Learning readiness)*

Activity B *Write the correct term for each description related to the nurse–client relationship.*

1. One who works with others to achieve a common goal.
_____

2. Manner in which a person best comprehends new information. _____

3. An intuitive awareness of what the client is experiencing, to perceive the client's emotional state and need for support. _____

4. The skills and concepts that the client and family must acquire to restore, maintain, or promote health.
_____

5. This relationship exists during the period when the nurse interacts with clients, sick or well, to promote or restore their health, help them cope with their illness, or assist them to die with dignity. _____

Activity C *Match the terms associated with nurse–client relationships given in Column A with their related explanations or definitions given in Column B.*

Column A

_____ 1. Kinesics

_____ 2. Paralanguage

_____ 3. Proxemics

_____ 4. Touch

_____ 5. Silence

Column B

a. Refers to the use of space when communicating.

b. Tactile stimulus produced by personal contact with another person or object.

c. Vocal sounds that communicate a message.

d. The art of remaining silent.

e. Body language.

Activity D *Briefly answer the following questions.*

1. What are the four basic roles of a nurse?

_____

_____

_____

2. Describe the two kinds of touch within the context of nursing.

_____

_____

_____

3. What factors can decrease a client's learning readiness? How should the nurse proceed?

_____

_____

_____

4. What is the role of a nurse as an educator? Give examples.

_____

_____

_____

5. What motivates clients to learn at an accelerated rate? What forces motivate clients to acquire new information?

_____

_____

_____

SECTION 2: APPLYING YOUR KNOWLEDGE

Activity E *Give rationale for the following questions.*

1. Why should both the nurse and the client participate in the working phase?

_____

_____

_____

2. What would be the best response by the nurse to a quiet and uncommunicative client?

_____

_____

_____

3. Why is empathetic listening important during nurse–client communication?

_____

_____

_____

4. Why should a nurse use affective touching cautiously?

_____

_____

_____

Activity F *Answer the following questions related to the nurse–client relationship.*

1. Which verbal and nonverbal communication techniques are effective with most American clients?

_____

_____

_____

2. Why is it important to acknowledge the "comfort zone" of a client? How can a nurse relieve a client's anxiety about physical closeness?

_____

_____

_____

3. How should the nurse respond when asked his or her opinion about treatment decisions by the clients or their family?

_____

_____

_____

4. What are the factors that interfere with a client's learning capacity? How can receptiveness to learning be increased?

_____

_____

_____

Activity G *Think over the following questions. Discuss them with your instructor or peers.*

1. Identify the options for communication with each type of client:
   - A client who has suffered a stroke, has expressive aphasia, and has lost use of his or her dominant hand
   - A non–English-speaking client
   - A client who has been deaf since birth
   - A client who has experienced significant hearing loss due to an occupational accident

2. A client diagnosed with a new onset of diabetes requires instruction on how to use a glucometer and self-administer insulin. What information will you need to gather in the learner assessment? How would you accommodate each style of learner: cognitive, affective, and psychomotor?

_____

_____

_____

_____

Activity H *Read the following case study. Use critical thinking skills to discuss and answer the questions that follow it.*

The nurse is caring for a 66-year-old female, several weeks postoperative from a right total hip replacement. The client is nearing the end of her rehabilitation stay. Before entering the client's room, the nurse checks on the unlicensed assistive personnel (UAP) to make sure the *delegated* task of taking vital signs has been completed. Before discharge, the nurse wants to assess the client's ability to complete her ADLs. The nurse, as *caregiver*, allows the client to complete as much as she can for herself and then provides some assistance with shoes and socks. The nurse reviews the exercise routine that the client must continue at home and *educates* her on the importance of continuing to take her medications as prescribed by her physician. The client is able to demonstrate hip precautions and appropriate ambulation with the walker.

As the nurse prepares to leave the room, the client asks to talk for a moment. The nurse pulls up a chair, leans forward, and focuses on the client. The nurse listens in silence as the client verbalizes her concern about going home. The client then asks the nurse, "Do you think I'm ready to go home?" The nurse asks the client how she feels about the tasks she has successfully completed and how hard she's worked and reminds her of the upcoming home evaluation. The nurse explains that the occupational therapist will practice ADLs with her at home and check to make sure her home is free of any hazards. The client thanks the nurse and says that she feels better. The nurse *collaborates* with physical therapist to discuss the client's ambulation and meets with the occupational therapist to discuss the client's home evaluation the next day. The nurse shares the client's concerns with the therapists. The nurse then confirms arrangements for the home health agency to follow the client after discharge.

1. What phases of the nurse–client relationship are demonstrated in the given case study?

_____

_____

_____

2. What verbal and nonverbal communication techniques are demonstrated in the nurse–client communication?

_____

_____

_____

3. What basic roles does the nurse perform in the case study in order to meet the client's needs? (Italicized words are clues.) Fill in the boxes in the concept map that follows.

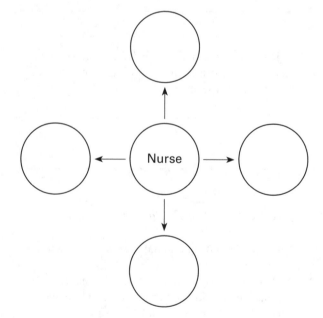

SECTION 3: GETTING READY FOR NCLEX

Activity I *Answer the following questions.*

1. The nurse is ready to do a dressing change on a client. Which of the following actions by the nurse would be appropriate to respect for the client's comfort zone and privacy? Select all that apply.
   1. Maintaining direct eye contact with the client
   2. Explaining the procedure beforehand to the client
   3. Ensuring that the client is properly draped
   4. Using affective touch
   5. Monitoring nonverbal communication

2. Which action by the nurse demonstrates an understanding of task-oriented touch? Select all that apply.
   1. Touching the forearm of a client when the client is anxious about a procedure
   2. Palpating a client's abdomen during an assessment
   3. Touching the hand of a client who is dying
   4. Touching a client's shoulder when he or she is upset
   5. Touching a client's wrist to count a radial pulse

3. A student nurse asks the nursing instructor, "When is it therapeutic to use silence with a client?" Which response(s) by the nursing instructor is appropriate? Select all that apply.
   1. To encourage a client's verbal communication
   2. To facilitate reaching the client's goals
   3. To ensure a client's comprehension before self-care
   4. To avoid overwhelming a client with new information
   5. To provide a time for the client to think and/or respond to a question
   6. To provide a sense of personal presence

4. During a nursing preceptor training session, a staff member asks the presenting nurse, "How does an affective learner best comprehend new information?" Which response by the presenting nurse is most appropriate?
   1. The learner listens to explanations.
   2. The learner likes to learn by doing.
   3. The learner prefers to read facts.
   4. The learner assimilates information that appeals to values.

5. A nursing student asks the nurse, "When is it appropriate to use personal space when interacting with a client?" Which response(s) by the nurse is appropriate? Select all that apply.
   1. When interviewing a client during the admission process
   2. During conversations that are not intended to be private
   3. During the physical assessment
   4. When sharing confidential information
   5. When participating in group interactions
   6. When giving a back rub

6. What action by the nurse would be most appropriate when dealing with older adults who lose the ability to hear at high-pitched ranges?
   1. Lower the voice pitch.
   2. Insert a stethoscope in client's ears.
   3. Use a magic slate or chalkboard.
   4. Ensure that the hearing aid is in good working order.

7. The nurse explains to the nursing student the working phase of the nurse–client relationship. Which statement by the nursing student demonstrates an understanding?
   1. "It's the exchange of names and a handshake."
   2. "It's when the client's immediate health problems have been resolved."
   3. "It's when the client assumes independent responsibility for self-care."
   4. "It's when a plan is mutually constructed to meet goals identified and put into action."

8. Which is the best strategy for the nurse to use when communicating with a client who has limited English proficiency (LEP)?
   1. Ask a family member to translate.
   2. Request a telephonic interpreter.
   3. Request a certified interpreter.
   4. Ask a bilingual staff member to interpret.

9. Which of the following terms reflects the principles a nurse would use when teaching an adult learner?
   1. Pedagogy
   2. Gerogogy
   3. Cybertexting
   4. Andragogy

10. The nurse is giving an in-service presentation to colleagues on how to better meet the educational needs of hospitalized clients. A colleague asks the nurse about teaching young adults who belong to "Generation Y," "Generation X," and "Net Generation" and what learning characteristics they might have. Which is the best response by the nurse? Select all that apply.
    1. They are technologically illiterate.
    2. They crave stimulation and quick responses.
    3. They prefer memorizing information and doing repetitive tasks.
    4. They expect immediate answers and feedback.
    5. They prefer visualizations and simulations.
    6. They like one instruction method to be provided for them.

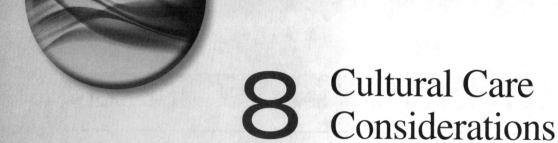

8 Cultural Care Considerations

LEARNING OBJECTIVES

1. Define terms related to culture.
2. List the five population groups delineated in the United States.
3. Differentiate race from ethnicity and culture.
4. Contrast stereotyping and generalization.
5. Describe how cultural background and practices influence actions and behaviors.
6. Name three views that societies use to explain illness or disease.
7. Discuss biocultural assessment.
8. Describe cultural assessment.
9. Explain the meaning and characteristics of transcultural nursing.
10. List at least five ways to demonstrate culturally competent nursing care.

SECTION 1: ASSESSING YOUR UNDERSTANDING

Activity A   *Fill in the blanks by choosing the correct word from the options given in parentheses.*

1. _____ provides a means for understanding people's values and beliefs, including those related to health practices. *(Ethnicity, Culture, Ethnocentrism)*

2. _____ refers to the activities governed by the rules of behavior that a particular cultural group avoids, forbids, or prohibits. *(Cultural blindness, Cultural imposition, Cultural taboos)*

3. _____ means the nurse understands his or her own worldview as well as the client's and how these worldviews affect nursing care. *(Cultural competence, Transcultural sensitivity, Cultural assessment)*

4. _____ refers to biologic differences in physical features, such as skin color, bone structure, and eye shape. *(Race, Culture, Ethnicity)*

Activity B   *Write the correct term for each of the following description.*

1. Assuming that all people in a particular cultural, racial, or ethnic group share the same values and beliefs, behave similarly, and are basically alike. _____

2. The belief that one's own ethnic heritage is the "correct" one and is superior to others. _____

3. An inability to recognize the values, beliefs, and practices of others because of strong ethnocentric preferences. _____

4. The care that fits a person's cultural values. _____

5. A person's ideas about what causes illness, the role of the sick person, how to restore health, and how one stays healthy. _____

Activity C   *In general, societies use three overall views to explain illness or disease. Match these views given in Column A with their related examples given in Column B.*

Column A

_____ 1. Biomedical or scientific perspective

_____ 2. Naturalistic or holistic perspective

_____ 3. Magico-religious perspective

Column B

a. Supernatural forces dominate.

b. Embraces a cause-and-effect philosophy of human body functions.

c. Espouses that human beings are only one part of nature; natural balance or harmony is essential for health.

Activity D *Briefly answer the following questions.*

1. What are the basic concepts that characterize culture?

_____

_____

_____

2. How do people demonstrate pride in their ethnic heritage?

_____

_____

_____

3. What is culture generalization? How does culture generalization assist healthcare providers to provide appropriate care?

_____

_____

_____

4. What is transcultural nursing? What are its characteristics?

_____

_____

_____

_____

SECTION 2: APPLYING YOUR KNOWLEDGE

Activity E *Give rationale for the following questions.*

1. Why is it important for the nurse not to equate skin color and other physical features with culture?

_____

_____

_____

2. Why is it important to evaluate biocultural ecology when providing healthcare?

_____

_____

_____

3. Why may it pose a challenge to supplement or restrict dietary consumption when providing health-related education to clients from culturally diverse populations?

_____

_____

_____

4. Why is caution needed when asking family members to interpret?

_____

_____

_____

5. How will recognizing that clients have different perceptions of time assist the nurse to provide more sensitive care?

_____

_____

_____

Activity F *Answer the following questions related to cultural care considerations.*

1. What general appearance and obvious physical characteristic components should the nurse evaluate when completing a biocultural assessment?

_____

_____

_____

2. What cultural elements should a nurse ask about or observe when performing a cultural assessment on a client?

_____

_____

_____

3. What are the recommendations that can help develop culturally sensitive nursing care?

_____

_____

_____

_____

_____

_____

Activity G *Think over the following questions. Discuss them with your instructor or peers.*

1. During an assessment on a Navajo client, the nurse is required to obtain the family members' health history. Because Navajos feel that no person has the right to speak for another, the client refuses to comment on family members' health problems. How would you respond?

_____

_____

_____

2. When assessing the health beliefs and practices of an older Hispanic adult, the nurse observes that the client uses a traditional folk healer to manage health problems. How would you respond?

_____

_____

_____

Activity H *Read the following case study. Use critical thinking skills to discuss and answer the questions that follow it.*

The nurse is caring for a 58-year-old male post–myocardial infarction. During report, the nurse learns that the client is part of the Appalachian culture. Before meeting the client, the nurse researches this particular culture. The nurse learns that this cultural group generally lives in rural areas, prefers isolation, and considers family to be extremely important. The nurse also learns that religion plays a strong role in their health/illness beliefs and that cardiovascular, respiratory, smoking, and alcohol issues are common health problems.

After completing the assessment, the nurse takes a few minutes to talk with the client and determine his individual needs. The client states that he wants his family members and preacher at his side while he is in the hospital. He requests that his wife and family be allowed extra visiting time because of the distance they must travel and also asks for privacy during his preacher's visits for prayer. The client talks about the difficulty of not being able to smoke. He informs the nurse that he enjoys smoking, that everyone in his family smokes, and that he's willing to cut down but not quit.

The nurse makes arrangements for the client's family to stay near the hospital and visit often and for the client's privacy when his preacher visits. The nurse then works with the client to set specific and realistic goals/outcomes that the client is willing and able to achieve for his plan of care.

1. What view(s) does the client use to explain his health/illness beliefs?

_____

_____

_____

2. How does the nurse incorporate the client's cultural beliefs into his plan of care?

_____

_____

_____

SECTION 3: GETTING READY FOR NCLEX

Activity I   *Answer the following questions.*

1. An older Asian female client continually agrees with the nurse even though they do not understand each other. What generalized cultural information would the nurse use to help provide appropriate cultural care for this client?
   1. The client considers it shameful to express her inability to understand the nurse.
   2. The client considers it disrespectful to disagree with the nurse.
   3. The client believes that disagreeing with the nurse would harm her spirit.
   4. The client believes that listening to the nurse nonjudgmentally is polite.

2. The nurse educator who is providing healthcare in-service instruction is asked about the biomedical or scientific perspective to explain illness and disease. Which statement by the nurse educator demonstrates an understanding of this view?
   1. This view is based on a cause-and-effect philosophy of human body function.
   2. This view is based on a belief that humans are only one part of nature.
   3. This view is based on a belief that supernatural forces dominate.
   4. This view is based on a belief that natural balance or harmony is necessary for health.

3. The nurse needs to communicate with a client who does not speak English. Which communication technique would be most appropriate for the nurse to use?
   1. Repeat the question without changing words.
   2. Look at the translator when asking questions.
   3. Speak slowly, using simple words and short sentences.
   4. Refer to an English or foreign language dictionary for bilingual words.

4. The nurse is caring for a group of culturally diverse clients. Which nursing action provides for culturally competent care for all individuals?
   1. Becoming familiar with physical differences among ethnic groups
   2. Learning to speak a second language
   3. Developing strategies to avoid cultural imposition
   4. Consulting the client about ways to solve health problems

5. Which of the following techniques would nurses use to facilitate interactions between themselves and their clients?
   1. Ask questions that can be answered with "yes" or "no."
   2. Sit within the client's comfort zone.
   3. Avoid making eye contact.
   4. Address clients by their first names.

6. The nurse is completing an admission on a new client. What does the nurse believe is the rationale for assessing the client's health beliefs and practices?
   1. To possess knowledge of health problems affecting a particular cultural group
   2. To accept each client as an individual
   3. To provide culturally competent care to the client
   4. To view the situation from the client's perspective

7. A nurse tells another nurse that the client admitted for surgery is of a different culture and most likely does not speak any English. What is this nurse engaged in?
   1. The nurse is generalizing about a culture.
   2. The nurse is stereotyping about a particular culture.
   3. The nurse is assuming ethnocentric traits.
   4. The nurse is imposing cultural characteristics.

8. Which of the following is the most important factor for the nurse to acknowledge when caring for a client of another culture?
   1. The nurse does not need to do a cultural assessment on most clients.
   2. The nurse must not judge a client's beliefs or practices.
   3. The nurse must explain that it is essential that the client follow the treatment plan.
   4. The nurse can only be concerned about the physical assessment and objective data.

9. Assessment includes the documentation of biologic differences in physical features, such as skin color, bone structure, and eye shape. What term should the nurse use to describe these biologic differences?
   1. Culture
   2. Ethnicity
   3. Race
   4. Minority

10. The nurse is completing a biocultural assessment made up of four areas. In what area would the nurse document the assessment of gait and range of motion?
    1. Physical appearance
    2. Mobility
    3. Behavior
    4. Body structure

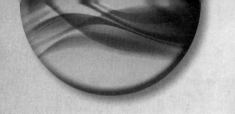

9 Complementary and Alternative Therapies

LEARNING OBJECTIVES

1. Differentiate between the terms *complementary therapy, alternative therapy*, and *integrative medicine*.
2. Give at least five reasons that individuals choose to use complementary and alternative therapies.
3. List four categories of complementary and alternative therapies that the National Center for Complementary and Alternative Medicine investigates.
4. Describe the basic beliefs of three examples of alternative whole medical systems: Ayurvedic medicine, Chinese medicine, and Native American medicine.
5. Identify four examples of practices that use the mind to promote or restore physical health.
6. Describe four examples of biologically based practices.
7. Name anatomic structures that are the focus of manipulative and body-based therapies and give examples of these therapies.
8. Describe techniques that are used in energy medicine.
9. Discuss the role nurses can play in relation to complementary and alternative therapies.

SECTION 1:   ASSESSING YOUR UNDERSTANDING

Activity A   *Fill in the blanks by choosing the correct word from the options given in parentheses.*

1. _____ therapy is one used in addition to conventional medical treatment. (*Complementary, Alternative, Allopathic*)

2. _____ has its roots in India and is the oldest system of medicine in the world. (*Acupuncture, Homeopathy, Ayurvedic*)

3. Chinese medicine proposes that health is the outcome of balancing _____, opposing forces that must remain equalized to maintain qi (or chi). (*prana and chakra, mind and body, yin and yang*)

4. _____ is one mind–body medicine used to help individuals overcome habits (such as smoking), relieve chronic pain, and extinguish irrational fears. (*Humor, Hypnosis, Biofeedback*)

5. _____ is the use of scents to alter emotions and biologic responses. (*Apitherapy, Shiatsu, Aromatherapy*)

6. _____ is a complementary health practice in which manual pressure is applied to the feet and hands. (*Reflexology, Massage therapy, Shiatsu*)

Activity B   *Write the correct term for each description.*

1. The Native Americans' medicine man (or woman) and spiritual figure with the extraordinary ability to heal. _____

2. Practitioners apply pressure to acupoints in various body meridians (energy channels) that correlate with an organ or its function to rebalance the body's energy and restore health. _____

3. Supplements that are microorganisms that exert beneficial health effects. _____

4. The medicinal use of bee venom. _____

5. Practitioners who perform spinal manipulation to treat neuromuscular disorders and a host of other diseases. _____

6. A mind–body technique in which the individual voluntarily controls one or more physiologic functions, such as body temperature, heart rate, blood pressure, and brain waves. _____

Activity C

Match the complementary and/or alternative therapy given in Column A to the associated feature or example given in Column B.

Column A

_____ **1.** Whole medical system

_____ **2.** Mind–body medicine

_____ **3.** Biologically based practices

_____ **4.** Manipulative and body-based therapies

_____ **5.** Energy medicine

_____ **6.** Conventional (allopathic) medicine

Column B

a. Uses techniques that rely on the power of the brain, emotions, social interactions, and spiritual factors to alter body functions or symptoms such as biofeedback, imagery, and spiritual healing.

b. Healing methods that focus on the structures and systems of the body, such as massage therapy, chiropractic, yoga, and tai chi.

c. Practices that embody traditional Western treatment of disease.

d. Techniques are used that claim to manipulate electromagnetic fields in the body, such as Reiki, acupuncture, and techniques involving magnets and electricity.

e. The belief that one's body has the power to heal itself and that healing involves the mind, body, and spirit (examples include Ayurvedic medicine, Chinese medicine, and homeopathy).

f. Use natural products such as dietary supplements, aromatherapy, and animal-derived extracts such as bee venom.

Activity D

Briefly answer the following questions.

1. Compare and contrast complementary therapy, alternative therapy, and integrated medicine.

_____

_____

_____

2. What are the mission of NCCAM?

_____

_____

_____

3. Why is the use of medicinal plants and herbs for therapy referred to as folk medicine?

_____

_____

_____

4. Which structures and systems of the body are the focuses of manipulative and body-based therapies?

_____

_____

_____

5. Why has the U.S. Food and Drug Administration warned against the use of Actra-Rx (Yilishen)?

_____

_____

_____

_____

_____

_____

SECTION 2: APPLYING YOUR KNOWLEDGE

Activity E *Provide rationale for the following questions.*

1. Why do individuals choose to use complementary or alternative therapies?

_____

_____

_____

2. Why is it important for clients to check labels on over-the-counter medications when taking herbal preparations?

_____

_____

_____

3. Why can't manufacturers of herbal preparations claim that their herbal product prevents or treats a disease?

_____

_____

_____

4. Why might tai chi be preferred by some clients rather than other forms of aerobic exercises?

_____

_____

_____

5. Why should the nurse and other healthcare providers tolerate or even support the use of complementary and alternative therapies if the practice is not dangerous or unhealthy?

_____

_____

_____

_____

_____

_____

_____

Activity F *Answer the following questions related to complementary and alternative therapies.*

1. A client asks how massage therapy can be of benefit to them. What information should the nurse provide?

_____

_____

_____

2. A client has heard about an herbal supplement and is considering using it as complementary therapy. The client is currently taking numerous medications. How should the nurse instruct the client?

_____

_____

_____

3. A client wants help in choosing between apitherapy and chiropractic treatments. The client is worried about the safety and the insurance coverage. Compare and contrast the two methods in terms of safety and insurance coverage.

_____

_____

_____

4. A client is curious about energy medicine. How would the nurse describe the techniques used in this type of complementary/alternative therapy?

_____

_____

_____

Activity G *Think over the following questions. Discuss them with your instructor or peers.*

1. The smell of the earth after a rain makes you feel happy. After a recent car accident, the smell of gas makes you break into a sweat. The two smells produce two different reactions. How do these smells elicit physiologic and psychological responses?

_____

_____

_____

2. Why has it become necessary for nurses to understand complementary and alternative therapies along with the allopathic system of medicine?

_____

_____

_____

_____

Activity H *Read the following case study. Use critical thinking skills to discuss and answer the questions that follow it.*

A 39-year-old male, a post–Iraq War veteran, is admitted to the Veteran's Hospital with a diagnosis of post-traumatic stress disorder (PTSD). The client has been having memory problems, flashbacks, hypervigilance, nightmares, insomnia, chronic anxiety, and mood swings. The client is admitted for evaluation and testing with treatment to follow on an outpatient basis. The client is discharged with the conventional medications for anxiety, depression, and insomnia along with orders for psychotherapy and behavioral therapy. In a follow-up outpatient visit, the client tells the nurse that he has continued with his traditional medications and therapies but has added some nontraditional complementary therapies for the treatment of his PTSD. One therapy includes the use of a technique in which the client can work with a machine that provides feedback to try to decrease his level of anxiety. He is also using another technique in which he uses his mind to visualize images of his body winning the battle over his anxiety and other symptoms. The client tells the nurse that he is also active in his church, believes that God is helping him daily, and has also added some vitamin and mineral supplements to his daily medication routine. The client feels he is making progress in the treatment of his PTSD and plans continue on his current treatment regimen.

1. How does the use of complementary and alternative medicine correlate with the nursing practice of holistic care (body, mind, and spirit)?

_____

_____

_____

2. What complementary therapies and biologic practice is the client using in addition to his traditional treatment plan? What risks do they hold for the client?

_____

_____

_____

3. What is the nurse's role when a client chooses to use a complementary or alternative therapy that has potential risks for harm?

_____

_____

_____

4. When documenting, what term does the nurse use to describe this combination of conventional medicine and complementary therapy?

_____

_____

_____

SECTION 3: GETTING READY FOR NCLEX

Activity I *Answer the following questions.*

1. A client chooses to use biofeedback to help him control his blood pressure along with the traditional/conventional treatment of medication. What term would the nurse use to describe the type of therapy that is being added to the client's traditional/conventional treatment?
   1. Integrative medicine
   2. Alternative therapy
   3. Allopathic medicine
   4. Complementary therapy

2. A nurse interviews a client and learns that the client is using alternative therapy to treat a sore back that has defied conventional therapy. Which rationale is most likely the one the client would give for using an alternative therapy.
   1. Desire to be more active in decision making and self-care
   2. Hope to relieve a chronic incurable back condition
   3. Provides a method for controlling healthcare costs
   4. Opposes traditional American health practices

3. An LPN is giving an in-service presentation to fellow colleagues because of a personal interest in alternative and complementary medicine. Which statement would be the nurse's best response when describing manipulative and body-based therapies?
   1. It's a therapy in which techniques are used to manipulate electromagnetic fields in the body.
   2. It's an alternative system of healing theory and practice that evolved from other cultures.
   3. It's a group of healing methods that focus on the structures and systems of the body, including bones and joints, the soft tissues, and the circulatory and lymphatic systems.
   4. It's the use of natural products such as dietary supplements, aromatherapy, and animal-derived extracts such as bee venom.

4. A client hospitalized for intractable pain asks the nurse if she can have the Reiki practitioner come to see her. Which of the following nursing actions is appropriate? Select all that apply.
   1. Communicate the client's request to the physician.
   2. Determine the reason the client feels the need for the Reiki practitioner.
   3. Make sure the Reiki practitioner is certified.
   4. Observe the practice to make sure of the client's safety.
   5. Facilitate the practitioner's visit.
   6. Recommend traditional medical care.

5. An LPN goes on a mission trip to India and learns techniques of Ayurvedic medicine. Which explanation would the nurse use to best describe the basic premise of this type of medicine to a client?
   1. It views disease as resulting from disharmony with Mother Earth, possession by an evil spirit, or violation of a taboo.
   2. Health is the outcome of balancing yin and yang, opposite forces that must remain equalized to maintain life's energy force.
   3. It helps individuals become unified with nature to develop a strong body, clear mind, and tranquil spirit.
   4. It corrects an imbalance between two attributes, such as motion and stillness or hot and cold, restoring harmony and health.

6. A nurse is using mind–body techniques in teaching a client how to overcome pain. The client chooses a technique that allows voluntary control of one or more physiologic functions, such as pain. When documenting this teaching, what term should the nurse use to describe this technique?
   1. Biofeedback
   2. Hypnosis
   3. Imagery
   4. Humor

7. A client asks the nurse about the use of aromatherapy as a complementary therapy to conventional medication for treatment of anxiety. Which statement is the most appropriate response?
   1. It is a technique that uses plants to treat diseases and disorders.
   2. It uses bee venom to treat inflammatory and neurologic conditions.
   3. It is the use of microorganisms that provide beneficial health effects.
   4. It is the use of scents to change emotions and biologic processes.

8. A client with multiple sclerosis has heard about using apitherapy in addition to conventional medical care for treatment of multiple sclerosis. The client asks the nurse to further explain apitherapy. Which of the following are appropriate responses by the nurse? Select all that apply.
   1. Physicians currently consider apitherapy a conventional treatment.
   2. Apitherapy uses bee venom that may induce the release of an anti-inflammatory and immunosuppressant hormone.
   3. Bee venom therapy is considered safe and effective.
   4. Apitherapy is an alternative that has been used for treating various inflammatory conditions of the joints and multiple sclerosis.
   5. Experiments with bee venom by the International Pain Institute have demonstrated relief of symptoms among volunteers.
   6. Further study is needed to validate the effectiveness of bee venom therapy.

9. The nurse is caring for a client who is using electromagnetic therapy as a complementary therapy for a broken leg. The nursing student asks the nurse to explain electromagnetic therapy. Which statement by the nurse would be the most appropriate response?
   1. In this method of healing, the practitioner transfers healing energy to the client by the laying on of hands.
   2. This is a healing therapy in which a needle is placed in one or more acupoints to unblock *qi*.
   3. This therapy promotes healing using electricity, magnets, or both.
   4. This therapy uses spinal manipulation as a generic method for curing neuromuscular disorders.

10. A nurse learns about the techniques of complementary medicine to assist clients in making informed choices. A client asks the nurse if she can use massage along with chemotherapy treatments for breast cancer. What would be the nurse's best response?
    1. "I would think about this, as it may interfere with the chemotherapy treatment."
    2. "I think it would be worth trying, especially since you said you ache after chemotherapy."
    3. "There are other therapies out there that might help you better."
    4. "I can't tell you that, as your doctor would have to approve."

10 End-of-Life Care

LEARNING OBJECTIVES

1. Define attitudes of society and healthcare workers toward death.
2. Discuss outcomes of informing a client about a terminal illness.
3. Explain how clients and families can maintain hopefulness during a terminal illness.
4. Name emotional reactions the dying client experiences.
5. Identify how the dying client can ensure that others carry out his or her wishes for terminal care.
6. Discuss the dilemma of physician-assisted suicide.
7. Describe physical phenomena that occur during the dying process.
8. Summarize psychological events that dying clients have reported.
9. Describe nursing management of the dying client and the family.

SECTION 1: ASSESSING YOUR UNDERSTANDING

Activity A *Fill in the blanks by choosing the correct word from the options given in parentheses.*

1. Physical effects of impending death include _____, in which peristalsis slows, causing gas and intestinal contents to accumulate. This buildup may stimulate the vomiting center, resulting in nausea and vomiting. (*renal impairment, gastrointestinal disturbances, musculoskeletal changes*)

2. The client can use _____ and determination to survive and prolong life, often referred to as the "will to live." (*will power, religious faith, inner resources*)

3. _____ is a painful yet normal reaction that helps clients to cope with loss and leads to emotional healing. (*Grieving, Coping, Accepting*)

4. _____ is one of the first signs of the client's worsening condition and of impending death. (*Cardiac dysfunction, Renal impairment, Central nervous system alteration*)

5. _____ may be prescribed by the physician to relieve the anxiety created by the feeling of suffocation caused by pulmonary edema in the dying client. (*An antidepressant, Pain medication, A sedative*)

Activity B *Write the correct term for each description.*

1. Treatment that reduces physical discomfort but does not alter a disease's progression. _____

2. Care that is arranged to provide periodic relief for the primary caregiver of the dying client. _____

3. Some clients seem to forestall dying when they feel that their loved ones are not yet prepared to deal with their death. _____

4. Care for terminally ill clients, who can live out their final days with comfort, dignity, and meaningfulness. _____

Activity C

Match the physical events that occur in a dying client given in Column A with the signs given in Column B.

Column A

_____ **1.** Renal impairment

_____ **2.** Musculoskeletal changes

_____ **3.** Pulmonary function impairment

_____ **4.** Peripheral circulation changes

Column B

a. The client loses urinary and rectal sphincter muscle control, causing incontinence of urine and stool.

b. The skin becomes pale or mottled, nail beds and lips may appear blue, and the client may feel cold.

c. Low cardiac output causes volume to diminish and toxic waste products to accumulate.

d. Failure of the heart's pumping function causes fluid to collect and breath sounds become moist.

Activity D

The following is a series of five reactions, in random order, experienced by dying clients when informed about their terminal illness. Write the correct sequence for the stages experienced by dying clients in the boxes.

1. Clients may displace feelings onto others, such as the physician, nurses, family, or even God. They may express feelings in less obvious ways, such as complaining about their care or blaming anyone and everyone for the slightest aggravation.

2. Dying clients accept their fate and make peace spiritually and with those to whom they are close. Clients may begin to detach themselves from activities and acquaintances and seek to be with only a small circle of relatives or friends.

3. A psychological coping mechanism in which a person refuses to believe certain information. Dying clients usually first deny that the diagnosis is accurate.

4. An attempt to postpone death. Usually, the clients make a secret bargain with God or some higher power. Clients attempt to negotiate a delay in dying until after a particularly significant event.

5. As clients realize the reality of their situation, they may mourn their potential losses, such as separation from their loved ones, the inability to fulfill their future goals, or loss of control.

☐→☐→☐→☐→☐

Activity E

Briefly answer the following questions that relate to this scenario.

An 85-year-old terminally ill client with lung cancer, fairly independent, has been living at home with his 81-year-old spouse as caregiver. Over the past few months, the client's condition has slowly begun to deteriorate. The client's spouse/caregiver is exhausted because the client's needs are more than she can manage. The client is no longer able to ambulate, is incontinent, and his pain management needs are not being met. The client's primary physician recommends either hospice home care or hospice institutionally based care.

1. Which hospice care setting would be most appropriate for this client and family and why?

_____

_____

_____

Activity F *Briefly answer the following questions.*

1. What have been the effects of technology and aggressive treatment on the attitude of healthcare workers towards death and dying?

_____

_____

_____

2. What is hospice care?

_____

_____

_____

3. What is a living will? How does it differ from a durable power of attorney?

_____

_____

_____

4. What factors should the nurse consider when caring for dying clients?

_____

_____

_____

5. How does the nurse facilitate and support the client's final decisions?

_____

_____

_____

SECTION 2: APPLYING YOUR KNOWLEDGE

Activity G *Give rationale for the following questions.*

1. Why does a nurse administer pain medications on a routine schedule for dying clients?

_____

_____

_____

2. Why would a physician prescribe a mild tranquilizer or antidepressant to the dying client?

_____

_____

_____

3. Why is it important for a nurse to be flexible and to interrupt physical care if and when the client indicates a need for companionship, support, and communication?

_____

_____

_____

4. Why does the nurse give oral care and ice chips to a dying client?

_____

_____

_____

5. Why should the nurse try to avoid unnecessary assessments and make frequent checks of the dying client?

_____

_____

_____

6. Why must the nurse convey a spirit of hopefulness to the dying client?

_____

_____

_____

Activity H   *Answer the following questions related to end-of-life care.*

1. When a family member is dying, how can the nurse promote family coping?

_____

_____

_____

2. What are the outcomes of being truthful with clients and honoring their right to know the seriousness of their condition?

_____

_____

_____

3. How does the nurse address spiritual distress with the dying client?

_____

_____

_____

_____

_____

_____

Activity I   *Think over the following questions. Discuss them with your instructor or peers.*

1. How will you prepare yourself to care for dying clients and their families?

_____

_____

2. How would client and family care differ for a client with an acute terminal illness and a chronic terminal illness?

_____

_____

_____

3. How would you respond to a family member experiencing anticipatory grieving who emotionally withdraws from the client?

_____

_____

_____

_____

_____

Activity J   *Read the following case study. Use critical thinking skills to discuss and answer the questions that follow it.*

A 54-year-old terminally ill client in the end stages of cancer chooses to remain at home with in-home hospice care. The client's family is supportive of the decision and wants their loved one surrounded by family and the familiarity of home. The nurse *spends* time listening to the client *mourn the loss* of plans made for the future. The nurse acknowledges the client's feelings, makes direct eye contact, and nods in response as the client talks of feeling *powerless* to help his loved one. The client's spouse *struggles* *to cope* with the eventual loss of his loved one. The nurse states, "It must be difficult to experience such feelings of helplessness," and sits with them to listen in silence as they continue to share their feelings and concerns. The nurse avoids giving advice or being critical and is empathetic to what they are experiencing. When the client states that she is *fearful about future pain*, the nurse reassures her and her family that pain relief and comfort measures will be provided.

As time passes, the client's condition deteriorates, and the nurse prepares the family for some of the physical changes they might observe as the client nears death. The client's heart rate decreases and her blood pressure begins to fall. The client's output decreases and her breath sounds become moist, with a noisy rattle, as she experiences periods of apnea. Although the client is unconscious, the nurse encourages the family to continue to talk to her. After several hours have passed, the spouse calls the family together to say their goodbyes. Once everyone has left, the spouse holds the client's hand, tells her how much he will miss her, and lets her know that he feels strong enough to go on. Within the hour, the client passes. The nurse provides time for the family to be alone with the client before completing her postmortem care.

1. How did the nurse provide support to the client, client's spouse, and family during their anticipatory grieving process?

_____

_____

_____

2. What actions by the nurse helped the family prepare for the impending death of their loved one?

_____

_____

_____

3. What physical events indicated the approaching death of the client?

_____

_____

_____

4. What psychological event occurred between the client and spouse prior to the client's death?

_____

_____

_____

5. Using the information from the given case study, identify additional nursing diagnoses for this client to place in the concept map that follows. (Italicized words are clues to the answer).

```
┌──────────────┐          ┌──────────────────┐          ┌──────────────┐
│              │      ↖   │ Reason for seek- │    ↗     │ Anticipatory │
└──────────────┘          │  ing healthcare: │          │   Grieving   │
                          │                  │          └──────────────┘
┌──────────────┐      ↙   │     Terminal     │    ↘     ┌──────────────┐
│              │          │  Illness—Cancer  │          │              │
└──────────────┘          └──────────────────┘          └──────────────┘
```

SECTION 3: GETTING READY FOR NCLEX

Activity K *Answer the following questions.*

1. What is the primary goal for pain control when caring for a client who is terminally ill?
   1. To relieve pain and provide sedation for the client
   2. To block pain without suppressing level of consciousness
   3. To reduce pain when it reaches an intense level
   4. To minimize pain that results in fear and anxiety

2. If all of the following interventions are feasible, which one is most appropriate for faciliting sleep for a terminally ill client?
   1. Playing the client's favorite music.
   2. Minimizing noise within the environment.
   3. Providing warm milk before bedtime.
   4. Using a dimly lit light in the room.

3. Which intervention is most appropriate for the nurse to perform when caring for a client who is unable to cough effectively and raise secretions?
   1. Give the client a drink of water.
   2. Pat the client on the back.
   3. Gently suction the client.
   4. Offer the client a throat lozenge.

4. When caring for a dying client, which nursing intervention is best for preventing the client's skin from breakdown?
   1. Massaging the client's body with oil
   2. Providing an adequate oral intake
   3. Giving the client a sponge bath twice a day
   4. Changing the client's position every 2 hours

5. In What position should a nurse place a client who is terminally ill following the administration of a tube feeding?
   1. Supine
   2. Prone
   3. Lateral oblique
   4. Semi-Fowler's

6. Which one of the following is an indication to the nurse that a terminally ill client is approaching death?
   1. The client becomes hypotensive.
   2. The client's skin becomes flushed.
   3. The client's urine appears pale.
   4. The client's bowel sounds are hyperactive.

7. When an unconscious client is in imminent potential for death, who is the person most responsible for determining the suitability of organs for transplantation?
   1. The client's attending physician
   2. The agency's pathologist
   3. The organ procurement officer
   4. The agency's risk manager

8. There is an order to administer metoclopramide (Reglan) 0.1 mg/kg IM 30 minutes before each tube feeding to prevent nausea. If the client weighs 110 lbs and the drug is supplied in 10 mg/2 mL vials, calculate the volume of a single dose?

9. Individuals of which religious group are most likely to withhold permission for a post-mortem examination (autopsy)?
   1. Those who are Amish
   2. Those who are Mormons
   3. Those who are Greek Orthodox
   4. Those who are Quakers

10. When caring for someone who is terminally ill, what resources the nurse consult regarding the client's choices for end-of-life care? Select all that apply.
    1. Last will and testament
    2. Living will
    3. Five Wishes document
    4. Durable power of attorney for healthcare

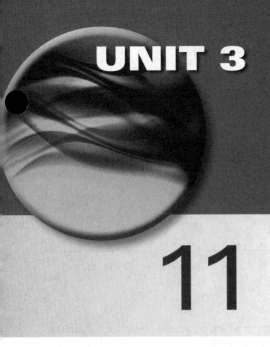
11 Pain Management

LEARNING OBJECTIVES

1. Define the term *pain*.
2. Compare nociceptive pain with neuropathic pain.
3. Give characteristics distinguishing acute from chronic pain.
4. Describe four phases of pain transmission.
5. Differentiate between pain perception, pain threshold, and pain tolerance.
6. Describe essential components of pain assessment.
7. Explain why assessing pain is difficult.
8. Give examples of tools for assessing the intensity of pain.
9. Discuss The Joint Commission's standards on pain assessment and pain management.
10. Explain pain management and list five techniques commonly used.
11. Name categories of drugs used to manage pain.
12. Describe methods of administering for analgesic drugs.
13. Discuss the issues of addiction, tolerance, and physical dependence associated with pain medication.
14. List examples of noninvasive techniques used to manage pain.
15. Identify two surgical procedures performed on clients with intractable pain.
16. List at least three nursing diagnoses besides Acute Pain and Chronic Pain that are common among clients with pain.
17. Discuss the nursing management of clients with pain.
18. Describe information pertinent to teaching clients and family about pain management.

SECTION 1: ASSESSING YOUR UNDERSTANDING

Activity A *Fill in the blanks by choosing the correct word from the options given in parentheses.*

1. _____ pain is subdivided into somatic and visceral pain. *(Neuropathic, Nociceptive, Chronic)*

2. It is speculated that some nondrug methods relieve pain by releasing _____ such as endorphins and enkephalins, which are natural morphine-like substances in the body that modulate pain transmission by blocking receptors for substance P. *(endogenous opiates, GABA, serotonin)*

3. _____ is a pain management technique that delivers bursts of electricity to the skin and underlying nerves. *(PENS, TENS, Acupuncture)*

4. _____ is a discomfort that has a short duration (from a few seconds to less than 6 months). It is associated with tissue trauma or some other recent identifiable etiology. *(Acute pain, Nociceptive pain, Neuropathic pain)*

5. _____ meals may help maximize intake in clients with drug-related or pain-related anorexia. *(Heavy; Protein-rich; Small, frequent)*

Activity B *Write the correct term for each description.*

1. The conscious experience of discomfort. _____

2. The point at which the pain-transmitting neurochemicals reach the brain, causing conscious awareness. _____

3. Discomfort that lasts longer than 6 months. _____

4. The amount of pain a person endures after the threshold has been reached. _____

5. A term used to describe discomfort that is perceived in a general area of the body but not in the exact site where an organ is anatomically located. _____

Activity C *Match the phases of pain transmission in Column A with the specific action that occurs in each of these phases in Column B.*

Column A

_____ 1. Transduction

_____ 2. Transmission

_____ 3. Perception

_____ 4. Modulation

Column B

a. The phase during which peripheral nerve fibers form synapses with neurons in the spinal cord. The pain impulses move from the spinal cord to sequentially higher levels in the brain.

b. The phase of pain impulse transmission during which the brain interacts with the spinal nerves in a downward fashion to alter the pain experience.

c. The conversion of chemical information in the cellular environment to electrical impulses that move toward the spinal cord. This phase is initiated by cellular disruption during which affected cells release various chemical mediators.

d. The phase of impulse transmission during which the brain experiences pain at a conscious level.

Activity D *Briefly answer the following question about the client situation given.*

A veteran with bilateral leg amputations complains to the nurse that he's experiencing itching and burning in his left foot.

Is this nociceptive or neuropathic pain and why?

_____

_____

_____

Activity E *Briefly answer the following questions.*

1. How do opioid and opiate medications differ in their action from nonopioid analgesic medications?

_____

_____

_____

2. List five general techniques for achieving pain management.

_____

_____

_____

3. List examples of adjuvant drugs used to manage pain.

_____

_____

_____

4. Explain why rhizotomy and cordotomy are effective treatments for intractable pain.

_____

_____

_____

Activity F *Label the phases of pain transmission in the given figure.*

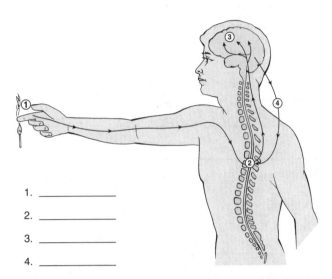

1. _____

2. _____

3. _____

4. _____

SECTION 2: APPLYING YOUR KNOWLEDGE

Activity G *Give rationale for the following questions.*

1. Why is the Wong-Baker FACES scale assessment tool best for specific types of clients?

_____

_____

_____

2. Why is risk for injury a concern for the client who is receiving narcotic analgesics?

_____

_____

_____

3. Why do older adults avoid taking opioid medications?

_____

_____

_____

4. Why do some nurses fear giving larger doses of narcotic analgesics when the client experiences tolerance?

_____

_____

_____

5. Why are drugs that are known to cause physical dependence discontinued gradually?

_____

_____

_____

Activity H *Answer the following questions related to pain management.*

1. A client requires an increased amount of opioid analgesic to achieve pain relief and fears addiction. How would the nurse explain the difference between addiction and tolerance?

_____

_____

_____

2. What are The Joint Commission's standards on pain assessment and pain management?

_____

_____

_____

3. Identify nursing responsibilities for pain management.

_____

_____

4. Identify nondrug interventions used to help manage pain.

_____

_____

_____

_____

Activity I *Think over the following questions. Discuss them with your peers or instructor.*

1. Discuss negative reactions that others may have to clients experiencing chronic pain.

_____

_____

_____

2. What factors can decrease a client's ability to cope with pain or lower pain tolerance?

_____

_____

_____

3. How does culture play a role in expressions of pain?

_____

_____

_____

_____

_____

_____

_____

Activity J *Read the following case study. Use critical thinking skills to discuss and answer the questions that follow it.*

The home health nurse visits a client who has had *low back pain* for the past 2 weeks. The nurse notes that the client is grimacing and holding her body stiffly. The nurse takes the client's vital signs, which appear slightly elevated from the last visit. The client indicates the location of the pain; the nurse examines the site in the lumbar/sacral area and finds no rashes or other abnormalities. The client describes the as sharp and intermittent and rates it as an 8 on a pain scale of 0 to 10. The nurse asks if the client has other symptoms or if anything makes the pain worse. The client replies that, at times, her right leg feels tingly and hurts when trying to bend over or bend down, walking is extremely painful. The client states the pain has been limiting her ability to get around the house, cook, clean, and do other *activities of daily living*. The nurse asks the client what she has been doing to relieve the pain. The client explains that she has tried hot baths, a heating pad, and ice packs, which provide only temporary relief. She informs the nurse that she frequently *sleeps in her recliner* to get relief from the pain; sitting well supported in a chair for short periods also seems to help, but sitting too long brings back the pain. The client states, "*I don't know what else to do.*" The client also states that she has been taking an occasional ibuprofen when the pain becomes too severe. The nurse explains that if the client takes the ibuprofen every 4 to 6 hours on a regularly scheduled basis, rather than just occasionally, she will experience more sustained pain control. The nurse reviews instructions, side effects, and precautions with the client for self-administering the ibuprofen. The client expresses her concern about becoming addicted to pain killers. The nurse educates the client on addiction as it relates to pain control and encourages the client to take the ibuprofen on a regular basis to relieve the pain. The nurse also recommends that the client see a physician to further explore the cause of the pain and tingling of the right leg. The client agrees and together they make an appointment to see the physician.

1. What components of a pain assessment did the nurse use when assessing the client's pain?

_____

_____

_____

2. What assessment tool did the nurse use to determine the intensity of the client's pain?

_____

_____

_____

3. What nonverbal cues of pain did the client demonstrate?

_____

_____

_____

4. What type of analgesic was the client using to relieve pain at home? How does this category of analgesic manage pain?

_____

_____

_____

5. What nondrug interventions did the nurse discover the client was using for pain relief? Are they established pain relief methods?

_____

_____

_____

6. How did the nurse provide for a more uniform level of pain relief with this client?

_____

_____

_____

7. Why shouldn't the client be concerned about becoming addicted to pain killers?

_____

_____

_____

8. Using the information from the given case study, identify nursing diagnoses to place in the following concept map for this client experiencing pain. (Italicized words are clues to the answers.)

Reason for seeking healthcare:

Low Back Pain

SECTION 3: GETTING READY FOR NCLEX

Activity K *Answer the following NCLEX-style questions.*

1. Which statement indicates a nurse's best understanding of why clients with acute pain cope better rather than chronic pain?
   1. Acute pain requires increasing drug therapy.
   2. Acute pain is nonspecific and generalized.
   3. The etiology of acute pain is unidentifiable.
   4. Pain diminishes with healing.

2. When caring for a client with pain, which of the following is an essential action by the nurse throughout the client's care?
   1. Giving assurance that pain management is a nursing and agency priority
   2. Giving assurance that pain relief will be immediate and effective
   3. Giving assurance that pain relief will be permanent
   4. Giving assurance that pain has a psychological basis and can be easily managed

3. When a client is receiving frequent administration of an opiate, which of the following is most important for the nurse to closely monitor?
   1. Respiratory rate
   2. Urinary output
   3. Mental status
   4. General appetite

4. The medical order for a client is morphine sulfate 4 mg IM q 4h prn pain. The drug is supplied in a 2 mL ampule that contains 10 mg. How much volume should the nurse administer? Record your answer to the nearest tenth. _____

5. To achieve a similar level of pain relief, what is the nurse's most accurate understanding when a parenteral dose of an analgesic is switched to an oral form?
   1. The oral dose will be lower than the parenteral dose.
   2. The oral dose will be higher than the parenteral dose.
   3. The administration of the oral dose will be less frequent than the parenteral dose.
   4. The administration of the oral dose will be more frequent than the parenteral dose.

6. When a nonsteroidal antiinflammatory drug (NSAID) is prescribed for an older adult, what teaching is most appropriate for the nurse to provide?
   1. Take the medication on a empty stomach.
   2. Avoid consuming milk with the medication.
   3. Take the medication when eating food.
   4. Avoid taking the medication with grapefruit juice.

7. Which of the following is the nursing standard for performing a pain assessment?
   1. Perform a pain assessment at the beginning and end of a shift.
   2. Perform a pain assessment once during the care of the client.
   3. Perform a pain assessment when vital signs are taken.
   4. Perform a pain assessment before administering an analgesic.

8. Which pain assessment tool is most appropriate to use when assessing the pain of a pediatric client?
   1. Using a numeric scale
   2. Using a word scale
   3. Using a linear scale
   4. Using a FACES scale

9. The nurse is correct in identifying which of the following clients at greatest risk for an adverse effect when administering opiate analgesia?
   1. A client with chronic obstructive lung disease.
   2. A client in traction following a fractured femur.
   3. A client who has Type 2 diabetes mellitus.
   4. A client who is passing a kidney stone.

10. Which of the following are nonverbal behaviors that suggest to a nurse that a client is in pain? Select all that apply.
    1. The client has become constipated.
    2. The client is eating poorly.
    3. The client moans frequently.
    4. The client is emotionally irritable.
    5. The client resists repositioning.
    6. The client requests family visitors.

12 Infection

SECTION 1: ASSESSING YOUR UNDERSTANDING

Activity A *Fill in the blanks by choosing the correct word from the options given in parentheses.*

1. _____ are physical barriers that prevent microorganisms from gaining entry or expel microorganisms before they multiply. *(Mechanical defense mechanisms, Chemical defense mechanisms, Electrical defense mechanisms)*

2. _____ bacteria grow and multiply in an atmosphere that lacks oxygen. *(Spirochetes, Aerobic, Anaerobic)*

3. _____ transmit rickettsial diseases. *(Humans, Arthropods, Microscopic worms)*

4. An infection that becomes widespread or systemic is called _____. *(localized infection, generalized infection, opportunistic infection)*

5. WBCs and other cells produce _____ in response to viral infection and other factors. This chemical protein appears to trigger infected cells to manufacture an antiviral protein and inhibit cell reproduction. *(lysozyme, immunoglobulins, interferon)*

6. _____ are nonpathogenic or remotely pathogenic microorganisms that take advantage of favorable situations and overwhelm the host. They commonly occur among immunocompromised clients. *(Nosocomial infections, Opportunistic infections, Reemerging infectious disease)*

Activity B *Write the correct term for each description.*

1. Destroy or incapacitate microorganisms with naturally produced biologic substances. Examples include enzymes, antibody substances, and secretions. _____

2. If microorganisms gain entry, sneezing, coughing, and vomiting can forcefully expel them. _____

3. Their primary function is phagocytosis, the ingestion of cells and foreign material, including microorganisms. _____

4. The ability of some bacteria to remain unaffected by antimicrobial drugs. _____

5. Occasionally, this type of microorganism is dormant in a living host, reactivates periodically, and causes infection to reoccur. _____

6. A bactericidal enzyme, capable of splitting the cell wall of some gram-positive bacteria. Present in tears, saliva, mucus, skin secretions, and some internal body fluids. _____

7. Infections acquired in the community setting that are infectious communicable diseases. In addition to general signs of systemic infection, these infections produce clusters of signs and symptoms that reflect dysfunction of the organs or tissues that the microorganisms have invaded. _____

Activity C *Match the six components of the chain of infection given in Column A with their characteristics given in Column B.*

Column A

_____ 1. Infectious agent

_____ 2. Reservoir

_____ 3. Portal of exit

_____ 4. Means of transmission

_____ 5. Portal of entry

_____ 6. Susceptible host

Column B

a. The route by which the infectious agent escapes from the reservoir. Examples include the respiratory, GI, or genitourinary tract; the skin and mucous membranes; and blood and other body fluids.

b. The person on or in whom the infectious agent will reside. Whether infection occurs depends on duration of exposure to the infectious agent and the person's ability to be compromised by or infected with disease.

c. Characteristics that must be present include the ability to move or be moved from one place to another, power to produce disease, an adequate number of agents, and the ability to invade a host.

d. The environment in which the infectious agent can survive and reproduce. It may be human, animal, or nonliving, such as contaminated food and water.

e. How the infectious agent is transferred or moved from its reservoir to the susceptible host. The five potential means are contact, droplet, airborne, vehicle, and vector.

f. How an infectious agent gains entrance into a susceptible host. Staphylococci, for example, can cause disease via the respiratory tract (pneumonia), skin (boils), blood (internal abscesses), or GI tract (food poisoning).

Activity D *Briefly answer the following questions.*

1. Which types of individuals are at increased risk for infection because their defenses are compromised in one or more ways?

_____

_____

_____

2. Describe how the skin and mucous membranes provide the first line of defense against microorganisms.

_____

_____

_____

3. How do antibodies work with other WBCs to defend the body from microorganisms?

_____

_____

_____

4. What is the difference between an emerging and reemerging infectious disease?

_____

_____

_____

5. Fever, which is the body's attempt to destroy the pathogen with heat, occurs in most people as an infection worsens. Which types of individuals may be an exception?

_____

_____

_____

SECTION 2: APPLYING YOUR KNOWLEDGE

Activity E *Give rationale for the following questions.*

1. Why are emerging and reemerging infectious diseases of serious concern?

_____

_____

_____

2. Why do nurses and other healthcare providers take precautions to control infection when caring for all clients regardless of diagnosis or infection status?

_____

_____

_____

3. Why is a WBC with a differential a more valuable source of information than a WBC without a differential?

_____

_____

_____

4. Why are hospitalized clients more susceptible to nosocomial infections?

_____

_____

_____

Activity F *Answer the following questions related to infection.*

1. What information will the nurse gather when performing an assessment on a client with a potential or actual infection?

_____

_____

_____

2. What are the postexposure recommendations following a needlestick injury?

_____

_____

_____

3. What actions will the nurse take to control the transmission of infection and prevent complications?

_____

_____

_____

4. Describe the medical management of a client with an infectious disorder.

_____

_____

_____

5. The initial localized reaction to an invading microorganism activates the inflammatory process; describe this process.

_____

_____

_____

6. What is the purpose of a culture and sensitivity test?

_____

_____

_____

Activity G *Think over the following questions. Discuss them with your instructor or peers.*

1. What community-acquired infections have you observed in your community?

_____

_____

_____

2. What were the signs and symptoms?

_____

_____

_____

3. How were these infections spread?

_____

_____

_____

4. Were some individuals more susceptible than others?

_____

_____

_____

Activity H

Read the following case study. Use critical thinking skills to discuss and answer the questions that follow it.

The hospital has just been informed that they will be receiving clients from another outlying hospital that is evacuating due to loss of power caused by localized flooding from hurricane conditions in the area. The nurse on the medical-surgical floor has just been notified that they will be receiving five of the incoming clients. The nurse identifies only two empty semiprivate rooms and one private room with negative air pressure flow that are available. The nurse receives a report that **Client A** has a diagnosis of cirrhosis with chronic hepatitis C. **Client B** has a diagnosis of a postsurgical amputation of the foot with a positive culture for *Staphylococcus aureus* wound infection. **Client C** is postoperative 1 day from a bowel resection with anastomosis. **Client D** has a diagnosis of active tuberculosis. **Client E** has a diagnosis of severe cellulitis with a positive culture for *S. aureus* and is on antibiotic therapy. Anticipating the arrival of these clients, the nurse prepares by reviewing transmission-based *precaution guidelines*, obtaining *vital signs* equipment, gathering *dressings and aseptic supplies*, and reviewing *medication orders*. As the first client arrives, the nurse enters the room, performs *hand hygiene*, and follows *appropriate precautions*.

1. Based on each client's diagnosis and information, which room(s) would you assign these clients to? Explain your rationale.

_____

_____

_____

2. What types of precautions are necessary to care for each of these client's appropriately?

_____

_____

_____

3. What types of infection(s) are represented in these clients?

_____

_____

_____

4. Using the information from the given case study and your text, identify six appropriate nursing actions/interventions when caring for a client with an infection or potential infection and place them in the concept map that follows.

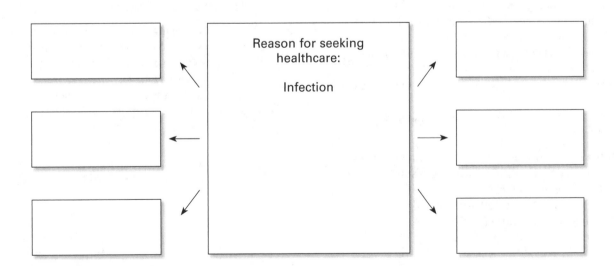

Reason for seeking healthcare:

Infection

SECTION 3: GETTING READY FOR NCLEX

Activity I   *Answer the following questions.*

1. What is the best explanation by a nurse for the fact that death from infections with multidrug-resistant microorganism is increased?
   1. Many pathogenic microorganisms are unaffected by antimicrobial drugs.
   2. Many pathogenic microorganisms react adversely with antimicrobial drugs.
   3. Antimicrobial drugs used for treating pathogens cause severe adverse effects.
   4. Antimicrobial drugs used for treating pathogens are still being developed.

2. What is the best nursing response when a client describes having periodic outbreaks of cold sores long after the initial infection of herpes simplex virus?
   1. Your particular viral strain is immune resistant.
   2. You never received proper antiviral therapy.
   3. Herpes virus remains dormant and reappears periodically.
   4. Recurrent outbreaks are due to a different viral strain.

3. What is the best nursing answer when someone asks about examples of community-acquired infections? Select all that apply.
   1. Tuberculosis
   2. Cystitis
   3. Meningitis
   4. Cholecystitis
   5. Influenza
   6. Appendicitis

4. When a nurse collects a stool specimen for ova and parasite examination, which action is most correct?
   1. The nurse places the entire specimen of feces in a cardboard container.
   2. The nurse takes a small amount of stool from the toilet bowl.
   3. The nurse takes a portion of stool to the laboratory while it is warm.
   4. The nurse refrigerates the specimen until the laboratory retrieves it.

5. What is the most effective method for preventing the transmission of infectious microorganisms?
   1. Covering the mouth when coughing
   2. Wiping the rectum well after toileting
   3. Eating nutritious meals each day
   4. Performing hand hygiene frequently

6. A physician orders penicillin G 300,000 Units IM q 6h. A multidose vial containing 1,000,000 Units of powdered penicillin G has been reconstituted to contain 250,000 Units/mL. Calculate the volume the nurse should administer per dose. Report the answer to the nearest tenth. _____

7. After administering an injection of penicillin in a physician's office for a confirmed case of streptococcal pharyngitis, how long should the nurse require the client to wait?
   1. 10 minutes
   2. 30 minutes
   3. 45 minutes
   4. 60 minutes

8. Which type of precautions is the nurse correct in using to prevent the transmission of pathogens from both recognized and unrecognized sources of infection?
   1. Contact precautions
   2. Droplet precautions
   3. Standard precautions
   4. Airborne precautions

9. Which of the following are situations in which the nurse should perform hand hygiene? Select all that apply.
   1. Before contact with every client
   2. After removing gloves
   3. When arriving home after work
   4. Before feeding clients
   5. Before preparing medications

10. Which of the following is an appropriate action when the nurse cares for a client on airborne precautions?
    1. Wear a gown when entering the room
    2. Don gloves after gowning
    3. Wear a mask when within 3 feet of client
    4. Wear a mask or use a particulate air filter respirator

13 Intravenous Therapy

LEARNING OBJECTIVES

1. Explain common indications for intravenous (IV) therapy.
2. Differentiate between crystalloid and colloid solutions and give examples of each.
3. Describe the difference between isotonic, hypotonic, and hypertonic solutions.
4. Explain the difference between whole blood, packed cells, blood products, and plasma expanders.
5. Describe nursing responsibilities for preparing IV solutions, selecting tubing, and selecting an infusion technique.
6. Identify nursing responsibilities when preparing the client for IV therapy.
7. Describe nursing actions involved in performing a venipuncture, including sites and devices commonly used.
8. Explain the equipment that must be replaced during IV therapy.
9. List complications of IV therapy and signs and symptoms for which the nurse monitors.
10. Explain how the nurse discontinues IV therapy.
11. Discuss the purpose of a medication lock.
12. Describe the nursing process for the client requiring IV therapy.
13. Discuss the purpose of total parenteral nutrition, and name one solution often administered concurrently.
14. Explain special considerations for blood transfusion therapy, including the equipment used, blood compatibility, and complications.

SECTION 1: ASSESSING YOUR UNDERSTANDING

Activity A *Fill in the blanks by choosing the correct word from the options given in parentheses.*

1. The nurse will select _____ to administer 1000 mL of 0.9% normal saline over 12 hours. (*primary tubing, secondary tubing, Y-administration tubing*)

2. The diameter of the venipuncture device always should be _____ that of the vein into which it will be inserted to reduce the potential for occluding blood flow. (*larger than, smaller than, equal to*)

3. Microdrip tubing, regardless of the manufacturer, delivers a standard volume of _____ drops (gtt)/mL. (*10, 15, 60*)

4. When an electronic infusion device is used to deliver IV solution, the rate is calculated in _____. (*milliliters per hour, drops per milliliter, drops per minute*)

5. _____ are nonblood solutions that pull fluid into the vascular space. They are used as an economical and virus-free substitute for blood and blood products when treating clients with hypovolemic shock. (*Plasma expanders, Packed red blood cells, Blood products*)

6. _____ is used when the client no longer needs continuous infusions, needs intermittent IV medication administration, or may need emergency IV fluids or medications. (*Macrodrip tubing, Microdrip tubing, Medication lock*)

Activity B *Write the correct term for each description.*

1. The nurse will select this type of tubing to administer a small volume of solution in a relatively short time through a port in the primary tubing. _____

2. A device that exerts positive pressure to infuse solutions. _____

3. The method for gaining access to the venous system by piercing a vein with one of a variety of devices. _____

4. The veins that are used for infusing IV fluids in infants. _____

5. The type of infusions that deliver solutions into a large central vein, such as the vena cava. _____

6. Administered when clients need fluid restoration as well as blood cells. _____

Activity C *Match the types of IV solution in Column A with their description in Column B.*

Column A

_____ **1.** Isotonic solutions

_____ **2.** Crystalloid solutions

_____ **3.** Hypotonic solutions

_____ **4.** Hypertonic solutions

_____ **5.** Colloid solutions

Column B

a. This type of solution is more concentrated (contains more dissolved substances) than plasma. Consequently, it draws fluid into the intravascular compartment from the more dilute areas in the cells and interstitial spaces.

b. This type of solution is used to replace circulating blood volume because the suspended molecules in the solutions pull fluid from other fluid compartments in the body. Examples include blood (whole blood and packed cells), blood products such as albumin, and solutions known as plasma expanders.

c. This type of solution contains fewer dissolved substances compared with plasma. Because the solution is dilute, the water in the solution passes through the semipermeable membrane of blood cells, causing them to swell.

d. This type of solution contains the same concentration of dissolved substances as is normally found in plasma. Because of its equal concentration to plasma, the solution causes no appreciable redistribution of body fluid on administration.

e. This type of solution consists of water and uniformly dissolved crystals such as salt (sodium chloride) or sugar (glucose, dextrose). Examples include 0.9% normal saline, 0.45% normal saline, and 10% dextrose in water.

Activity D *Briefly answer the following questions.*

1. Describe the indications for intravenous therapy.

_____

_____

_____

2. What are the nursing responsibilities for preparing intravenous solutions?

_____

_____

_____

3. When is filtered tubing used?

_____

_____

_____

4. What are the selection criteria for a venipuncture site?

_____

_____

_____

5. What circumstances would require inserting a central venous access device? Why is a chest x-ray required following insertion?

_____

_____

_____

6. What is the purpose of total parenteral nutrition?

_____

_____

_____

SECTION 2: APPLYING YOUR KNOWLEDGE

Activity E *Give rationale for the following questions.*

1. Why do tubing manufacturers design the drop size to deliver large-sized drops (macrodrip tubing) and small-sized drops (microdrip tubing)?

_____

_____

_____

2. Why must the nurse elevate the solution 18 to 24 inches above the infusion site when infusing an IV solution by gravity?

_____

_____

_____

3. Why is venipuncture in the foot avoided?

_____

_____

_____

4. Why are midline and midclavicular catheters considered peripheral venous access devices?

_____

_____

_____

5. Why are packed red blood cells preferred over whole blood in clients with congestive heart failure?

_____

_____

_____

6. Why is a lipid emulsion sometimes administered concurrently with total parenteral nutrition?

_____

_____

_____

Activity F *Answer the following questions related to intravenous therapy.*

1. Identify the nursing responsibilities when preparing a client for IV therapy.

_____

_____

_____

2. Which healthcare providers may insert a central venous access device?

_____

_____

_____

3. Identify the appropriate time frames to replace IV equipment.

_____

_____

4. What complications should the nurse monitor for when caring for a client with IV therapy?

_____

_____

_____

5. What are the possible complications of a blood transfusion?

_____

_____

_____

Activity G   *Think over the following questions. Discuss them with your peers or instructor.*

1. Discuss the nursing interventions indicated for a client receiving IV therapy with a nursing diagnosis of Risk for Imbalanced Fluid Volume related to the rate of infusion that exceeds circulatory capacity.

_____

_____

_____

2. Discuss the nursing interventions indicated for a client receiving IV therapy with a nursing diagnosis of Risk for Infection secondary to venipuncture and presence of a venous access device.

_____

_____

_____

3. Discuss the nursing care required for a client receiving total parenteral nutrition.

_____

_____

_____

Activity H   *Read the following case study. Use critical thinking skills to discuss and answer the questions that follow it.*

A client is scheduled for a total knee arthroplasty, and the nurse is preparing him for surgery. The nurse reviews the order for an IV of 1000 mL of lactated Ringer's (LR) solution to infuse over 8 hours. The nurse explains to the client the purpose of the ordered procedure and gathers the equipment. The nurse starts the IV in the client's left antecubital fossa and uses an electronic infusion device to infuse the solution. The physician has discussed the procedure with the client and indicated that he may need to receive blood after the surgery if blood loss is significant. The client is typed and cross-matched in advance of his surgical procedure. The client's blood is type O.

1. What are the necessary items that the nurse would gather to start the IV?

_____

_____

_____

2. What type of solution is LR and why is it appropriate for this client?

_____

_____

_____

3. At what rate per hour would the nurse infuse this solution?

_____

_____

_____

4. Why would the nurse choose the antecubital fossa as the venipuncture site?

_____

_____

_____

5. If the client requires blood postoperatively, what would be his best option?

_____

_____

_____

6. The client's spouse has a blood type of AB. Can she donate blood for her spouse? Why or why not?

_____

_____

_____

SECTION 3: GETTING READY FOR NCLEX

Activity I *Answer the following NCLEX-style questions.*

1. What is the best reason for closely monitoring older adults who are receiving IV therapy?
1. Older adults their defense mechanisms are less efficient
2. Older adults are prone to circulatory overload
3. Older adults have lower fluid requirements
4. Older adults prefer oral fluid replacements

2. When a client is receiving blood, which of the following nursing actions is essential to determine if chilling is the result of an emerging complication or of infusing cold blood?
1. Comparing the client's pre-infusion temperature with one during a chill
2. Documenting the client's temperature after the completion of the blood transfusion
3. Documenting the temperature of the blood before administering the blood transfusion
4. Comparing the client's temperature with the temperature of the blood

3. For which client is it appropriate for the nurse to consult the physician about initiating total parenteral nutrition?
1. A client who is consuming 50% of all meals
2. A client who professes to be a vegan
3. A client whose oral intake will be restricted for a week
4. A client whose admitting diagnosis is liver cancer

4. Which of the following nursing actions is most appropriate when the nurse observes that a venipuncture site is red, warm, and painful.
1. Report the findings to the physician.
2. Change the site of the IV infusion.
3. Elevate the site above the client's head.
4. Slow the rate of the IV infusion.

5. Which of the following assessments is the best indication that the client has an adequate fluid volume?
1. The client's blood pressure is 90/56.
2. The client's skin tents over the sternum.
3. The client's urine output is 2700 mL.
4. The client's respirations sound moist and gurgly.

6. If an IV of 1000 mL was started at 8:00 AM and is infusing at 125 mL/hr, at what time should the nurse expect that the infusion will be completed?
1. 12:00 noon
2. 2:00 PM
3. 4:00 PM
4. 8:00 PM

7. A nurse is accurate in identifying which IV solution as one that will transfer fluid from the intravascular space to the interstitial and intracellular spaces?
1. 0.9% saline solution
2. Ringer's solution
3. 3% saline solution
4. 0.45% saline solution

8. Fill in the blank with the rate that the nurse should set an electronic infusion device so that 1000 mL of IV solution infuses in 10 hours? The container of solution has macrodrip tubing. _____

9. Which of the following is the best reason the nurse can provide that a client requires a central venous catheter?
1. Client has 0.9% normal saline ordered.
2. Client will be receiving total parenteral nutrition (TPN).
3. Client will be receiving infusions of albumin.
4. Client has an infusion order for platelets.

10. A client with type A positive blood requires a transfusion. Which of the following is the nurse correct in identifying as compatible blood types? Select all that apply.
1. Type A positive
2. Type A negative
3. Type AB positive
4. Type AB negative
5. Type O positive
6. Type O negative

14 Perioperative Care

LEARNING OBJECTIVES

1. Describe why surgical procedures may be performed.
2. Differentiate the phases of perioperative care.
3. Outline preoperative assessments needed to identify surgical risk factors.
4. List components of a preoperative teaching plan.
5. Describe physical preparation of the client for surgery.
6. List preoperative medications that may be ordered.
7. Discuss psychosocial preparation of the client for surgery, including strategies for alleviating clients' preoperative anxiety.
8. Compare types of anesthesia.
9. Describe the roles and functions of the surgical team members.
10. Describe nursing management of the intraoperative client.
11. Discuss assessments needed to prevent postoperative complications.
12. Describe standards of care, nursing diagnoses, and common interventions for general surgical clients in the later postoperative period.

SECTION 1: ASSESSING YOUR UNDERSTANDING

Activity A Fill in the blanks by choosing the correct word from the options given in parentheses.

1. The _____ begins with admission to the recovery area and continues until the client receives a follow-up evaluation at home or is discharged to a rehabilitation unit. (*preoperative phase, intraoperative phase, postoperative phase*)

2. The _____ is a physician who has completed 2 years of residency in anesthesia. (*anesthesiologist, anesthetist, first assistant*)

3. Healing by _____ occurs when the wound layers are sutured together so that wound edges are well approximated. This type of incision usually heals in 8 to 10 days, with minimal scarring. (*primary intention, secondary intention, tertiary intention*)

4. Interruption of blood supply secondary to prolonged pressure, nerve injury related to prolonged pressure, postoperative hypotension, dependent edema, and joint injury may result from _____ in the OR. (*hypothermia, poor body alignment, malignant hyperthermia*)

5. Postoperative pain reaches its peak between _____ hours after surgery. (*6 and 12, 12 and 36, 36 and 48*)

6. _____ occurs when the wound completely separates and organs protrude. (*Wound infection, Wound evisceration, Wound dehiscence*)

7. The _____ assists the surgical team by handing instruments to the surgeon and assistants, preparing sutures, receiving specimens for laboratory examination, and counting sponges and needles. (*scrub nurse, circulating nurse, anesthetist*)

Activity B Write the correct term for each description.

1. Danger of aspiration from saliva, mucus, vomitus, or blood exists until the client is fully awake and can swallow without difficulty. This equipment must be kept at the client's bedside until the danger of aspiration no longer exists. _____

2. This phase begins with the decision to perform surgery and continues until the client reaches the operating area. _____

3. This member of the surgical team may be an RN, a licensed practical or vocational nurse (LPNs/LVNs), or a surgical technologist who assist the surgeon and first assistant. _____

4. The approximation of wound edges is delayed secondary to infection. When the wound is drained and cleaned of infection, the wound edges are sutured together. The resulting scar is wider than that with primary intention. _____

5. Separation of wound edges without the protrusion of organs. _____

6. This member of the surgical team assists in the surgical procedure and may be involved with the client's preoperative and postoperative care. He or she may be another physician, a surgical resident, or an RN who has appropriate approval and endorsement from the American Operating Room Nurses (AORN) and the American College of Surgeons. _____

Activity C *Match the preoperative medications given in Column A with the corresponding benefits given in Column B.*

Column A

_____ **1.** Anticholinergics

_____ **2.** Antiemetic drugs

_____ **3.** Histamine-2 receptor antagonists

_____ **4.** Narcotics

_____ **5.** Sedatives

_____ **6.** Tranquilizers

Column B

a. Decrease gastric acidity and volume.

b. Decrease respiratory tract secretions, dry mucous membranes, and interrupt vagal stimulation.

c. Reduce nausea, prevent emesis, and enhance preoperative sedation.

d. Reduce preoperative anxiety, slow motor activity, and promote induction of anesthesia.

e. Decrease the amount of anesthesia needed, help reduce anxiety and pain, and promote sleep.

f. Promote sleep, decrease anxiety, and reduce the amount of anesthesia needed.

Activity D *Consider the following figure.*

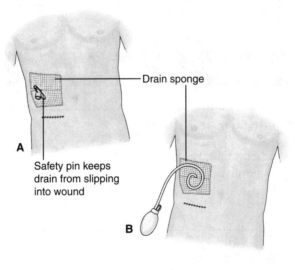

Drain sponge

A

Safety pin keeps drain from slipping into wound

B

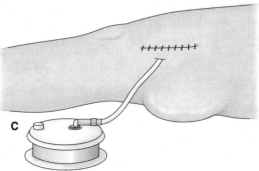

C

1. Identify the types of surgical drains.

   A. _____

   B. _____

   C. _____

2. What are the assessments a nurse should perform when assessing a wound?

   _____

   _____

   _____

Activity E *Briefly answer the following questions.*

1. Identify the basic elements of a nursing preoperative assessment.

   _____

   _____

   _____

2. The nurse identifies if the client is at risk for complications during or after surgery based on what general risk factors?

   _____

   _____

3. What is the purpose of adequate preoperative teaching/ learning?

   _____

   _____

   _____

4. What is included in the physical preparation of a client for surgery?

   _____

   _____

   _____

5. Describe the responsibilities of the circulating nurse.

   _____

   _____

   _____

6. What factors may lead to hypoxia postoperatively?

   _____

   _____

   _____

SECTION 2: APPLYING YOUR KNOWLEDGE

Activity F *Give rationale for the following questions.*

1. Why is it best to teach clients about their surgical procedure and expectations during the preoperative period?

   _____

   _____

   _____

2. Why should a client sign a surgical consent form or operative permit before surgery? What does it indicate?

   _____

   _____

   _____

3. Why is the air filtered and a positive pressure maintained in the surgical suite?

   _____

   _____

   _____

4. Why must shock be detected early and treated promptly in the postoperative phase?

   _____

   _____

   _____

5. Why are antiembolism stockings used postoperatively?

_____

_____

_____

6. Why must the nurse inspect dressings frequently and check under the bedding of the client postoperatively?

_____

_____

_____

_____

Activity G _Answer the following questions related to perioperative care._

1. What assessments will the nurse perform on a client admitted for surgery?

_____

_____

_____

2. What information will the nurse include in preoperative teaching?

_____

_____

_____

3. Describe the differences between general anesthesia and regional anesthesia.

_____

_____

_____

4. Describe psychosocial preparation for the client.

_____

_____

_____

5. Describe nursing management of the intraoperative client.

_____

_____

_____

6. Identify the minimum standards of care for the general surgical client.

_____

_____

_____

Activity H _Think over the following questions. Discuss them with your instructor or peers._

1. A client complains of discomfort and does not want to perform deep breathing and coughing exercises, use the incentive spirometer, or ambulate. How will you proceed? What education will you provide?

_____

_____

_____

2. A client who has undergone surgery is unable to expel gas or have a bowel movement. What nursing interventions would you implement? If the nursing interventions are not effective, what would you do?

_____

_____

_____

3. A client is receiving pain medication postoperatively. What safety measures would you implement to prevent client injury?

_____

_____

_____

4. A client is being discharged following a surgical procedure. What information will you need to provide to the client and/or the family?

_____

_____

_____

Activity I

Read the following case study. Use critical thinking skills to discuss and answer the questions that follow it.

A 58-year-old client with a history of *diabetes* is admitted to an outpatient surgical center for a routine endoscopy. Prior to admission, the client was given instructions for preprocedure bowel preparation that needed to be completed the day before. The client was also instructed to remain nothing by mouth (NPO) after midnight. The client has brought her spouse with her. Upon admission, the nurse weighs the client and orients her to the room. The client is 5 ft in height and *weighs 220 lb*.

1. What types of information would the nurse gather in the preprocedural assessment of this client?

_____

_____

_____

2. What type of anesthesia/sedation would typically be used for this client? How would it be administered?

_____

_____

_____

3. What are the nursing implications for this type of anesthesia/sedation?

_____

_____

_____

4. Using the information from the given case study, identify two surgical/procedural risk factors and potential complications from them. (Italicized words are potential clues.)

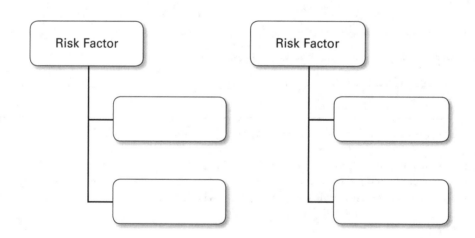

SECTION 3: GETTING READY FOR NCLEX

Activity J *Answer the following questions.*

1. A client is hospitalized for a surgical procedure. During the assessment, the nurse notes that the client has not carried out a specific portion of the preoperative instructions. Which of the following nursing interventions should the nurse perform?
   1. Suggest an alternative recommendation to the instruction.
   2. Notify the surgeon.
   3. Document on the client's chart.
   4. Ask the client to implement the instructions and appear for the surgery later.

2. A nurse applying for a position in the local hospital asks the interviewing nurse what the responsibilities of a circulating nurse would be. What would be the interviewing nurse's most appropriate response?
   1. The circulating nurse obtains and opens wrapped sterile equipment
   2. The circulating nurse prepares sutures for the surgeon
   3. The circulating nurse hands instruments to the surgeon and assistants
   4. The circulating nurse assists with putting the client to sleep

3. The nurse explains to the student nurse the factors that may promote anxiety for a client undergoing a surgical procedure. Which factors would the nurse be most likely to include? Select all that apply.
   1. Decreased mobility
   2. Unfamiliar environment
   3. Unclear expectations
   4. Decreased alertness
   5. Postoperative pain

4. A nurse needs to care for a client during the immediate postoperative period. Which of the following factors predisposes the client to hypoxia?
   1. Pooling of secretions in the lungs
   2. Fluid and electrolyte loss
   3. Physical and psychological trauma
   4. Increased mobility

5. A nurse explains to a client who underwent surgery the rationale for using caution when changing the wound dressings. What would be the nurse's most appropriate explanation?
   1. Caution is needed to prevent damaging new tissue
   2. Caution is needed to minimize causing pain to the client
   3. Caution is needed to promote faster wound healing
   4. Caution is needed to avoid wound infection

6. What does weight gain during the postoperative period signify?
   1. Urine retention
   2. Fluid accumulation
   3. Healthy recovery
   4. Paralytic ileus

7. Which of the following preoperative medications causes decreased respiratory tract secretions, dry mucous membranes, and interrupts vagal stimulation?
   1. Histamine$_2$-receptor antagonists
   2. Antianxiety drugs
   3. Anticholinergics
   4. Sedatives

8. Which type of anesthesia describes a state in which the client is free of pain, fear, and anxiety and can tolerate unpleasant procedures while maintaining independent cardiorespiratory function and the ability to respond to verbal commands and tactile stimulation?
   1. General anesthesia
   2. Regional anesthesia
   3. Epidural block
   4. Procedural sedation

9. Which of the following postoperative complications results from saliva, mucus, vomitus, or blood, making its way into the lungs as a result of difficulty in swallowing or a client's inability to expectorate oral secretions?
   1. Aspiration
   2. Hypoxia
   3. Shock
   4. Hemorrhage

10. A client asks the nurse about the healing of the surgical wound. The nurse explains the stages of healing, with one stage lasting 21 days to at least several months, allowing for increased wound strength through physiologic processes. What stage is the nurse referring to?
    1. The inflammatory stage.
    2. The proliferative phase.
    3. The maturation phase.
    4. The approximation phase.

15 Disaster Situations

LEARNING OBJECTIVES

1. Define disaster and give two general examples.
2. Identify three categories of human disasters that may result from acts of terrorism.
3. Name three methods by which a radiologic disaster could be created.
4. Explain the difference between external and internal radiation contamination.
5. Name three substances used to prevent or reduce radiologic organ damage.
6. List possible indications of a bioterrorism attempt.
7. Name three biologic agents likely to be used as weapons of mass destruction.
8. List possible indications of a chemical terrorism attempt.
9. Name four types of chemical agents that may be used to create a human disaster.
10. List four triage categories that emergency workers use to prioritize victims' need for treatment.
11. Provide examples of collaborative problems and nursing diagnoses that the nurse may be required to manage following a disaster.

SECTION 1: ASSESSING YOUR UNDERSTANDING

Activity A *Fill in the blanks by choosing the correct word from the options given in parentheses.*

1. _____ is a disaster caused by pathogens or their toxins that cause harm to humans and other living species. (*Biologic disaster, Radiologic disaster, Chemical disaster*)

2. _____ is a disease that develops from the neurotoxin produced by *Clostridium botulinum*, which is generally food-borne. There have been no reports of person-to-person transmission. (*Anthrax, Botulism, Smallpox*)

3. Laboratory studies suggest that _____, a new antiviral agent, may be effective against smallpox. (*cidofovir, doxycycline, ciprofloxacin*)

4. Detection of _____ is difficult because most agents are liquids that vaporize quickly with either no odors or odors that may be attributed to other substances. (*biologic disasters, radiologic disasters, chemical disasters*)

5. Exposure to _____ leads to tearing, coughing, bronchospasms, and laryngospasms with airway obstruction from localized swelling. (*biologic toxins, respiratory toxins, radiologic toxins*)

6. _____ occurs from exposure to fallout on the skin, hair, and clothing. (*Prussian blue, External radiologic contamination, Internal radiologic contamination*)

Activity B *Write the correct term for each description.*

1. The American Red Cross defines this as "a threatening . . . event of such destructive magnitude and force as to dislocate people, separate family members, damage or destroy homes, and injure or kill people." _____

2. A spore-forming bacterium known as *Bacillus anthracis*, which causes disease when inhaled, ingested, or introduced into nonintact skin. It is treated fairly successfully with fluoroquinolones. _____

3. A solid salt or volatile liquid chemical that causes death in minutes. The gas that forms with release is colorless and may have a faint odor of "bitter almonds." _____

4. This type of contamination occurs when fallout enters an open wound, is inhaled via contaminated air, or is consumed through contaminated food and water. _____

5. The greatest potential for lethality occurs with paralysis of the respiratory muscles. If large numbers of people were to become acutely ill simultaneously as a consequence of bioterrorism, the numbers of ventilators available in any particular agency would likely become exhausted quickly. _____

6. A highly contagious disease caused by the variola virus. _____

Activity C *Match the antidotes or medications given in Column A with the conditions they treat in Column B.*

Column A

_____ **1.** Prussian blue

_____ **2.** Pralidoxime chloride

_____ **3.** Potassium iodide

_____ **4.** Diethylenetriamine pentaacetate (DTPA)

_____ **5.** Atropine sulfate

_____ **6.** Amyl nitrite, sodium nitrite, and sodium thiosulfate

Column B

a. Prevents radioactive iodine from reaching the thyroid gland by saturating the gland with nonradioactive iodine. The person must take it as soon as possible up to 24 hours after exposure. It limits or protects only the thyroid gland; it does not interfere with radiologic effects on other organs.

b. Reactivates acetylcholinesterase with exposure to nerve agents.

c. A dye used to treat internal contamination with ingested radioactive cesium. The dye promotes the excretion of cesium by trapping it in the intestine and preventing its absorption.

d. An injectable salt or inhalant spray that contains calcium (Ca-DTPA) or zinc (Zn-DTPA) and is used to treat internal contamination with radioactive substances such as plutonium.

e. May be administered alone or together as an antidote for cyanide poisoning.

f. Counteracts excess acetylcholine at muscarinic sites with exposure to nerve agents.

Activity D *Briefly answer the following questions.*

1. Identify three types of human disasters.

_____

_____

_____

2. How can radiologic disasters occur?

_____

_____

_____

3. What are indications of bioterrorism?

_____

_____

_____

4. How can smallpox be distinguished from chickenpox?

_____

_____

_____

5. What are the indications of a chemical terrorism?

_____

_____

_____

6. What are the early signs of botulism?

_____

_____

_____

SECTION 2:   APPLYING YOUR KNOWLEDGE

Activity E   *Give rationale for the following questions.*

1. Why do terrorists exploit actual or potential human disasters?

_____

_____

_____

2. How can radiologic disasters cause life-threatening consequences when injury is not caused by penetrating or blunt trauma?

_____

_____

_____

3. Why are anthrax, botulism, and smallpox likely to be used in bioterrorist warfare?

_____

_____

_____

4. Why are tetracyclines not used initially to treat anthrax infections?

_____

_____

_____

5. How could a person who was not directly exposed to a radiologic disaster exhibit signs and symptoms of radiologic contamination?

_____

_____

_____

Activity F   *Answer the following questions related to disaster situations.*

1. What is the most immediate concern when dealing with a radiologic disaster?

_____

_____

_____

2. Describe the isolation precautions for smallpox.

_____

_____

_____

3. What are the supportive measures that should be taken with exposure to a nerve agent?

_____

_____

_____

4. Describe the signs and symptoms of cyanide poisoning.

_____

_____

_____

5. What measures should be taken with exposure to chlorine or phosgene?

_____

_____

_____

6. Describe the decontamination process for exposure to a vesicant.

_____

_____

_____

Activity G *Think over the following questions. Discuss them with your instructor or peers.*

1. There has been an accidental explosion at a chemical plant near your facility. You have been assigned to triage the victims. Describe the precautions you would take and the care you would provide to each of the following victims:
   - Casualty A—This victim was close to the blast and has sustained partial and full-thickness burns over 85% of the body, respirations are shallow, and pulse is thready.
   - Casualty B—This victim has an obvious fracture to the left forearm and some tearing from exposure to the chemicals. This victim has no coughing and states no difficulty breathing.
   - Casualty C—This victim has no tearing, coughing, or difficulty breathing. The victim has some minor lacerations and is emotionally distraught; Casualty A is this person's spouse.
   - Casualty D—This victim was not exposed to the blast but was exposed to the chemicals escaping from the receptacles. The victim has no obvious signs of trauma but is repeatedly coughing and gasping for breath.

   _____

   _____

   _____

Activity H *Read the following case study. Use critical thinking skills to discuss and answer the questions that follow it.*

The nurse and healthcare/emergency response team are involved in a mock disaster drill for a potential biologic threat. The drill begins with the notification that the local Research Laboratory Center has a lab research worker who has accidentally been exposed to the smallpox virus by handling a contaminated object that contained the live virus. The nurse and team have been called to immediately help contain the situation.

1. What types of precautions/safety measures are required to care for this client?

   _____

   _____

   _____

2. According to the given case study, arrange the following symptoms for smallpox in order of progression/development.
   A. The rash appears on tongue and mouth and develops on face, spreading to extremities, and becomes fluid-filled papules with an area resembling a "navel."
   B. Scabs have resolved.
   C. Onset of high fever, headache, body aches, malaise
   D. Pustules begin to crust and scab.
   E. No evidence of symptoms
   F. Papules become pustules round and firm, as though embedded with pellets.
   G. Scabs are shed over a 3-week period, leaving scars.

   ☐ → ☐ → ☐ → ☐ → ☐ → ☐ → ☐

3. What is the treatment for smallpox?

   _____

   _____

4. When should the vaccine be given, and under what conditions is the vaccine rendered useless?

   _____

   _____

   _____

5. What action must the team of healthcare providers take to protect the public in relationship to this case of accidental exposure?

   _____

   _____

   _____

6. For what community population is the vaccine contraindicated?

_____

_____

_____

7. If this were a bioterrorist attack, what type of delivery method would most likely be used to affect the highest number of individuals?

_____

_____

_____

SECTION 3: GETTING READY FOR NCLEX

Activity I   _Answer the following questions._

1. Of the following observations, which one is most indicative to a nurse that a chemical agent has been released in act of terrorism?
1. There are numerous dead animals in the immediate area.
2. A body of water appears to have a peculiar color.
3. Loud sirens are being sounded within the community.
4. First responders are gathering in the nearby vicinity.

2. When caring for a client exposed to cyanide, which of the following antidotes that the nurse administers is an inhalant that converts cyanide into a nontoxic substance?
1. Methemoglobin
2. Sodium nitrite
3. Amyl nitrite
4. Sodium thiosulfate

3. What is the best rationale for a nurse moving a victim of a common respiratory toxin to higher ground immediately?
1. Toxic respiratory agents are carried on air currents to the lower ground.
2. Toxic respiratory agents toxic vapors stay close to the ground.
3. Toxic respiratory agents are always released close to the ground.
4. Heavy and solid respiratory toxins cannot move higher.

4. Which of the following should the nurse advocate for limiting external contamination following exposure to radiation?
1. Remove all or at least outer clothing before entering a shelter
2. Drinking only bottled water rather than tap water
3. Covering the nose and mouth with some type of cloth
4. Avoiding consumption of exposed fresh food

5. Which of the following substances will a nurse most likely distribute to protect the thyroid from the effects of radiation?
1. Prussian blue
2. Potassium iodide
3. Cesium 127
4. Atropine sulfate

6. Which of the following is the best advice the nurse can give persons who may be infected with anthrax?
1. Wear a mask to avoid transmitting droplets.
2. Cover skin lesions with a transparent dressing.
3. Caution others to avoid touching skin lesions.
4. Isolate yourself by staying indoors out of drafts.

7. Which is the usual site for the nurse to administer a smallpox vaccination?
1. Deltoid
2. Lateral thigh
3. Abdomen
4. Outer buttocks

8. When participating in a mock triage of disaster victims, if the nurse assessed a person as having multisystem trauma, in which category would the person be placed?
1. Immediate
2. Delayed
3. Minimal
4. Expectant

9. What nursing action is appropriate for disaster victims who fall into a minimal triage category?
1. Provide treatment to decrease congestion of victims
2. Delegate assistive personnel to attend to minor injuries
3. Reassess the victim at frequent intervals
4. Stabilize victim with life-threatening problems

10. Which of the following are nursing actions that can restore survivors' ability to cope with a disaster? Select all that apply?
1. Provide information about the disaster
2. Censure those who are acting hysterically
3. Listen to victims recount their experiences
4. Reunite family members or friends

16 Caring for Clients With Fluid, Electrolyte, and Acid–Base Imbalances

LEARNING OBJECTIVES

1. List three chemical substances that are components of body fluid.
2. Name the two main fluid locations in the human body and two subdivisions.
3. Give the average fluid intake per day for adults.
4. List four ways in which the body normally loses fluid.
5. Identify five processes by which water and dissolved chemicals are relocated in the body.
6. Name three mechanisms that help regulate fluid and electrolyte balance.
7. List two types of fluid imbalance.
8. Explain the difference between hypovolemia and dehydration.
9. Explain hemoconcentration and hemodilution.
10. Identify assessment findings of and nursing interventions for hypovolemia.
11. List and identify the differences in three types of edema.
12. Identify assessment findings of and nursing interventions for hypervolemia.
13. Explain third-spacing and medical techniques for relocating this fluid.
14. List factors that contribute to electrolyte loss and excess.
15. Name four electrolyte imbalances that pose a major threat to well-being.
16. Discuss the nursing management of clients with electrolyte imbalances.
17. Discuss the role of acids and bases in body fluid.
18. Explain pH and identify the normal range of plasma pH.
19. Identify two chemicals and two organs that play major roles in regulating acid–base balance.
20. Give the names of two major acid–base imbalances and subdivisions of each.
21. List three components of arterial blood gas findings used to determine acid–base imbalances.
22. Discuss the nursing management of clients with acid–base imbalances.

SECTION 1: ASSESSING YOUR UNDERSTANDING

Activity A *Fill in the blanks by choosing the correct word from the options given in parentheses.*

1. _____ can occur with severe renal failure; severe burns; administration of potassium-sparing diuretics; overuse of potassium supplements, salt substitutes or some diet sodas, or potassium-rich foods; crushing injuries; Addison's disease; and rapid administration of parenteral potassium salts. (*Hypercalcemia, Hypernatremia, Hyperkalemia*)

2. _____ are substances that carry an electrical charge when dissolved in fluid. (*Electrolytes, Acids, Bases*)

3. About 60% of the adult human body is water. Most body water is located in _____. (*intravascular fluid, intracellular fluid, interstitial fluid*)

4. The power to draw water toward an area of greater concentration is referred to as _____. *(filtration, tonicity, osmotic pressure)*

5. Hypovolemia results in _____, a high ratio of blood components in relation to watery plasma, which increases the potential for blood clots and urinary stones and compromises the kidney's ability to excrete nitrogen wastes. *(hemodilution, hypervolemia, hemoconcentration)*

6. _____ is associated with parathyroid gland tumors, multiple fractures, Paget's disease, hyperparathyroidism, excessive doses of vitamin D, prolonged immobilization, some chemotherapeutic agents, and certain malignant diseases. *(Hypercalcemia, Hyperkalemia, Hypernatremia)*

7. In healthy adults, oral fluid intake averages about 2500 mL/day; however, it can range between _____, with a similar volume of fluid loss. *(1800 and 3000 mL/day, 2000 and 3000 mL/day, 1500 and 3500 mL/day)*

8. Normal plasma pH is _____, or slightly alkaline. *(7 which is neutral, 7.35 to 7.45, 1 to 14)*

Activity B *Write the correct term for each description.*

1. Positively or negatively charged substances. _____

2. As excess fluid volume is distributed to the interstitial space, indentations in the skin after compression may be noted. This type of edema usually does not occur, however, until there is a 3-L excess in the intravascular volume. _____

3. The concentration of substances in blood. _____

4. Causes include profuse watery diarrhea, excessive salt intake without sufficient water intake, high fever, decreased water intake, excessive administration of solutions that contain sodium, excessive water loss without an accompanying loss of sodium, and severe burns. _____

5. Positively charged ion. _____

6. This electrolyte imbalance may result from renal failure, Addison's disease, excessive use of antacids or laxatives that contain magnesium, and hyperparathyroidism. _____

7. The main tool for measuring blood pH, CO_2 content $(PaCO_2)$, and bicarbonate. _____

8. Negatively charged ion. _____

Activity C *Match the terms given in Column A with their related descriptions given in Column B.*

Column A

_____ **1.** Osmosis

_____ **2.** Filtration

_____ **3.** Passive diffusion

_____ **4.** Facilitated diffusion

_____ **5.** Active transport

Column B

a. Promotes the movement of fluid and some dissolved substances through a semipermeable membrane according to pressure differences.

b. Certain dissolved substances require assistance from a carrier molecule to pass through a semipermeable membrane.

c. The movement of water through a semipermeable membrane from a dilute area to a more concentrated area.

d. Requires an energy source, a substance called adenosine triphosphate (ATP), to drive dissolved chemicals from an area of low concentration to an area of higher concentration.

e. A physiologic process by which dissolved substances (e.g., electrolytes) move from an area of high concentration to an area of lower concentration through a semipermeable membrane.

Activity D *Briefly answer the following questions.*

1. What are the mechanisms of fluid loss?

_____

_____

_____

2. Describe the difference between hypovolemia and dehydration.

_____

_____

_____

3. Describe conditions that place the client at risk for developing hyponatremia?

_____

_____

_____

4. What are causes of hypervolemia?

_____

_____

_____

5. What is third-spacing? What is it associated with?

_____

_____

_____

6. What is responsible for electrical potentials that develop across cell membranes and perhaps for the degree of cell membrane permeability?

_____

_____

_____

7. What two signs can be used to assess for hypocalcemia?

_____

_____

_____

SECTION 2: APPLYING YOUR KNOWLEDGE

Activity E   _Give rationale for the following questions._

1. Why is dehydration the most common fluid imbalance in older adults?

_____

_____

2. How do colloids contribute to fluid concentration and act as a force for attracting water?

_____

_____

3. Why is the forehead or sternum used to assess fluid status in older adults?

_____

_____

_____

4. Why should potassium never be administered in a concentrated strength by IV?

_____

_____

5. Why are older adults at risk for developing electrolyte imbalances?

_____

_____

6. Why must the client be closely monitored when administering magnesium sulfate IV?

_____

_____

Activity F   _Answer the following questions related to fluid, electrolyte, and acid–base imbalances._

1. How do chemical regulators in the body maintain acid–base balance?

_____

_____

_____

2. What conditions place the client at risk for developing hypomagnesemia?

_____

_____

_____

3. How do the lungs and kidneys facilitate the ratio of bicarbonate to carbonic acid?

_____

_____

_____

4. Describe the medical management of third-spacing.

_____

_____

_____

5. Identify the types and subtypes of acid–base imbalances.

_____

_____

_____

Activity G *Think over the following questions. Discuss them with your instructor or peers.*

1. Laboratory results for your client include elevated hematocrit and blood cell counts, and the urine specific gravity is high. Your client has been experiencing excessive thirst. What do these assessment findings indicate? What nursing assessments and interventions are indicated?

_____

_____

_____

2. Assessment of your client reveals an elevated BP, an increased breathing effort, and pitting edema. Laboratory results include a decreased blood cell count, a decreased hematocrit, and the urine specific gravity is low. What nursing assessments and interventions are indicated?

_____

_____

_____

Activity H *Read the following case study. Use critical thinking skills to discuss and answer the questions that follow it.*

A client has presented to the ER with complaints of fatigue, *nausea*, *vomiting*, weakness, and a *poor appetite*. The client's current medications include furosemide (Lasix) 40 mg po daily, one multivitamin po daily, digoxin 0.25 mg po daily, and docusate (Colace) 100 mg po as needed. The nurse observes some slight *confusion* in the client and a *decreased* *respiratory rate*. The client states that he has been taking an occasional glass of water with a teaspoon of baking soda for his upset stomach. The client's ECG results show a flattened T wave, ST segment depression, and a U wave. The nurse prepares to take vital signs while awaiting the results from the lab for electrolytes and ABGs.

1. Are the client's symptoms indicative of a fluid or electrolyte imbalance? Give your rationale.

_____

_____

_____

2. Why did the physician order ABGs?

_____

_____

_____

3. As the nurse, how would you care for or manage this client?

_____

_____

_____

4. Using the information from the given case study, identify five additional nursing diagnoses for the concept map below. (Italicized words are clues to the answer.)

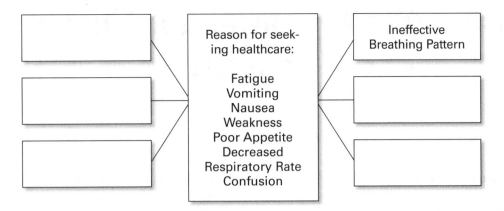

SECTION 3: GETTING READY FOR NCLEX

Activity I   *Answer the following questions.*

1. For which of the following conditions would the nurse anticipate administering salt tablets?
   1. Mild deficits of serum sodium
   2. Severe deficits of serum magnesium
   3. Mild deficits of serum potassium
   4. Severe deficits of serum calcium

2. If a client's parathyroid glands were accidentally removed during a procedure, which condition should the nurse prepare for?
   1. Hypomagnesemia
   2. Hyperkalemia
   3. Hypernatremia
   4. Hypocalcemia

3. A client is having a problem with the absorption of calcium. Which vitamin deficiency would the nurse anticipate in this client?
   1. Vitamin A
   2. Vitamin B
   3. Vitamin C
   4. Vitamin D

4. Which of the following points should a nurse include in the teaching plan for clients who have a potential for hypovolemia?
   1. Avoid consuming alcohol and caffeine.
   2. Increase intake of dried peas and beans.
   3. Increase intake of milk and dairy products.
   4. Avoid table salt or food containing sodium.

5. For which of the following categories of medications should the nurse monitor a client for lowered serum sodium and potassium levels?
   1. Diuretics
   2. Analgesics
   3. Antibiotics
   4. Sedatives

6. When the nurse reviews arterial blood gas results on several clients, which one indicates a normal blood pH?
   1. 7.35 to 7.45
   2. 6.35 to 6.45
   3. 7 to 8
   4. 8.35 to 8.45

7. When caring for a client who is dehydrated, the nurse can anticipate that a client may manifest which of the following? Select all that apply.
   1. Labored breathing
   2. Postural hypotension
   3. Dark yellow urine
   4. Bounding pulse
   5. Elevated temperature
   6. Flushed skin

8. When a nurse collects data, which sign or symptom is the first one to occur in hypovolemia?
   1. Low blood pressure
   2. Increased thirst
   3. Low urine specific gravity
   4. Mild confusion

9. A physician orders furosemide 40 mg oral solution bid for a client who has difficulty swallowing tablets. Calculate the dose the nurse should administer for a supplied dose of 10 mg/mL.

10. Which of the following conditions can the nurse anticipate causing respiratory alkalosis?
    1. Uncontrolled diabetes
    2. Rapid breathing
    3. Chronic respiratory disease
    4. Prolonged vomiting

17 Caring for Clients in Shock

LEARNING OBJECTIVES

1. Define shock.

2. Name four general categories of shock.

3. Identify the subcategories of distributive shock.

4. List pathophysiologic consequences of shock.

5. Name the three stages of shock.

6. Identify three physiologic mechanisms that attempt to compensate for shock.

7. Discuss signs and symptoms manifested by clients in shock.

8. Name three diagnostic measurements used when monitoring clients in shock.

9. Give three medical approaches for treating shock.

10. List complications of shock.

11. Discuss the nursing management of clients with shock.

SECTION 1: ASSESSING YOUR UNDERSTANDING

Activity A *Fill in the blanks by choosing the correct word from the options given in parentheses.*

1. In _____, the most common type of shock, the volume of extracellular fluid is significantly diminished, primarily because of lost or reduced blood or plasma. *(hypovolemic shock, distributive shock, cardiogenic shock)*

2. In shock, the partial pressure of oxygen in arterial blood falls below _____. *(40 mm Hg, 60 mm Hg, 80 mm Hg)*

3. _____ is the pressure of the blood in the right atrium or venae cavae. It distinguishes relationships among hemodynamic variables in shock: venous return, quality of right ventricular function, and vascular tone. *(Pulmonary artery pressure, Arterial blood gas, Central venous pressure)*

4. Drugs with _____ increase peripheral vascular resistance and raise BP. *(alpha-adrenergic activity, beta-adrenergic activity, cholinergic activity)*

5. In shock, the pulse pressure tends to _____ as the falling systolic pressure nears the diastolic pressure. *(widen, narrow, falter)*

6. Capillary filling longer than 3 seconds and cyanosis, especially of the nail beds, lips, and earlobes, indicate _____. *(fluid deficiency, electrolyte deficiency, oxygen deficiency)*

Activity B *Write the correct term for each description.*

1. A life-threatening condition that occurs when arterial blood flow and oxygen delivery to tissues and cells are inadequate. This condition develops as a consequence of one of three events: (1) blood volume decreases, (2) the heart fails as an effective pump, or (3) peripheral blood vessels massively dilate. _____

2. The type of shock that is sometimes called normovolemic shock because the amount of fluid in the circulatory system is not reduced, yet the fluid circulation does not permit effective tissue perfusion. _____

3. The diagnostic measurement that is used because left ventricular function is more pertinent to circulation than the right. Knowing fluid pressures on the left side of the heart is more meaningful. _____

4. The category of drugs that are the main medications used to treat shock. _____

5. A body cavity that when filled with fluid, air, or tissue can lead to obstructive shock. _____

6. Drugs in this category increase heart rate and improve the force of heart contraction. _____

Activity C   *Match the physiologic mechanisms of compensation in Column A with their specific effects in Column B.*

Column A

_____ 1. Catecholamines (epinephrine and norepinephrine)

_____ 2. Aldosterone

_____ 3. Glucocorticoids

_____ 4. Angiotensin II

_____ 5. Antidiuretic hormone (also known as vasopressin)

Column B

a. Help(s) the body respond to stress by secreting cortisol.

b. Causes sodium and water to be reabsorbed by the kidney to raise blood pressure.

c. Low blood volume stimulates secretion which promotes reabsorption of water that the kidneys would ordinarily excrete.

d. Increase heart rate, myocardial contractility, and dilate bronchi.

e. Raises blood pressure by constricting arterioles.

Activity D   *The steps of cellular hypoxia are in random order. Arrange the steps in proper sequence.*

1. Sodium and water enter the cells, potassium exits the cell, and the cells eventually rupture.

2. Pyruvic and lactic acid increases, causing metabolic acidosis.

3. A decreased amount of oxygen reaches the cells.

4. Lysosomes leak enzymatic fluid and contribute to further cellular destruction.

5. Hypoxic cells are forced to switch to anaerobic metabolism.

6. Without an energy source, the sodium-potassium pump is ineffective.

☐→☐→☐→☐→☐→☐

Activity E   *Differentiate among the types of distributive shock based on the given criteria.*

	Occurrence	Causes	Physiologic Response
Neurogenic shock			
Septic shock			
Anaphylactic shock			

Activity F   *Briefly answer the following questions.*

1. What situations can cause hypovolemic shock?

_____

_____

2. Following cellular hypoxia, as the decompensation stage progresses, coagulation defects occur. Describe these events.

_____

_____

3. What is often the first sign of inadequate oxygen delivery to the tissues?

_____

_____

_____

4. What cardiovascular changes occur during the decompensation phase of shock?

_____

_____

_____

5. How are respirations affected during shock?

_____

_____

_____

SECTION 2:   APPLYING YOUR KNOWLEDGE

Activity G *Give rationale for the following questions.*

1. Why is the use of PASGs or MAST controversial?

_____

_____

_____

2. Why does the systolic and diastolic blood pressure fall during shock?

_____

_____

_____

3. Why is activity restricted to total rest during shock?

_____

_____

_____

4. Why would a client's recovery from shock be tenuous?

_____

_____

_____

Activity H *Answer the following questions that relate to caring for clients in shock.*

1. How are pulse rate, volume, and rhythm used to identify the severity of shock and estimate the approximate reduction in blood volume?

_____

_____

_____

2. What factors lead to decreased urine output during shock?

_____

_____

_____

3. What changes are seen in the skin during shock?

_____

_____

_____

4. Describe nursing management of clients with impending or actual shock.

_____

_____

_____

5. What are the criteria for diagnosing systemic inflammatory response syndrome (SIRS)?

_____

_____

_____

Activity I
Think over the following questions. Discuss them with your peers or instructors.

A client is brought into the emergency department with acute hemorrhagic blood loss. Blood pressure is 85/45 mm Hg, heart rate 118 beats/minute, respirations 30 breaths/minute, oxygen saturation 93%, and temperature 97.7° F. Skin is cool; the client drifts in and out of consciousness. A Foley catheter is inserted; there is no urine return.

1. What type of shock is the client experiencing?
2. What stage of shock is the client experiencing?
3. What are the priority medical interventions?
4. What are the priority nursing diagnoses?
5. What are the priority nursing interventions?

SECTION 3: GETTING READY FOR NCLEX

Activity J
Answer the following questions.

1. A client in shock has been prescribed dopamine, a vasopressor. Which of the following would be the best time for the nurse to initiate the administration of dopamine?
   1. Before fluid therapy
   2. After fluid therapy
   3. While urine output is normal
   4. When systolic pressure is normal

2. Which of the following clients would the nurse anticipate developing hypovolemic shock?
   1. A client with a spinal cord injury
   2. A client recovering from surgery
   3. A client prescribed an antibiotic
   4. A client having a heart attack

3. Which of the following is the most important nursing assessment when caring for a client at risk for cardiogenic shock?
   1. Monitor the client's urine output.
   2. Check the client's temperature.
   3. Listen to the client's lung sounds.
   4. Review hematologic lab results.

4. When the nurse uses a pulse oximeter and notes that the SpO_2 level is above 90%, what is the most likely measurement of PaO_2?
   1. 20 mm Hg
   2. 40 mm Hg
   3. 60 mm Hg
   4. 80 mm Hg

5. Which of the following characteristics is the major reason older adults are more likely to develop hypovolemic shock than younger adults?
   1. Older adults are less active than other adults.
   2. Older adults have more cardiac disorders.
   3. Older adults have a lower fluid volume.
   4. Older adults have more respiratory diseases.

6. Which of the following is the most accurate understanding by a nurse for the etiology undlerlying obstructive shock?
   1. Endotoxins trigger the release of vasodilating chemicals.
   2. Mast cells release massive amounts of histamine.
   3. The volume of blood into and out of the heart is reduced.
   4. The vasomotor center in the medulla decreases vascular resistance.

7. When caring for a client receiving an infusion of dopamine (Intropin), which assessment is most important for the nurse to monitor?
   1. Heart rate
   2. Level of consciousness
   3. Peripheral reflexes
   4. Blood pressure

8. Which of the following should the nurse report immediately when caring for a client receiving an IV infusion of dopamine?
   1. Infiltration of IV fluid
   2. Rapid, deep respirations
   3. Twitching of skeletal muscles
   4. Increased bowel sounds

9. The physician orders 0.2 mg of epinephrine (Adrenalin) subcutaneously stat when a client experiences an allergic reaction. Calculate how much volume the nurse should administer if the medication is supplied in a dose of 1 mg/mL.

10. A nurse is present at a sports event during which a terrorist bomb explodes causing traumatic injuries to spectators. Which of the following is the most appropriate nursing method for controlling hemorrhage when a client receives a laceration in a lower extremity?
    1. Apply PASG (pneumatic antishock garment).
    2. Apply direct pressure to the location of the injury.
    3. Elevate the extemity higher than the heart.
    4. Wrap the extremity with an item of clothing.

18 Caring for Clients With Cancer

LEARNING OBJECTIVES

1. Discuss the pathophysiology and etiology of cancer.
2. Differentiate benign and malignant tumors.
3. Name factors that contribute to the development of cancer.
4. Identify the warning signs of cancer.
5. Describe ways to reduce risks of cancer.
6. Explain methods for diagnosing cancer.
7. Describe systems for staging and grading malignant tumors.
8. Differentiate various treatments and methods for managing cancer.
9. Discuss various adverse effects that occur with cancer treatments and methods used to treat those effects.
10. Describe emotions associated with the diagnosis of cancer.
11. Clarify nursing care required for clients experiencing cancer and cancer treatments.

SECTION 1: ASSESSING YOUR UNDERSTANDING

Activity A *Fill in the blanks by choosing the correct word from the options given in parentheses.*

1. The nursing specialty related to care of clients with cancer is _____. (*oncology nursing, chemotherapy, metastasis nursing*)

2. A surgical procedure when the entire tumor cannot be removed but as much of it as possible is removed is referred to as _____. (*cytoreductive surgery, primary treatment, salvage surgery*)

3. _____ carcinogens include prolonged exposures to sunlight, radiation, and pollutants. (*Chemical, Environmental, Unavoidable*)

4. _____ surgery may be done after extensive surgery to correct defects caused by the original surgery. (*Mohs, Laser, Reconstructive*)

Activity B *Write the correct term for each description.*

1. When tumors are confined and have not invaded vital organs, the surgery is more likely to be curative. _____

2. These types of carcinogens are believed to account for 75% of all cancers. Examples include tobacco, asbestos, coal dust, pesticides, and formaldehydes. _____

3. When radioisotopes are used to treat cancer, these three safety principles must always be kept in mind. _____

4. Surgery that helps to relieve uncomfortable symptoms or prolong life. _____

5. Specialized tests that identify specific proteins, antigens, hormones, genes, or enzymes that cancer cells release. _____

6. A type of surgery that involves shaving off one thin layer of skin at a time. Each layer is examined microscopically. Surgery ends when all cells look normal. _____

Activity C *Match the terms in Column A with their related descriptions in Column B.*

Column A

_____ **1.** Neoplasms (tumors)

_____ **2.** Carcinomas

_____ **3.** Lymphomas

_____ **4.** Leukemias

_____ **5.** Sarcomas

_____ **6.** Benign

_____ **7.** Malignant

Column B

a. Cancers originating from organs that fight infection.

b. Not invasive or spreading; remain at their site of development.

c. New growths of abnormal tissue.

d. Invasive and capable of spreading; likely to metastasize.

e. Cancers originating from organs that form blood.

f. Cancers originating from epithelial cells.

g. Cancers originating from connective tissue, such as bone or muscle.

Activity D *Compare the nonsurgical treatments of cancer based on the given criteria.*

Treatment	Location/Source	Method	Outcome
External radiation therapy			
Internal radiation therapy			
Chemotherapy			
Stem cell transplantation			
Immunotherapy			
Hyperthermia			
Photodynamic therapy			
Gene therapy			

Activity E *Briefly answer the following questions.*

1. Describe the difference between normal and abnormal cell growth.

2. How can malignant cancers metastasize?

3. How do cancer cells develop?

4. What is laser surgery?

5. What is the TNM classification grading system?

6. Explain cell differentiation and how it relates to prognosis.

SECTION 2:   APPLYING YOUR KNOWLEDGE

Activity F   *Give rationale for the following questions.*

1. How are genetic factors linked to cancer?

_____

_____

_____

2. When a malignant tumor is removed, why is a lymph node dissection usually done, along with a wide excision of the tumor?

_____

_____

_____

3. Why are the lungs, liver, and kidneys most affected by chemical carcinogens?

_____

_____

_____

4. How is diet related to cancer?

_____

_____

_____

5. Why are epithelial tissue, hair follicles, and bone marrow most susceptible to the adverse effects of chemotherapy? Which common adverse effects are associated with this susceptibility?

_____

_____

_____

Activity G   *Answer the following questions related to caring for the client with cancer.*

1. How is the immune system a factor in the prevention or development of cancer?

_____

_____

_____

2. What are the seven warning signals of cancer?

_____

_____

_____

3. What are healthy lifestyle habits that reduce the risk of cancer?

_____

_____

_____

Activity H   *Think over the following questions. Discuss them with your instructor or peers.*

1. A client is receiving sealed brachytherapy. What precaution would you take to protect the client, yourself, and others who may come in contact with the client?

_____

_____

_____

2. A client is receiving chemotherapy. What are priority nursing diagnoses for this client? What will you include in client and family teaching?

_____

_____

_____

3. A client has been diagnosed with cancer and has a poor prognosis. What psychosocial nursing diagnoses would you anticipate? What nursing interventions would you use to provide support for the client and the client's family?

_____

_____

_____

_____

_____

_____

_____

_____

SECTION 3: GETTING READY FOR NCLEX

Activity I   *Answer the following questions.*

1. When advising a client on diet modifications to reduce the risk of cancer, the nurse is correct in recommending which of the following?
1. "Increase your intake of red meat."
2. "Decrease your intake of dietary fiber."
3. "Increase your intake of processed meat."
4. "Increase your intake of cruciferous vegetables."

2. Which of the following instructions does the nurse provide to clients receiving radiation therapy?
1. Report when there is difficulty with swallowing.
2. Report when there are mood swings.
3. Report when there is a loss of appetite.
4. Report when there are sleep disorders.

3. The nurse is explaining the client's upcoming surgery for cancer, stating that liquid nitrogen is used to freeze and destroy cancer cells. The nurse is describing what kind of surgery?
1. Electrosurgery
2. Laser
3. Cryosurgery
4. Chemosurgery

4. Which of the following is a nursing intervention when managing clients receiving radiation therapy?
1. Monitor clients for signs of bone marrow suppression.
2. Monitor clients for dehydration.
3. Monitor clients for insufficient urine output.
4. Monitor clients for signs of increased blood sugar levels.

5. Which of the following safety measures must the nurse implement to minimize radiation effects when working with clients who have just undergone treatment with radioisotopes?
1. Wear a special uniform to block radiation.
2. Do not attend the client for the first 14 hours.
3. Wear a face mask and gloves.
4. Limit time spent with the client.

6. Which of the following is an important nursing intervention when managing clients receiving a bone marrow transplant?
1. Monitor clients for signs of elevated urine specific gravity.
2. Monitor clients for signs of infection.
3. Monitor clients for signs of elevated blood urea nitrogen.
4. Monitor clients for signs of elevated blood pressure.

7. A client asks the nurse about the stage of the recently diagnosed malignant tumor. The client states: "My doctor told me it is T1, NO, MX." What is the nurse's best response?
1. "The tumor is connected to another organ."
2. "The tumor is small with no evidence of metastasis at this time."
3. "The tumor is small but does not have well-defined margins."
4. "The tumor is well-differentiated and will respond well to treatment."

8. The nurse practitioner is concerned that a client has not had regular checkups as a means of catching any abnormalities early. Which of the following is an early warning sign and symptom of cancer?
1. Fibrocystic breast disease
2. Yeast infection
3. Stasis ulcers
4. A change in a wart or mole

9. A client tells the nurse that the physician wants to examine the tumor density, shape, size, volume, and location as well as looking at the blood vessels that feed the tumor. The client asks what is the test that does this. The nurse correctly states that it is which of the following tests?

1. A nuclear scan.
2. A computed tomography.
3. An ultrasound test.
4. A fluoroscopy examination.

10. A client is being treated with radiation therapy and develops thrombocytopenia. What nursing intervention has the highest priority?

1. Advise the client to shave with an electric razor.
2. Avoid using soap and friction on the irradiated area.
3. Keep the client's lips moist with lip balm.
4. Tell the client to wear loose cotton clothing.

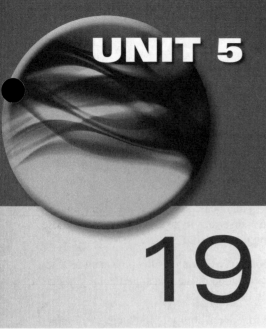

UNIT 5

CARING FOR CLIENTS WITH RESPIRATORY DISORDERS

19 Introduction to the Respiratory System

LEARNING OBJECTIVES

1. Describe the structures of the upper and lower airways.
2. Explain the normal physiology of the respiratory system.
3. Differentiate respiration, ventilation, diffusion, and perfusion.
4. Describe oxygen transport.
5. Define forces that interfere with breathing, including airway resistance and lung compliance.
6. Identify elements of a respiratory assessment.
7. List diagnostic tests that may be performed on the respiratory tract.
8. Discuss preparation and care of clients having respiratory diagnostic procedures

SECTION 1: ASSESSING YOUR UNDERSTANDING

Activity A   *Fill in the blanks by choosing the correct word from the options given in parentheses.*

1. _____ secreted from the nasal mucosa traps small particles. *(Mucus, Conchae, Cilia)*

2. The _____ transports air from the laryngeal pharynx to the bronchi and lungs. *(trachea, oropharynx, nasopharynx)*

3. Stimulating the carina causes _____. *(sneezing, coughing, aspiration)*

4. The _____ are extensions of the nasal cavity located in the surrounding facial bones. *(frontal sinuses, sphenoidal sinuses, paranasal sinuses)*

5. The _____ contains the adenoids and openings of the eustachian tubes. *(nasopharynx, oropharynx, laryngeal pharynx)*

6. The _____ are paired elastic structures enclosed by the thoracic cage that contain the alveoli. *(bronchi, lungs, vocal cords)*

7. _____ are discrete sounds that result from the delayed opening of deflated airways. *(Crackles, Wheezes, Friction rubs)*

Activity B   *Write the correct term for each description.*

1. These fine hairs move the mucus to the back of the throat. This movement helps prevent irritation to and contamination of the lower airway. _____

2. This is an important structure in the larynx; it is a cartilaginous valve flap that covers the opening to the larynx during swallowing. _____

3. These cells are located within the epithelium of the alveoli; they destroy foreign material such as bacteria. _____

4. These bones change the flow of inspired air to moisturize the air and to warm it better. _____

5. The area of the pharynx that contains the tongue.
_____

6. The ratio that indicates the effectiveness of airflow within the alveoli and the adequacy of gas exchange within the pulmonary capillaries. _____

Activity C *Match the diagnostic tests in Column A with the corresponding descriptions in Column B.*

Column A

_____ **1.** Arterial blood gases

_____ **2.** Pulmonary function studies

_____ **3.** Sputum studies

_____ **4.** Pulse oximetry

_____ **5.** Pulmonary angiography

_____ **6.** Lung scans

_____ **7.** Chest x-rays

_____ **8.** Bronchoscopy

Column B

a. Examined for pathogenic microorganisms and cancer cells; culture and sensitivity tests are done to diagnose infections and prescribe antibiotics.

b. A radioisotope study that allows the physician to assess the arterial circulation of the lungs, particularly to detect pulmonary emboli.

c. Measure the functional ability of the lungs.

d. Determine the blood's pH; oxygen-carrying capacity; and levels of oxygen, CO_2, and bicarbonate ion.

e. Allows for direct visualization of the larynx, trachea, and bronchi.

f. Used for diagnostic purposes, such as to diagnose lung cancer, COPD, and pulmonary edema.

g. A noninvasive method that uses a light beam to measure the oxygen content of hemoglobin (SaO_2).

h. Used to screen for asymptomatic disease and to diagnose tumors, foreign bodies, and other abnormal conditions.

Activity D *Identify elements of respiratory physiology based on the criteria given.*

	Definition	Mechanics
Respiration		
Ventilation		
Diffusion		
Perfusion		

Activity E *Answer the following questions using the given figure.*

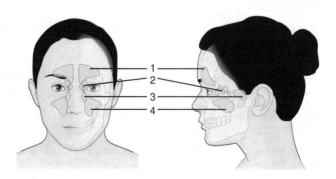

1. Identify and label the paranasal sinuses shown on the figure.

   1. _____

   2. _____

   3. _____

   4. _____

2. Which sinuses are the largest and the most accessible to treatment?

   _____

   _____

   _____

Activity F *Briefly answer the following questions.*

1. Describe the flow of air once it enters the right and left mainstem bronchi.

   _____

   _____

   _____

2. Where is the site of oxygen and CO_2 exchange?

   _____

   _____

   _____

3. What does alveolar respiration determine?

   _____

   _____

   _____

4. How do the lungs and kidneys compensate for acid–base imbalances?

   _____

   _____

   _____

5. What would be the indications for a thoracentesis?

   _____

   _____

   _____

SECTION 2: APPLYING YOUR KNOWLEDGE

Activity G *Give rationale for the following questions.*

1. Why is aspiration of foreign objects more likely in the right mainstem bronchus and right upper lung?

   _____

   _____

   _____

2. Why are older adults at a greater risk from respiratory disease?

   _____

   _____

   _____

3. Why may it be necessary to collect sputum on successive days?

   _____

   _____

   _____

4. Why must the nurse determine if the client has any allergies, particularly to iodine, shellfish, or contrast dye with a pulmonary angiography?

   _____

   _____

   _____

Activity H *Answer the following questions related to caring for clients with respiratory disorders.*

1. Which forces can interfere with breathing, including airway resistance and lung compliance?

_____

_____

_____

2. Describe the transport of gases.

_____

_____

_____

3. What are the neurologic control mechanisms of ventilation?

_____

_____

_____

4. What is included in the assessment of the client's respiratory history?

_____

_____

_____

5. What is included in a physical assessment of the respiratory system?

_____

_____

_____

_____

Activity I *Think over the following questions. Discuss them with your instructor or peers.*

1. You are preparing a client for a therapeutic thoracentesis at the bedside. Describe the preprocedural and postprocedural nursing care required.

_____

_____

_____

2. You are preparing a client for a bronchoscopy. Describe the preprocedural and postprocedural nursing care required.

_____

_____

_____

3. You are performing a physical assessment on a client and detect crackles that were not noted on the previous assessment. You ask the client to cough and listen again. The crackles are still present. What does this indicate? What further nursing assessments and interventions would you initiate?

_____

_____

_____

SECTION 3: GETTING READY FOR NCLEX

Activity J *Answer the following questions.*

1. When caring for older adults, it is important that the nurse remember that the alveolar walls become thinner and contain fewer capillaries. What is the impact of this change?
   1. The client's lungs have decreased elasticity.
   2. Gas exchange is decreased as a result.
   3. The lungs become increasingly stiff.
   4. There are decreased number of alveoli.

2. During the physical examination of a client, which of the following methods does the examiner use to palpate for tactile or vocal fremitus?
   1. The examiner uses the palmar surface of the fingers and hands.
   2. The examiner asks client to repeat "11" while moving his or her hands.
   3. The examiner performs percussion of the neck wall.
   4. The examiner observes vibrations when the client remains quiet.

3. A new nurse is preparing a client for a thoracentesis. As the nurse positions the client, which of the following demonstrates the nurse's knowledge of correct positioning for this procedure?
   1. The client sits at the side of the bed.
   2. The client lies on the affected side.
   3. The client lies flat on the back.
   4. The client lies down with the head raised.

4. A client asks the nurse why a sputum specimen is needed. Which of the following provides the correct explanation?
   1. "Sputum is collected to see if there are any foreign bodies present."
   2. "Sputum is examined to see if there are any cancer cells."
   3. "Sputum is needed as a first step in identifying pulmonary emboli."
   4. "Sputum is indicative of an inflammatory process in the lungs."

5. During the physical examination of a client, the nurse auscultates breath sounds. Which of the following would the nurse correctly identify as normal?
   1. Sounds heard over the trachea—medium pitched
   2. Sounds heard between the trachea and upper lungs—loud
   3. Sounds heard over the lung fields—quiet and low pitched
   4. Sounds that are discrete—continuous and musical

6. When examining the posterior pharynx and tonsils, which of the following objective data does the nurse note?
   1. Difficulty in sneezing
   2. Suppressed gag reflex
   3. Deformities
   4. Inflammation

7. A client who is seen in a clinic states that a cold seems to have progressed into the sinuses, with increased pressure and pain as well as an increased feeling of congestion. What explanation for this can the nurse provide?
   1. Mucus is easily trapped in the frontal sinuses when experiencing an infection.
   2. The lining of the sinuses is continuous with the mucous membrane lining of the nasal cavity.
   3. The number of sinuses makes it difficult to prevent infection from occurring.
   4. The sinuses lighten the weight of the skull but cannot prevent mucus from accumulating.

8. A client is seen in the emergency room for complaints of shortness of breath. The physician orders arterial blood gases. The nurse expects to see which of the following lab values if the pH level is within normal range?
   1. 7 to 7.49
   2. 7.35 to 7.45
   3. 7.5 to 7.6
   4. 7.55 to 7.65

9. Which of the following nursing activities is most important when a client comes back from a respiratory test?
   1. Avoid repeating information about postprocedure expectations.
   2. Assess for signs of respiratory distress following invasive procedures.
   3. Be sure that explanations are detailed and exhaustive.
   4. Teach the family about respiratory disease.

10. A client has undergone thoracentesis and has been ordered to undergo a chest x-ray. Which of the following would the nurse identify as the rationale for the x-ray when speaking with the client?
    1. It evaluates pulmonary edema.
    2. It will help rule out emphysema.
    3. It will assess for any cardiac distress.
    4. It will check for pneumothorax.

20 Caring for Clients With Upper Respiratory Disorders

LEARNING OBJECTIVES

1. Describe nursing care for clients experiencing infectious or inflammatory upper respiratory disorders.
2. Discuss assessment data required to provide nursing care to clients with structural disorders of the upper airway.
3. Describe airway problems a client may experience following trauma or obstruction to the upper airway.
4. Identify risk factors that contribute to the development of laryngeal cancer.
5. Identify the earliest symptoms of laryngeal cancer.
6. Discuss treatments for laryngeal cancer.
7. Describe measures used to promote alternative methods of communication for clients with a laryngectomy.
8. Discuss psychosocial issues that clients may experience following a laryngectomy.
9. Relate treatment modalities for clients experiencing short-term or long-term problems with airway management.
10. Identify possible reasons for and nursing management of a tracheostomy.
11. Explain why a client may require endotracheal intubation.

SECTION 1: ASSESSING YOUR UNDERSTANDING

Activity A *Fill in the blanks by choosing the correct word from the options given in parentheses.*

1. Chronic adenoidal infections can result in acute or chronic infections in the _____. *(middle ear, inner ear, outer ear)*

2. If drainage of clear fluid is observed following a nasal fracture, a Dextrostix is used to determine the presence of glucose, which is diagnostic for _____ and suggests a fracture in the cribriform plate. *(hemorrhage, mucus, cerebrospinal fluid)*

3. Expectoration of bloody sputum is called _____. *(hemoptysis, epistaxis, rhinorrhea)*

4. _____ is usually the earliest symptom of laryngeal cancer. *(A lump in the throat, Persistent hoarseness, Dysphagia)*

5. The physician specifies the amount of air to be injected into the cuffed tracheostomy tube, usually to achieve a pressure between _____. *(10 and 15 mm H_2O, 20 and 25 mm H_2O, 30 and 35 mm H_2O)*

6. _____ is a nursing intervention frequently used to promote maximum lung expansion and improve oxygen exchange. *(Application of oxygen, Positioning in semi-Fowler's position, Monitoring ABGs)*

Activity B *Write the correct term for each description.*

1. A deviated septum, nasal polyps, and hypertrophied turbinates are common causes of this condition. _____

2. The universal sign for choking. _____

3. A high-pitched, harsh sound during respiration, indicative of airway obstruction. _____

4. Characterized by frequent, brief episodes of respiratory standstill during sleep. _____

5. Spasm of the laryngeal muscles, resulting in narrowing of the larynx. _____

6. These two devices are kept at the bedside at all times following a tracheostomy. _____

Activity C *Match the terms in Column A with their related descriptions in Column B*

Column A

_____ 1. Tracheotomy

_____ 2. Tracheostomy

_____ 3. Endotracheal tube

_____ 4. Positive pressure ventilator

_____ 5. Negative pressure ventilator

_____ 6. Airway pressure release ventilation

Column B

a. Inserted through the mouth or nose into the trachea to provide a patent airway for clients who cannot maintain an adequate airway on their own.

b. Exert a pulling or sucking force on the external chest.

c. A surgical opening into the trachea into which a tracheostomy or laryngectomy tube is inserted.

d. Promotes spontaneous breathing in a ventilated client; this is accomplished through the use of extended periods of CPAP.

e. The surgical procedure that makes an opening into the trachea.

f. Inflate the lungs by pushing air into the airway.

Activity D *Compare the following upper airway illnesses using the given criteria.*

	Description	Cause	Symptoms	Treatment
Rhinitis				
Sinusitis				
Pharyngitis				
Tonsillitis and adenoiditis				
Peritonsillar abscess				
Laryngitis				

Activity E *Briefly answer the following questions.*

1. What observations and assessments will the nurse make that are specific for the client following sinus surgery?

_____

_____

_____

2. What complications can occur following pharyngitis caused by group A streptococci?

_____

_____

_____

3. What interventions may the nurse initiate independently to control bleeding for epistaxis?

_____

_____

_____

4. What are the symptoms of obstructive sleep apnea?

_____

_____

_____

5. Which carcinogens are associated with laryngeal cancer?

_____

_____

_____

6. What are indications for an endotracheal tube?

_____

_____

_____

SECTION 2: APPLYING YOUR KNOWLEDGE

Activity F *Give rationale for the following questions.*

1. Why should clients taking prescription medications consult their physician before taking over-the-counter medications for an upper respiratory ailment?

_____

_____

_____

2. Why should the head of the bed be elevated 45° when the client is fully awake after a tonsillectomy and adenoidectomy?

_____

_____

_____

3. How does sleep apnea cause serious side effects that affect the cardiopulmonary system?

_____

_____

_____

4. What are the benefits of ice packs or ice collars?

_____

_____

_____

5. How can the creation of a new opening following a tracheostomy cause a life-threatening situation?

_____

_____

_____

Activity G *Answer the following questions related to caring for clients with upper respiratory disorders.*

1. What are the risk factors for sleep apnea?

_____

_____

2. Describe the physical changes associated with a total laryngectomy.

_____

_____

_____

3. Why is a humidified mist collar usually necessary following a tracheostomy?

_____

_____

_____

4. What is the nursing management for the client with an endotracheal tube?

_____

_____

_____

5. Describe a tracheoesophageal puncture.

_____

_____

_____

Activity H *Think over the following questions. Discuss them with your instructor or peers.*

1. A client who has undergone a total laryngectomy is disturbed by the appearance of the tracheostomy and is refusing visitors. What interventions could you use to facilitate the client's acceptance of body changes and promote social interaction?

_____

_____

_____

2. The client with a tracheostomy has copious secretions. What guidelines will you follow to perform suctioning?

_____

_____

_____

3. You are in a restaurant when the person at the next table stands up and is observed to be clutching and grabbing at the neck/throat and is trying to speak but cannot. What actions will you take?

_____

_____

_____

_____

_____

_____

_____

_____

_____

SECTION 3: GETTING READY FOR NCLEX

Activity I *Answer the following questions.*

1. Which of the following is an important preventive factor that the nurse should teach a client with rhinitis?
   1. Not to blow the nose.
   2. Consume small doses of ice chips.
   3. Not to lift objects weighing more than 5 to 10 lb.
   4. Wash hands frequently.

2. Which of the following signs may be revealed in a visual examination if the client has a tonsillar infection caused by group A streptococci?
   1. White patches on the tonsils
   2. Hemorrhage in the tonsils
   3. Hypertrophied tonsils
   4. Bleeding in the tonsils

3. A nurse caring for a client undergoing drainage of a peritonsillar abscess places an ice collar near the client's throat. What is the best explanation for this action?
   1. The ice collar reduces swelling and pain.
   2. The ice collar will help the client to swallow fluids.
   3. The ice collar will reduce the risk of respiratory infection.
   4. The ice collar will prevent excessive bleeding.

4. A client is seen by a physician for a potential diagnosis of laryngeal cancer. Which of the following signs does the nurse expect to see in this client?
   1. Bacterial infection
   2. Persistent hoarseness
   3. Aphonia
   4. Peritonsillar abscess

5. What does a nurse assess postoperatively in a client with a nasal fracture?
   1. Allergic reaction
   2. Airway obstruction
   3. Extreme sense of smell
   4. Stridor

6. Which of the following symptoms should a nurse assess in a client when implementing interventions for trauma to the upper airway?
   1. Pain when talking
   2. Burning in the throat
   3. Increased nasal swelling
   4. Presence of laryngospasm

7. A client is admitted to a surgical care unit from the post anesthesia care unit with a new tracheostomy. What is the nurse's priority action?
   1. Encourage the client to engage in self care.
   2. Help the client to communicate needs.
   3. Keep the airway patent.
   4. Prevent the onset of infection.

8. Following a laryngectomy, the client uses a method of speech involves a throat vibrator (held against the neck) that projects sound into the mouth, causing words to be formed with the mouth. The nurse recognizes this as what type of alternative speech?
   1. Tracheoesophageal puncture (TEP)
   2. Esophageal speech
   3. Artificial (electric) larynx
   4. Speech therapy

9. For a client recovering from sinus surgery, which of the following actions should the nurse recommend for a postoperative period of 10 to 14 days?
   1. Lift 15- to 20-lb dumbbells daily to strengthen arms.
   2. Avoid doing the Valsalva maneuver.
   3. Blow the nose frequently.
   4. Remain in a cool environment.

10. A client comes to the doctor's office stating that he has a lump in his throat and is afraid that it is cancer. Which initial question by the nurse addresses the earliest symptom of laryngeal cancer?
    1. "Do you smoke or have you ever smoked?"
    2. "Do you have a burning in your throat?"
    3. "Do you have swollen lymph nodes?"
    4. "Did you notice a persistent cough?"

21 Caring for Clients With Lower Respiratory Disorders

LEARNING OBJECTIVES

1. Describe infectious and inflammatory disorders of the lower respiratory airway.
2. Identify critical assessments needed for a client with an infectious disorder of the lower respiratory airway.
3. Define disorders classified as obstructive pulmonary disease.
4. Discuss strategies for preventing and managing occupational lung diseases.
5. Describe the pathophysiology of pulmonary hypertension.
6. List risk factors associated with the development of pulmonary embolism.
7. Discuss conditions that may lead to acute respiratory distress syndrome.
8. Differentiate acute and chronic respiratory failure.
9. Explain the difficulties associated with early diagnosis of lung cancer.
10. Describe nursing assessments required for a client who experiences trauma to the chest.
11. Explain the purpose of chest tubes after thoracic surgery.
12. Describe preoperative and postoperative nursing management for clients undergoing thoracic care.

SECTION 1: ASSESSING YOUR UNDERSTANDING

Activity A *Fill in the blanks by choosing the correct word from the options given in parentheses.*

1. Inflammation of the mucous membranes that line the major bronchi and their branches characterizes _____. *(pneumonia, acute bronchitis, pleurisy)*

2. _____ is an abnormal collection of fluid between the visceral and parietal pleurae. *(Pleurisy, Pleural effusion, Lung abscess)*

3. _____ is an acute respiratory disease of relatively short duration. *(Lung abscess, Empyema, Influenza)*

4. _____ is the initial infection of a bacterial infectious disease primarily caused by *M. tuberculosis*. *(Primary tuberculosis, Secondary tuberculosis, Tertiary tuberculosis)*

5. _____ usually involves reactivation of the initial infection. The person already has had an immune response, and thus the lesions that form tend to remain in the lungs. *(Primary tuberculosis, Secondary tuberculosis, Tertiary tuberculosis)*

6. _____ is the collapse of alveoli. It may involve a small portion of the lung or an entire lobe. When alveoli collapse, they cannot perform their function of gas exchange. *(Bronchiectasis, Atelectasis, Chronic bronchitis)*

7. _____ is an inherited multisystem disorder that affects infants, children, and young adults. It obstructs the lungs and pancreas, leading to major lung infections. *(Emphysema, Asthma, Cystic fibrosis)*

8. _____ is associated with factors such as upper respiratory infections, emotional upsets, and exercise. *(Nonallergic asthma, Allergic asthma, Mixed asthma)*

9. _____ are a common injury and may result from a hard fall or a blow to the chest. The injuries are not usually considered serious unless accompanied by other injuries. *(Rib fractures, Penetrating wounds, Blast injuries)*

10. Gunshot and stab wounds are common types of _____ to the lungs; they can potentially affect cardiopulmonary function and may be life threatening. *(fracture injuries, blast injuries, penetrating wounds)*

11. When symptoms of _____ occur, they include chest pain, chest wall bulging, difficulty swallowing, dyspnea, and orthopnea. Symptoms are related to pressure on other chest structures. *(lung cancer, mediastinal tumors, flail chest)*

Activity B   *Write the correct term for each of the following descriptions.*

1. Most commonly gives rise to acute bronchitis. _____

2. This lower respiratory disorder refers to an acute inflammation of the parietal and visceral pleurae. _____

3. These applications may provide some topical comfort for pleurisy. _____

4. Type of pneumonias referred to as *typical pneumonias*. _____

5. Found in clients with COPD and is characterized by chronic infection and irreversible dilatation of the bronchi and bronchioles. _____

6. Prolonged (or extended) inflammation of the bronchi, accompanied by a chronic cough and excessive production of mucus for at least 3 months per year for 2 consecutive years. _____

7. This type of asthma occurs in response to allergens, such as pollen, dust, spores, and animal dander. _____

8. Components include chest physical therapy (including postural drainage, percussion, and vibration) two to four times daily, deep-breathing and coughing exercises, nebulized treatments, and medications. _____

9. Silicosis and asbestosis are in a category of these lower respiratory disorders, which result in the lungs having a decreased volume and inability to expand completely. _____

10. Occurs when two or more adjacent ribs fracture in multiple places and the fragments are free floating. This affects the stability of the chest wall and results in impairment of chest-wall movement. _____

11. The name for the three conditions that predispose a person to clot formation: venostasis, disruption of the vessel lining, and hypercoagulability. _____

12. It remains the number one cause of cancer-related deaths among men and women in the United States. _____

Activity C   *Given in Column A are obstructive pulmonary diseases. Match these disorders with their associated assessment findings in Column B.*

Column A

_____ 1. Bronchiectasis

_____ 2. Atelectasis

_____ 3. Chronic bronchitis

_____ 4. Emphysema

_____ 5. Asthma

_____ 6. Cystic fibrosis

Column B

a. The earliest symptom is a chronic cough productive of thick, white mucus, especially when rising in the morning and in the evening. Bronchospasm may occur during severe bouts of coughing.

b. Typified by paroxysms of shortness of breath, wheezing, and coughing as well as the production of thick, tenacious sputum.

c. Shortness of breath with minimal activity is called exertional dyspnea and often is the first symptom of this condition. As the disease progresses, breathlessness occurs even at rest. A chronic cough invariably is present and productive of mucopurulent sputum. Inspiration is difficult because of the rigid chest cage, and the chest is characteristically barrel shaped.

d. Clients experience a chronic cough with expectoration of copious amounts of purulent sputum and possible hemoptysis. The coughing worsens when the client changes position. Clients also experience fatigue, weight loss, anorexia, and dyspnea.

e. The three major reasons to suspect this disorder in children are (1) respiratory symptoms, (2) failure to thrive, and (3) foul-smelling, bulky, greasy stools.

f. Small areas may cause few symptoms. With larger areas, cyanosis, fever, pain, dyspnea, increased pulse and respiratory rates, and increased pulmonary secretions may be seen. Although crackling may be auscultated over the affected areas, usually, breath sounds are absent.

Activity D *To determine peak flow, the nurse instructs the client in the use of a peak flow meter. The following steps are in a jumbled order. Arrange the steps in the correct order in the boxes that follow.*

1. Form a tight seal around the mouthpiece with lips.
2. Note the reading.
3. Sit upright in bed or chair or stand and inhale as deeply as possible.
4. Exhale forcefully and quickly.
5. Monitor the peak flow readings according to the three zones.
6. After 2 to 3 weeks of asthma therapy, determine your best or usual individual peak flow.
7. Repeat these steps two more times; write the highest of the three numbers in the asthma record.
8. Depending on the zone, take actions as instructed by healthcare providers.

☐→☐→☐→☐→☐→☐→☐→☐

Activity E *Briefly answer the following questions.*

1. Describe the signs and symptoms of acute bronchitis.

2. What are the causes of pneumonia in addition to microorganism infection?

3. What are the signs and symptoms of pneumonia?

4. What are the assessment findings for a lung abscess?

5. How is TB most commonly transmitted? Does exposure always result in illness?

6. Describe the surgical treatment of tuberculosis.

7. Describe the treatment for bronchiectasis.

8. Describe the nursing interventions indicated for management of chronic bronchitis.

9. What are the dietary indications when cystic fibrosis affects the digestive system?

10. Identify the assessment findings for pulmonary arterial hypertension.

11. What is the treatment for respiratory failure?

SECTION 2: APPLYING YOUR KNOWLEDGE

Activity F *Give rationale for the following questions.*

1. Why is a sputum culture and sensitivity ordered with lower respiratory infections?

_____

_____

_____

2. Why is pleurisy so painful?

_____

_____

_____

3. Why is treatment of tuberculosis with medication less than ideal? How are these issues addressed?

_____

_____

_____

4. How does emphysema prevent the proper exchange of oxygen and CO_2 during respiration?

_____

_____

_____

5. Why is oxygen cautiously administered to clients with emphysema?

_____

_____

_____

6. How does absence of the protein CF transmembrane conductance regulator (CFTR) result in the symptoms of cystic fibrosis?

_____

_____

_____

7. Why are anticoagulants used in the treatment of pulmonary emboli?

_____

_____

_____

8. Why are thrombolytics used in the treatment of pulmonary emboli?

_____

_____

_____

9. Why has the incidence of lung cancer markedly increased since the early 1980s?

_____

_____

_____

10. Why does lung cancer have a high mortality rate?

_____

_____

_____

11. Why are all penetrating wounds to the chest considered serious?

_____

_____

_____

Activity G *Answer the following questions related to caring for clients with lower respiratory disorders.*

1. Describe the pathophysiology of pneumonia.

_____

_____

_____

2. What are typical assessment findings with pleurisy?

_____

_____

_____

3. What are the typical assessment findings with a pleural effusion?

_____

_____

_____

4. Describe the medical and surgical management of empyema.

_____

_____

_____

5. What are the signs and symptoms of tuberculosis?

_____

_____

_____

6. Nursing management of atelectasis focuses on prevention; what are the nursing interventions indicated to assist with the prevention of atelectasis?

_____

_____

_____

7. Describe the pathophysiology of asthma.

_____

_____

_____

8. Describe the medical management for primary pulmonary arterial hypertension. Describe the medical management for secondary pulmonary arterial hypertension.

_____

_____

_____

9. What are the symptoms of pulmonary edema? What type of treatment does pulmonary edema require?

_____

_____

_____

10. What signs and symptoms are seen with impending respiratory failure?

_____

_____

_____

11. Why would a thoracotomy be performed?

_____

_____

_____

12. Describe the care for a chest tube.

_____

_____

_____

Activity H *Think over the following questions and then discuss them with your instructor or peers.*

1. Your client is diagnosed with bacterial pneumonia. What nursing assessments and interventions are indicated?

_____

_____

_____

2. You have volunteered to administer the influenza vaccine at a local clinic. Which types of clients will you advise against receiving the vaccine?

_____

_____

_____

3. Your client is diagnosed with asthma. What education will you provide to assist the client in managing the symptoms?

_____

_____

_____

4. Your client is diagnosed with emphysema. What strategies will you teach the client to slow the disease progression?

_____

_____

_____

Activity I *Read the following case study. Use critical thinking skills to discuss and answer the questions that follow it.*

The local community hospital is experiencing an influenza epidemic. Various local schools have closed for several days due to the high number of students and staff sick with the flu. The hospital has set up a separate area to assist those clients presenting with *the signs and symptoms* of influenza and is providing immunizations and FluMist to the public for a minimal cost. Nurses at the hospital are providing free educational in-service programs about influenza and the precautions to take for prevention.

1. What are the signs and symptoms of influenza in order of progression? The stages below are in a jumbled order. Indicate the correct sequence of the answers in the boxes that follow.
  1. Duration of fever may persist for 3 days; other symptoms usually continue for 7 to 10 days, although cough may persist longer.
  2. Sudden, abrupt onset of fever and chills, severe headache, and muscle aches
  3. Incubation period 1 to 4 days
  4. Respiratory symptoms, sneezing, sore throat, dry cough, nasal discharge, anorexia, and weakness
  5. Period of contagion is 1 day before symptoms begin through 5 days after onset of illness.

  □ → □ → □ → □ → □

2. What type of precautions must the nurse take when caring for these clients in the hospital?

_____

_____

_____

3. What contraindications must the nurse be aware of when administering FluMist?

_____

_____

_____

4. What is the reason that flu immunization does not provide protection for several years?

_____

_____

_____

5. Concept Map: Using the information from the given case study, identify four nursing diagnoses with "related to" statements for the client experiencing influenza. (Italicized words are clues to the answers.)

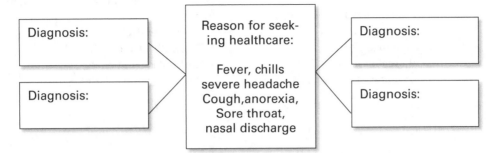

Diagnosis:		

Diagnosis:		

Reason for seeking healthcare:

Fever, chills severe headache Cough, anorexia, Sore throat, nasal discharge

Diagnosis:		

Diagnosis:		

SECTION 3: GETTING READY FOR NCLEX

Activity J *Answer the following questions.*

1. A client presents at the clinic with complaints that are symptomatic of acute bronchitis. What symptom does the nurse expect to assess in this client?
  1. Nonproductive cough
  2. Labored breathing
  3. Anorexia
  4. Gastric ulceration

2. Which of the following should the nurse include in the teaching plan for a client with acute bronchitis?
  1. Advise the client to avoid coughing as much as possible.
  2. Encourage the client to consume adequate calories.
  3. Inform the client to wash hands frequently.
  4. Teach the client to rest in a semi-Fowler's position.

3. An adult client with cystic fibrosis is hospitalized with an acute respiratory infection. A nursing intervention is to provide chest physical therapy at least every 12 hours. When is the best time to perform this procedure?
  1. After the client has had adequate rest.
  2. At least two hours after a meal.
  3. Right before breakfast and dinner.
  4. When the client is experiencing a bronchospasm.

4. Which of the following would be the most appropriate nursing intervention when caring for a client with a fractured rib?
  1. Apply immobilization device after examination by physician.
  2. Discourage taking deep breaths if breathing is painful.
  3. Advise against using analgesics and regional nerve blocks.
  4. Encourage increased fluid intake if pulmonary contusion exists.

5. A client with COPD asks the nurse about the purpose of pursed lip breathing. What is the nurse's best response?
  1. "Pursed lip breathing controls respiratory rate and depth, slowing expiration."
  2. "Pursed lip breathing increases the strength of muscles used for breathing."
  3. "Pursed lip breathing prevents the accumulation of secretions."
  4. "Pursed lip breathing will make you more comfortable."

6. When caring for a client with influenza, which action by the nurse is most important?
  1. Maintain airborne transmission precautions
  2. Advise to client to remain on complete bed rest
  3. Administer oxygen as ordered
  4. Observe for signs of respiratory distress

7. When reviewing clients' medical history, the nurse is looking for factors that may predispose a client to the development of tuberculosis. Which of the following is a contributing factor?
  1. Exposure to toxic gases
  2. Obstruction by tumor
  3. Congenital abnormalities
  4. Malnutrition

8. When assessing a client with tuberculosis, the nurse recognizes which of the following sign/symptom as a characteristic of the latter stage of the disease?
  1. Fatigue
  2. Hemoptysis
  3. Anorexia
  4. Weight loss

9. When reviewing a client's medical record, the nurse recognizes that which of the following signs is indicative of asthma?
   1. Production of abnormally thick, sticky mucus in the lungs
   2. Faulty transport of sodium in lung cells
   3. Paroxysms of shortness of breath
   4. Altered electrolyte balance in the sweat glands

10. A client comes to an urgent care clinic with pleurisy. The nurse is most correct in anticipating that which of the following will be the most common complaint from the client?
   1. Thick, green sputum
   2. Pain with each breath
   3. Hot flashes with chills
   4. Petechiae on the chest

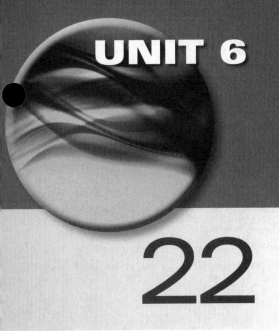

UNIT 6

CARING FOR CLIENTS WITH CARDIOVASCULAR DISORDERS

22 Introduction to the Cardiovascular System

LEARNING OBJECTIVES

1. Describe the normal anatomy and physiology of the cardiovascular system.
2. Identify and describe focus assessment criteria when caring for a client with cardiovascular problems.
3. List common diagnostic tests used to evaluate the client with suspected heart disease.
4. Discuss the nursing management of a client undergoing cardiovascular diagnostic tests.

SECTION 1: ASSESSING YOUR UNDERSTANDING

Activity A   *Fill in the blanks by choosing the correct word from the options given in parentheses.*

1. The _____ consists of muscle tissue and is the force behind the heart's pumping action. *(epicardium, myocardium, endocardium)*

2. During a _____ state, the myocardial cells are at rest. This occurs during diastole, before an impulse is generated. *(polarized, depolarized, repolarized)*

3. _____ carry oxygenated blood from the heart. *(Arteries, Veins, Valves)*

4. _____ refers to contraction of the atria and ventricles during the cardiac cycle. *(Systole, Conduction, Diastole)*

5. The heart rate _____ when receptors are stimulated by the cholinergic neurotransmitter acetylcholine released from parasympathetic nerve fibers. *(increases, pauses, decreases)*

6. Taking blood pressure with the client in the lying, sitting, and standing positions is referred to as _____. *(pulse deficit, pulse pressure, orthostatic vital signs)*

7. The first normal heart sound, referred to as _____, is heard with the closing of the mitral and tricuspid valves. *(S_1 ["lub"], S_2 ["dub"], S_3 [gallop])*

8. _____ are caused by turbulent blood flow through diseased heart valves. *(Murmurs and clicks, Atrial and ventricular gallops, Friction rubs)*

Activity B   *Write the correct term for each description.*

1. Ions realign themselves in their original position and wait for another electrical impulse. _____

2. These vessels return deoxygenated blood to the heart. _____

3. Refers to relaxation of the atria and ventricle during the cardiac cycle. _____

4. The heart rate and force of contraction increase when receptors are stimulated by adrenergic neurotransmitters released by this type of nerve fiber. _____

5. The amount of blood pumped per contraction of the heart. _____

6. The characteristics that are assessed when the nurse palpates a pulse. _____

7. The heart sound associated with the closing of the aortic and pulmonic valves. _____

8. This occurs when blood is not pumped efficiently. When blood has nowhere else to go, the extra fluid enters the tissues. _____

9. Distention of this vein usually indicates increased fluid volume and pressure in the right side of the heart.

_____

Activity C   *Match the heart valves given in Column A to their related location or function given in Column B.*

Column A

_____ **1.** Atrioventricular (AV) valves

_____ **2.** Tricuspid valve

_____ **3.** Bicuspid valve

_____ **4.** Semilunar valves

_____ **5.** Pulmonic valve

_____ **6.** Aortic valve

Column B

a. The valve between the right ventricle and pulmonary artery.

b. The valve between the right atrium and right ventricle.

c. The two valves that prevent blood from flowing back into the ventricles after the heart contracts.

d. The two valves that separate the atria from the ventricles. They prevent blood from returning to the atria when the ventricles contract.

e. The valve between the left atrium and left ventricle (also known as the mitral valve).

f. The valve between the left ventricle and aorta.

Activity D   *The cardiopulmonary circulation is given in a jumbled order. Indicate the correct order of events by filling in the boxes with the correct sequence.*

1. Blood travels into the right ventricle and is pumped into the pulmonary artery.

2. The left ventricle pumps the blood through the aorta to all the body's cells and tissues.

3. The pulmonary veins bring the oxygenated blood into the left atrium.

4. The lungs exchange the oxygen in inspired air for the CO_2 in the venous blood. The CO_2 is transferred into the alveoli and exhaled.

5. The right atrium fills with blood, and the tricuspid valve opens.

6. The oxygenated blood flows out of the left atrium through the bicuspid (mitral) valve and into the left ventricle.

7. The largest veins, the inferior vena cava and superior vena cava, bring venous (deoxygenated) blood from all areas of the body into the right atrium.

8. The pulmonary artery branches to deliver venous blood to the right and left lungs.

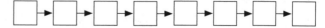

Activity E *Compare the following diagnostic tests based on the criteria.*

Diagnostic Test	Description	Purpose
Radiography		
Radionuclide studies		
Magnetic resonance imaging (MRI)		
Echocardiography		
Transesophageal echocardiography (TEE)		
Electrocardiography		
Ambulatory ECG (Holter monitoring)		
Exercise electrocardiography (Stress test)		
Cardiac catheterization		
Arteriography		
Angiocardiography		
Aortography		
Peripheral arteriography		

Activity F *The conduction system sustains the electrical activity of the heart. Label the locations of each part of the conduction system.*

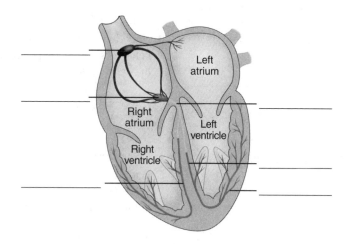

Activity G *Briefly answer the following questions.*

1. Describe the structure and function of the pericardium.

_____

_____

_____

2. Describe the function of the chordae tendineae and papillary muscles.

_____

_____

_____

3. Describe the structure and function of capillaries.

_____

_____

_____

4. What type of pain may be indicative of cardiovascular problems?

_____

_____

_____

5. How is a pulse deficit determined?

_____

_____

_____

6. What characteristics of respiration are included in the nursing assessment?

_____

_____

_____

SECTION 2: APPLYING YOUR KNOWLEDGE

Activity H *Give rationale for the following questions.*

1. Why is the myocardium the first tissue of the body to receive oxygen-rich blood?

_____

_____

2. Why are cells resistant to electrical stimulation during the refractory period?

_____

_____

_____

3. Why is the family medical history an important feature of the health history?

_____

_____

_____

4. How do the client's general appearance, nonverbal behaviors, and body position contribute to assessment of the cardiovascular system?

_____

_____

_____

5. Why is it important to compare the information on a heart monitor with palpation of the pulse and/or auscultation of the apical heart rate?

_____

_____

_____

6. Why are cardiovascular problems exhibited as crackles in the lungs?

_____

_____

_____

Activity I *Answer the following questions related to the cardiovascular system.*

1. What is the normal sequence of events in the conduction system of the heart?

_____

_____

_____

2. What information is obtained during a history assessment of the cardiovascular system?

_____

_____

_____

3. What information is obtained during the nursing assessment of the skin?

_____

_____

_____

_____

4. How are mental status changes related to cardiovascular problems?

_____

_____

_____

5. How do baroreceptors regulate the heart rate?

_____

_____

_____

6. How do chemoreceptors regulate the heart rate?

_____

_____

_____

_____

Activity J *Think over the following questions. Discuss them with your instructor or peers.*

1. A client is scheduled for an MRI. What questions will you need to ask the client to make sure he or she is a candidate for this type of procedure? How will you prepare the client for this diagnostic test? What medications may you need to administer?

_____

_____

_____

2. A client is scheduled for a cardiac catheterization. What preprocedure care activities will you perform? What are the postprocedure guidelines you should follow? What discharge instructions will you provide?

_____

_____

_____

SECTION 3:   GETTING READY FOR NCLEX

Activity K *Answer the following questions.*

1. What is the best reason for the nurse to ask if a client is allergic to seafood prior to undergoing cardiac diagnostic tests?
   1. A seafood allergy can contribute to cardiac symptoms.
   2. A seafood allergy may indicate an allergy to contrast media.
   3. A seafood allergy interacts with many cardiac medications.
   4. A seafood allergy is a biomarker for several cardiac disorders.

2. When a nurse assesses a client, what is the most significant manifestation of ischemia?
   1. Peripheral edema
   2. Thready pulse
   3. Fever
   4. Pain

3. Which type of cuff is best for the nurse to use to ensure an accurate measurement?
   1. A cuff with a width is that is 80% of the mid-arm circumference.
   2. A cuff bladder that is 40% of the mid-arm circumference.
   3. A cuff that is connected to a mercury manometer.
   4. A cuff that is connected to an aneroid manometer.

4. What is the most likely manifestation of cerebral insufficiency when the nurse assesses a client with a history of a cardiac disorder?
   1. Distended neck veins
   2. Bounding carotid pulse
   3. Faint heart sounds
   4. Mental confusion

5. Which of the following technologies is best when the nurse needs to send ECG information in real time on a client who is distant from a cardiac monitor?
   1. Holter monitor
   2. Cardiac pacemaker
   3. Cardiac telemetry
   4. Coronary arteriography

6. What is the best nursing approach during the care of a client who has decreased perfusion to the brain secondary to vascular disease?
   1. Repeat explanations as necessary.
   2. Give the client pamphlets to read.
   3. Communicate with the client's family.
   4. Avoid explanations that are complex.

7. When the nurse assesses heart sounds, which location is best for hearing an S1 sound?
   1. At the heart's apex
   2. In the midsternal area
   3. Left of the sternum in the 2nd intercostal space
   4. Right of the sternum in the 2nd intercostal space

8. When the nurse instructs a client about exercise electrocardiography, which is the best explanation for its purpose?
   1. The test can show how the heart responds to the stress of activity.
   2. The test can show which coronary arteries may be narrowed.
   3. The test can help diagnose how well the cardiac valves function.
   4. The test helps to image the beating heart from a device in the esophagus.

9. Which one of the following assessment findings should the nurse report immediately after a client returns from a heart catheterization?
   1. Tenderness over the catheter insertion site
   2. Sharp pain in the extremity used for catheter insertion
   3. A palpated lump where the catheter was inserted
   4. Capillary refill <2 seconds in the toes on the side of catheterization

10. Following a cardiac catheterization which nursing instruction is most appropriate in the client's immediate post-procedural recovery?
    1. Keep the leg straight and temporarily avoid movement.
    2. Flex the hip and moderately exercise the cannulated leg.
    3. Refrain from consuming fluids or eating solid food.
    4. Resume usual activities of living after being discharged.

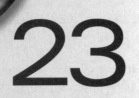

23 Caring for Clients With Infectious and Inflammatory Disorders of the Heart and Blood Vessels

LEARNING OBJECTIVES

1. Identify three organisms that cause infectious conditions of the heart.
2. List four inflammatory conditions of the heart.
3. Describe treatment for inflammatory and infectious heart disorders.
4. Discuss the nursing management of clients with infectious or inflammatory heart disorders.
5. Name three types of cardiomyopathy.
6. Differentiate between thrombophlebitis and thromboangiitis obliterans.
7. List three interventions that reduce the risk of thrombophlebitis.
8. Discuss the nursing management of clients with inflammatory disorders of peripheral blood vessels.

SECTION 1: ASSESSING YOUR UNDERSTANDING

Activity A *Fill in the blanks by choosing the correct word from the options given in parentheses.*

1. The inflammatory symptoms of _____ are believed to be induced by antibodies originally formed to destroy the group A beta-hemolytic streptococcal microorganisms. *(rheumatic carditis, infective endocarditis, myocarditis)*

2. Treatments for _____ involve initially prescribed high doses of an intravenous (IV) antibiotic to which the organism is susceptible. Antibiotic therapy extends at least 2 to 6 weeks. If a heart valve has been severely damaged and drug therapy does not adequately support the failing heart, valve replacement may be necessary. *(infective endocarditis, pericarditis, myocarditis)*

3. The _____ is the most common location of vegetations and microbial deposits. *(mitral valve, aortic valve, pulmonary valve)*

4. Treatment of _____ depends on the underlying cause. A myocardial infarction must be ruled out. Rest, analgesics, antipyretics, nonsteroidal anti-inflammatory drugs, and sometimes corticosteroids are prescribed. Pericardiocentesis may be necessary when cardiac output is severely reduced. *(rheumatic carditis, infective endocarditis, pericarditis)*

5. Black longitudinal lines called _____ can be seen in the nails; this is a sign associated with infective endocarditis. *(Roth's spots, Janeway lesions, splinter hemorrhages)*

6. _____ cardiomyopathy has symptoms of exertional dyspnea, dependent edema in the legs, ascites, and hepatomegaly. *(Dilated, Hypertrophic, Restrictive)*

7. Most commonly, blood clots develop deep in the lower extremities; they are referred to as _____. *(thromboangiitis obliterans, Buerger's disease, deep vein thrombosis)*

8. Monitoring of prothrombin time (PT) is important for clients taking the oral anticoagulant warfarin (Coumadin) for venous thrombosis; PT should be _____ times the control value (12 to 15 seconds) to achieve the therapeutic effect of anticoagulant therapy. *(1.5 to 2.5, 3.0 to 3.5, 3.5 to 4.5)*

Activity B *Write the correct term for each description.*

1. Inflammation can be a primary condition or a secondary condition. The inflammation can occur with or without effusion. _____

2. Treatment of this condition generally involves IV antibiotics. Penicillin is the drug of choice for group A streptococci unless contraindicated because of an allergy. Bed rest may be indicated, depending on the client's condition. Aspirin is used to control the formation of blood clots around heart valves. Steroids are used to suppress the inflammatory response. _____

3. This type of cardiomyopathy is associated with syncope or near-syncopal episodes, which the client may describe as "graying out." Clients also may feel fatigued, become short of breath, and develop chest pain. _____

4. This atypical heart sound may be the first abnormal sign detected in any type of cardiomyopathy. _____

5. Thrombi in the extremities that become mobile and move in the venous circulation to the lungs. _____

6. Painful nodules that may appear on the pads of the fingers and toes with infective endocarditis. _____

7. Inflammation of blood vessels associated with clot formation and fibrosis of the blood vessel wall. It affects primarily the small arteries and veins of the legs. It occasionally involves the arms. _____

Activity C *Match the inflammatory disorders in Column A with their symptoms in Column B.*

Column A

_____ 1. Rheumatic carditis

_____ 2. Infective endocarditis

_____ 3. Myocarditis

_____ 4. Pericarditis

Column B

a. Clients may complain of sharp stabbing or squeezing chest discomfort that resembles a myocardial infarction; sitting up, however, relieves the pain. Accompanying manifestations include a low-grade fever, tachycardia, dysrhythmias, dyspnea, malaise, fatigue, and anorexia.

b. The heart rate is rapid and the rhythm may be abnormal. A red, spotty rash (referred to as erythema marginatum) appears on the trunk but disappears rapidly, leaving irregular circles on the skin. Joints may become swollen, warm, red, and painful. Central nervous system manifestations result in chorea.

c. The client is dyspneic or complains of heaviness in the chest. One chief characteristic is precordial pain. Moving and breathing deeply worsen the pain; sitting upright and leaning forward relieve it. A pericardial friction rub (a scratchy, high-pitched sound) is a diagnostic sign. Heart sounds are difficult to hear because the accumulating fluid muffles them.

d. A heart murmur may be present from malfunctioning valves. Petechiae (tiny, reddish hemorrhagic spots on the skin and mucous membranes) are signs of embolization. Pronounced weakness, anorexia, and weight loss are common.

Activity D *Compare the following procedures based on the given criteria.*

Procedure	Purpose of Procedure
Ventriculomyomectomy	
Pericardiocentesis	

Procedure	Purpose of Procedure
Pericardiostomy	
Pericardiectomy	
Decortication	
Venography	
Impedance plethysmography (IPG)	
Thrombectomy	
Vena caval filter	
Vena caval plication	

Activity E

The steps to perform an assessment of pulsus paradoxus are listed in a jumbled order. Write the correct sequence for the assessment in the following boxes provided.

1. Note when the first BP sound (Korotkoff) is heard.

2. Measure the difference in millimeters of mercury between the first BP sound heard during expiration and the first BP sound heard during both inspiration and expiration.

3. Ask the client to breathe normally throughout the assessment.

4. Deflate the cuff slowly, noting that sounds are audible during expiration but not inspiration.

5. Continue to deflate the cuff until BP sounds are heard during both inspiration and expiration.

6. Inflate the BP cuff 20 mm Hg above systolic pressure.

☐→☐→☐→☐→☐→☐

Activity F

Briefly answer the following questions.

1. How does a blood clot form? Why do signs of swelling, redness, warmth, and tenderness develop?

2. What factors predispose clients to clot formation?

3. Describe the medical and surgical treatment of thrombophlebitis.

4. Describe methods for preventing venous stasis and thrombophlebitis.

5. What is involved in the medical and surgical management of thromboangiitis obliterans?

6. Which type of microorganisms cause infective endocarditis? Where are these microorganisms commonly found?

Activity G *Give rationale for the following questions.*

1. Why does rheumatic carditis lead to cardiac complications such as a heart murmur, congestive heart failure, and pericarditis?

_____

_____

_____

2. Why are clients with a history of rheumatic fever told to take prophylactic antibiotics before any invasive procedure?

_____

_____

_____

3. Why does infective endocarditis lead to complications such as a murmur, congestive heart failure, and emboli?

_____

_____

_____

4. Why does myocarditis result in complications such as congestive heart failure, tachycardia, and dysrhythmias?

_____

_____

_____

5. Why does pericarditis result in cardiac tamponade and respiratory symptoms?

_____

_____

_____

6. Why has infective endocarditis among older adults increased?

_____

_____

_____

SECTION 2: APPLYING YOUR KNOWLEDGE

Activity H *Answer the following questions related to caring for clients with infection and inflammatory disorders of the heart and blood vessels.*

1. What information will the nurse include in teaching clients with infectious and inflammatory heart disorders?

_____

_____

_____

2. How will the nurse instruct a client required to perform Buerger-Allen exercises?

_____

_____

_____

3. What information is included in teaching for clients with cardiomyopathy?

_____

_____

4. Describe the nursing assessments indicated for a client with thrombophlebitis.

_____

_____

_____

5. What are possible assessment findings for a client with thromboangiitis obliterans?

_____

_____

_____

6. What information is included in teaching clients with thrombophlebitis?

_____

_____

Activity I   *Think over the following questions. Discuss them with your instructor or peers.*

1. Your client has been diagnosed with thrombophlebitis. What nursing interventions will you use to prevent complications and promote comfort? What precautions will you need to take with the interventions you identified?

_____

_____

_____

2. Your client is diagnosed with pericarditis. Describe the nursing assessments and intervention to detect and limit the effects of decreased cardiac output. What equipment will you keep at the bedside in the event of cardiac tamponade? What nursing assessments and interventions are indicated following a pericardiocentesis?

_____

_____

_____

SECTION 3:   GETTING READY FOR NCLEX

Activity J   *Answer the following questions.*

1. When collecting data during a nursing assessment of a client with infective endocarditis, which of the following is most suggestive of its etiology?
   1. The client had varicella (chickenpox) as a child.
   2. The client experienced pharygnitis that went untreated.
   3. The client has a family history of cardiac disorders.
   4. The client has had recurrent respiratory infections.

2. When caring for a client with myocarditis that develops tachycardia, what is the most appropriate nursing action?
   1. Place the client in supine position
   2. Encourage deep breathing
   3. Assess the client's level of pain
   4. Administer supplemental oxygen

3. When a nurse assess the heart sounds of a client, which one is most suggestive of cardiac pathology?
   1. A loud S1 at the heart's apex during systole
   2. A rumbling sound during heart contractions
   3. A splitting of the S2 sounds in the pulmonic area
   4. A sound that is synchronous with the apical pulse

4. What is the best nursing technique for augmenting heart sounds?
   1. Have the client sit and lean forward
   2. Tell the client to refrain from talking
   3. Turn off all electrical equipment
   4. Auscultate through the client's back

5. Which nursing instruction is best for a client who has a history of thrombi in the deep veins of the legs?
   1. Tell the client to wear supportive athletic shoes.
   2. Advise the client for walk about frequently.
   3. Suggest the client restrict dietary sodium.
   4. Recommend sitting at periods during the day.

6. When a client is prescribed warfarin (Coumadin), the nurse's dietary teaching should include limiting or eating consistent amounts of foods that contain which vitamin to prevent interfering with the medication's therapeutic effect?
   1. Vitamin A
   2. Vitamin B
   3. Vitamin D
   4. Vitamin K

7. Calculate the amount of warfarin (Coumadin) the nurse should administer to a client whose physician has prescribed 7 1/2 mg p.o. daily. The warfarin is supplied in 5 mg tablets.

_____

8. Before administering warfarin (Coumadin) to a client, which laboratory test results should be evaluated?
   1. PT and PTT
   2. PTT and INR
   3. PT and INR
   4. Bleeding time

9. Place the following heart valves in the sequence in which blood travels from the right side of the heart through and out the left side of the heart.
   1. Aortic valve
   2. Tricuspid valve
   3. Mitral valve
   4. Pulmonic valve

10. What category of medications should the nurse inform clients with a history of infective endocarditis that they must take prophylactically for a lifetime prior to undergoing various procedures such as teeth cleaning?
    1. Anticoagulants
    2. Antibiotics
    3. Steroids
    4. Diuretics

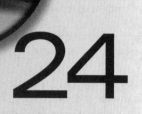

24 Caring for Clients With Valvular Disorders of the Heart

LEARNING OBJECTIVES
1. List five disorders that commonly affect heart valves.
2. Discuss assessment findings common among clients with valvular disorders.
3. Name three diagnostic tests used to confirm valvular disorders.
4. Identify consequences of valvular disorders.
5. Name five categories of drugs used to treat valvular disorders.
6. Give two examples of treatments other than drug therapy to correct valvular disorders.
7. Discuss nursing management of clients with valvular disorders.

SECTION 1: ASSESSING YOUR UNDERSTANDING

Activity A *Fill in the blanks by choosing the correct word from the options given in parentheses.*

1. _____ is a narrowing of the opening in the aortic valve when the valve cusps become stiff and rigid. It is a common valvular disorder in the United States, especially among older adults. *(Aortic stenosis, Aortic regurgitation, Mitral stenosis)*

2. Medical management of mitral stenosis may include a daily _____, dipyridamole (Persantine), or other oral anticoagulant to avoid clot formation. *(aspirin, beta-blocker, cardiac glycoside)*

3. _____ occurs when the mitral valve does not close completely. *(Mitral stenosis, Mitral regurgitation, Aortic stenosis)*

4. If pulmonary congestion occurs with mitral regurgitation, the client will develop _____. *(shortness of breath and moist lung sounds, edema of the feet and ankles, nausea and vomiting)*

5. _____ occurs when valve cusps enlarge, become floppy, and bulge backward into the left atrium. *(Mitral stenosis, Aortic stenosis, Mitral valve prolapse)*

Activity B *Write the correct term for each description.*

1. In young adults, aortic stenosis usually is a later consequence of this type of defect in which the valve has two instead of three cusps. _____

2. Can result from damage to the valve cusps or papillary muscles. _____

3. Occurs when the aortic valve does not close tightly and blood can leak backwards into the left ventricle. _____

4. Mitral stenosis is primarily a sequela of this inflammatory heart condition. _____

5. Medical management of mitral regurgitation often includes this type of medication, which reduces afterload. _____

Activity C *Match the diagnostic tests in Column A with their descriptions in Column B.*

Column A	Column B
_____ **1.** Chest radiograph	**a.** Reflects the large mass and force of the contracting muscle.
_____ **2.** Echocardiogram	**b.** Ventricular enlargement is evident.
_____ **3.** Electrocardiogram	**c.** The pressure of blood in the left ventricle is higher than usual.
_____ **4.** Left-sided cardiac catheterization	**d.** Validates the ventricular thickening and diminished transvalvular size.

Activity D *Give the purpose for the following procedures.*

Procedure	Purpose of procedure
Balloon valvuloplasty	
Annuloplasty	
Intra-aortic balloon pump	
Cardioversion	
Commissurotomy	
Implantation of a biologic or prosthetic valve	

Activity E *Briefly answer the following questions.*

1. In addition to age-related changes and congenital defects, what are other causes of aortic stenosis?

_____

_____

_____

2. A stiff, calcified aortic valve cannot open properly and needs more force to push blood through its narrowed opening. What is the body's response? How can this lead to left-sided heart failure?

_____

_____

_____

3. Describe the medical and surgical management of aortic regurgitation.

_____

_____

_____

4. What are pharmacologic considerations with administration of beta-blockers?

_____

_____

_____

5. How does mitral stenosis result in pulmonary hypertension and the potential for pulmonary edema? What are the effects on the client?

_____

_____

_____

6. What changes in heart sounds occur in mitral stenosis?

_____

_____

_____

SECTION 2: APPLYING YOUR KNOWLEDGE

Activity F *Give rationale for the following questions.*

1. Why do clients with aortic stenosis develop symptoms of dyspnea and fatigue with activity, dizziness, fainting, and angina? Why is heart pulsation displaced and carotid pulse weak?

_____

_____

_____

2. Why do clients with aortic regurgitation experience angina?

_____

_____

_____

3. How can mitral stenosis lead to arterial emboli?

_____

_____

_____

4. Why do some clients with mitral regurgitation remain asymptomatic or develop symptoms gradually over years?

_____

_____

_____

5. Why do clients with mitral regurgitation develop hypertension and tachycardia?

_____

_____

_____

6. Why are clients with mitral valve prolapse syndrome advised to avoid caffeine and alcohol? What dietary recommendations are made?

_____

_____

_____

Activity G *Answer the following questions related to caring for clients with valvular disorders of the heart.*

1. Describe the medical and surgical management of aortic stenosis.

_____

_____

_____

2. What are signs and symptoms of aortic regurgitation?

_____

_____

_____

3. How can mitral stenosis lead to right-sided heart failure?

_____

_____

_____

4. What happens when the mitral valve becomes incompetent?

_____

_____

_____

5. Describe the assessment finding for mitral valve prolapse.

_____

_____

_____

6. Describe the medical management of mitral valve prolapse.

_____

_____

_____

Activity H *Think over the following questions. Discuss them with your instructor or peers.*

1. Your client is diagnosed with aortic stenosis. What nursing assessments and interventions are indicated to ensure adequate cardiac output and tissue perfusion?

_____

_____

_____

2. Your client is at risk for developing signs and symptoms of pulmonary congestion. What nursing assessments and interventions are indicated to detect and reduce the effects of pulmonary congestion?

_____

_____

_____

SECTION 3: GETTING READY FOR NCLEX

Activity I *Answer the following questions.*

1. For which one of the following signs or symptoms would a client with mitral stenosis contact healthcare personnel early in the disorder?
   1. Dyspnea on exertion
   2. Changes in heart sounds
   3. Enlargement of the abdomen
   4. Neck vein distension

2. When a client with aortic stenosis asks the nurse about the cause of the disorder, which of the following responses is most accurate?
   1. Aortic stenosis usually occurs following a streptococcal infection.
   2. Aortic stenosis usually occurs as an atypical immune response.
   3. Aortic stenosis is usually a result of age-related changes.
   4. Aortic stenosis usually results when blood leaks from the valve.

3. What nursing intervention is best for managing activity intolerance experienced by a client with a valvular disorder?
   1. To assume a supine position.
   2. Caution the client against lifting heavy objects.
   3. Intersperse periods of activity with rest.
   4. Instruct the client to consume more carbohydrates.

4. Which of the following dietary choices should the nurse tell the client on a sodium restricted diet to avoid? Select all that apply.
   1. Canned soup
   2. Processed meats
   3. Fresh spinach
   4. Barbecue sauce
   5. Canned peaches
   6. Pepperoni pizza

5. Which side effect is most important for the nurse to instruct the client who takes clopidogrel (Plavix) to report?
   1. Bleeding
   2. Headache
   3. Constipation
   4. Tinnitus

6. Which assessment is the nurse most likely to detect when a client with a valvular disorder experiences a decrease in cardiac output?
   1. Bradycardia
   2. Dizziness
   3. Weight gain
   4. Flushed skin

7. After instructing a client with a valvular disorder to avoid medications that are cardiac stimulants, which category of drugs, if identified by the client, is the best evidence that the client has understood the nurse's teaching?
   1. Drugs classifed as antiinflammatory
   2. Drugs classified as antianginals
   3. Drugs classified as decongestants
   4. Drugs classified as sulfonamides

8. If a client is on fluid restrictions, which of the following should the nurse inform the client must be counted as part of a client's fluid intake? Select all that apply.
   1. Ripe banana
   2. Applesauce
   3. Ice cream
   4. Gelatin

9. What is the most appropriate nursing action when a client with mitral prolapse experiences chest pain.
  1. Instruct the client to breathe deeply and rapidly for 3 to 5 minutes.
  2. Instruct the client to lie flat and elevate the legs for 3 to 5 minutes.
  3. Tell the client to walk briskly for about 3 to 5 minutes.
  4. Tell the client to restrain from activity for 3 to 5 minutes.

10. Which of the following symptoms caused by increased catecholamines will a client with mitral valve prolapse syndrome report to the nurse? Select all that apply.
  1. Tachycardia
  2. Breathlessness
  3. Thirst
  4. Blurred vision
  5. Polyuria
  6. Palpitations

25 Caring for Clients With Disorders of Coronary and Peripheral Blood Vessels

LEARNING OBJECTIVES

1. Distinguish between arteriosclerosis and atherosclerosis.
2. List risk factors associated with coronary artery disease and discuss which can be modified.
3. Describe the symptoms, diagnosis, treatment, and nursing management of coronary artery disease.
4. Discuss the symptoms, diagnosis, treatment, and nursing management of myocardial infarction.
5. Discuss the symptoms, diagnosis, treatment, and nursing management of peripheral vascular diseases such as peripheral artery disease, Raynaud's disease, thrombosis, phlebothrombosis, embolism, and venous insufficiency.
6. Discuss the symptoms, diagnosis, and treatment of varicose veins.
7. Describe nursing management of clients undergoing surgery for varicose veins.
8. Discuss the symptoms, diagnosis, treatment, and nursing management of clients with an aortic aneurysm.

SECTION 1: ASSESSING YOUR UNDERSTANDING

Activity A   Fill in the blanks by choosing the correct word from the options given in parentheses.

1. _____ refers to the loss of elasticity or hardening of the arteries that accompanies the aging process. (*Atheroma, Arteriosclerosis, Atherosclerosis*)

2. _____ is an area of tissue that dies from inadequate oxygenation. (*Ischemia, An infarct, A thrombosis*)

3. _____ is characterized by periodic constriction of the arteries that supply the extremities. The disorder is most common in young women; symptoms often develop after exposure to cold. (*Raynaud's disease, A thrombus, An embolus*)

4. _____ is the development of a clot within a vein without inflammation. (*A thrombus, Phlebothrombosis, An embolus*)

5. Mild fever and pain, swelling, and tenderness of the affected extremity (and possibly a positive Homans' sign) are signs and symptoms of _____. (*an arterial occlusion, a deep vein thrombosis, an embolus*)

6. _____ is a peripheral vascular disorder in which the flow of venous blood is impaired through deep or superficial veins (or both). The condition usually affects the lower extremities, most often the medial aspect of the leg or around the ankle. (*Venous insufficiency, Varicose veins, Aneurysm*)

7. Legs feel heavy and tired, particularly after prolonged standing; activity or elevation of the legs relieves the discomfort. These are symptoms of _____. (*an aneurysm, a thrombus, varicose veins*)

Activity B   Write the correct term for each description.

1. A condition in which the lumen of arteries fills with fatty deposits called plaque. _____

2. Refers to arteriosclerotic and atherosclerotic changes in the coronary arteries supplying the myocardium.

   _____

3. A radiologic test that produces x-rays of the coronary arteries using an electron beam. _____

4. Occurs when there is prolonged total occlusion of coronary arterial blood flow. _____

5. The most common cause of a myocardial infarction.

   _____

6. A medically supervised program that combines exercise and educational activities to speed recovery and reduce or prevent recurring episodes following a significant cardiac event. _____

7. Dilated, tortuous veins. _____

8. A stretching and bulging of an arterial wall. _____

Activity C *Match the diagnostic tests of peripheral blood vessels in Column A to their descriptions in Column B.*

Column A

_____ **1.** Phlebography

_____ **2.** Doppler ultrasonography

_____ **3.** Plethysmography

_____ **4.** Photoplethysmography

_____ **5.** Air plethysmography

Column B

a. Measures volume changes in the venous or arterial system.

b. Used to detect abnormalities in peripheral blood flow.

c. A diagnostic test for venous pathology; measures light that is not absorbed by hemoglobin and consequently is reflected back to the machine.

d. Measures venous pressure by filling a cuff with air after it is applied to the calf while the client is supine with the legs elevated. When the client stands, the pressure is measured again and venous pressure increases, indicating an increased volume of venous reflux.

e. Identifies the point of obstruction in thrombosis using a contrast dye; also known as arteriography or venography.

Activity D *Compare the following procedures based on the following criteria.*

Procedure	Purpose	Description
Percutaneous transluminal coronary angioplasty (PTCA)		
Atherectomy		
Coronary artery bypass graft (CABG)		
Transmyocardial revascularization (TMR)		

Activity E *Briefly answer the following questions.*

1. What are contributing factors to hyperlipidemia?

_____

_____

_____

2. How can atherosclerosis contribute to the development of a blood clot?

_____

_____

_____

3. What are typical symptoms associated with coronary artery disease?

_____

_____

_____

4. Describe the treatment for coronary artery disease.

_____

_____

_____

5. What interventions will the nurse perform to relieve symptoms of angina?

_____

_____

_____

6. What activities may assist the client in aborting an attack associated with Raynaud's disease?

_____

_____

_____

7. Describe the treatment for a venous thrombus.

_____

_____

_____

_____

8. What types of treatments may be ordered to promote venous circulation for a client with venous insufficiency?

_____

_____

_____

9. What is the treatment for an aneurysm?

_____

_____

_____

SECTION 2: APPLYING YOUR KNOWLEDGE

Activity F   _Provide the rationale for the following questions._

1. Why are women who have coronary artery disease (CAD) often misdiagnosed?

_____

_____

_____

2. Why do clients with CAD experience angina pectoris?

_____

_____

_____

3. Why are coronary stents usually placed following a percutaneous transluminal coronary angioplasty?

_____

_____

_____

4. Why is troponin considered the gold standard for determining heart damage in the early stages of a myocardial infarction? What other isoenzymes are cardiac specific?

_____

_____

5. Why is the goal for administering thrombolytics a "door to needle" time of 30 minutes? What is the alternative for clients who are not candidates for thrombolytic therapy?

_____

_____

_____

6. Why do symptoms of localized edema, dermatitis, discoloration, and venous stasis ulcers occur with venous insufficiency?

_____

_____

_____

7. How can an aneurysm lead to shock or death?

_____

_____

_____

Activity G   *Answer the following questions related to disorders of coronary and peripheral blood vessels.*

1. Describe the significance of low-density lipoproteins and high-density lipoproteins in coronary artery disease.

_____

_____

_____

2. What events follow a myocardial infarction that restores some of the lost blood flow and damage to the myocardial tissue?

_____

_____

_____

3. What treatment is indicated in the symptomatic management following a myocardial infarction?

_____

_____

_____

4. What conditions or situations commonly precipitate the development of a thrombosis in the venous system?

_____

_____

_____

5. What are the signs and symptoms of an arterial thrombus?

_____

_____

_____

6. What is the treatment for an arterial thrombus?

_____

_____

_____

7. How do varicose veins develop?

_____

_____

_____

Activity H   *Think over the following questions. Discuss them with your instructor or peers.*

1. Your client states that she is at risk for coronary artery disease because of heredity factors and asks what behavior changes she can make to reduce her risk. What educational information would you provide?

_____

_____

_____

2. A client is diagnosed in the emergency department with an acute myocardial infarction. You took the client's medical history and knew that thrombolytic therapy is absolutely contraindicated. What are the possible reasons this client cannot receive thrombolytics?

_____

_____

_____

3. Your client is ready for discharge following percutaneous transluminal coronary angioplasty. What discharge information will you provide?

_____

_____

_____

4. Your client has been admitted with a deep vein thrombosis. What are the nursing assessments and interventions indicated?

_____

_____

_____

SECTION 3: GETTING READY FOR NCLEX

Activity I *Answer the following questions.*

1. Which one of the following is the chief indication to the nurse that a client may have coronary artery disease?
   1. Heart palpitations
   2. Hypertension
   3. Chest pain
   4. Syncope

2. When the nurse reviews the results of a client's lipid profile, which one is most associated with coronary artery disease?
   1. Elevated high density lipoprotein (HDL)
   2. Elevated low density lipoprotein (LDL)
   3. Low triglycerides
   4. Low total cholesterol

3. Which of the following is a nurse most accurate in identifying as reversible coronary artery disease risk factors? Select all that apply.
   1. Genetic predisposition
   2. Lifelong obesity
   3. Cigarette smoking
   4. Diabetes mellitus
   5. Sedentary lifestyle
   6. Male gender

4. Which dietary change can the nurse advocate as being best for reducing the risk for coronary artery disease?
   1. Eat 4 servings of green vegetables per day
   2. Drink 3 glasses of whole milk per day.
   3. Consume fatty fish at least twice a week.
   4. Use lemon juice instead of salt for seasoning

5. Which side effects can the nurse anticipate may occur after applying a transdermal patch of nitroglycerin to a client with coronary artery disease? Select all that apply.
   1. Vomiting
   2. Headache
   3. Hypotension
   4. Irregular pulse
   5. Shortness of breath
   6. Flushed skin

6. Which of the following signs and symptoms when assessed by the nurse is associated more with a myocardial infarction rather than angina pectoris? Select all that apply.
   1. Substernal discomfort
   2. Crushing chest pain
   3. Evidence of diaphoresis
   4. Feeling nauseous

7. When a nurse interviews a client with Raynaud's disease, which one of the following is the most classic sign of the disorder?
   1. The hands are cyanotic and painful when cold.
   2. There is pain and tenderness when the leg is dorsiflexed.
   3. One leg is swollen and warmer than the other.
   4. The skin of the hands is shiny and taut.

8. What is the most appropriate nursing instructions when teaching a client methods for reducing the consequences of varicose veins? Select all that apply.
   1. Wear thigh high support stockings.
   2. Elevate the legs as much as possible.
   3. Avoid sitting with the knees crossed.
   4. Take baths rather than showers.

9. What nursing assessment is most indicative that a client has an abdominal aortic aneurysm?
   1. Bowel sounds are diminished or absent.
   2. A pulsating mass is felt in the abdomen.
   3. The abdomen is distended and tender.
   4. Feces is pencil-shaped when eliminated.

10. Which one of the following is the nurse correct in identifying as the drug of choice for dissolving a clot within a coronary artery?
    1. heparin (Calciparin)
    2. warfarin (Coumadin)
    3. alteplase (Activase)
    4. enoxaparin (Loveinox)

26 Caring for Clients With Cardiac Dysrhythmias

LEARNING OBJECTIVES

1. Name and describe common cardiac dysrhythmias.
2. Identify medications to control or eliminate dysrhythmias.
3. Explain the purpose and advantages of elective cardioversion.
4. Explain when defibrillation is used to treat dysrhythmias.
5. Discuss the purpose for implanting an automatic internal cardiac defibrillator.
6. Name various types of artificial pacemakers and the purpose for their use.
7. Describe nursing management of the client with a dysrhythmia treated by drug therapy, elective cardioversion, defibrillation, or pacemaker insertion.

SECTION 1:   ASSESSING YOUR UNDERSTANDING

Activity A   *Fill in the blanks by choosing the correct word from the options given in parentheses.*

1. A _____ is a conduction disorder that results in an abnormally slow or rapid heart rate or one that does not proceed through the conduction system in the usual manner. _____ *(dysrhythmia, sinus bradycardia, sinus tachycardia)*

2. In _____, several areas in the right atrium initiate impulses resulting in disorganized, rapid activity. *(atrial flutter, atrial fibrillation, heart block)*

3. In _____, the atrial impulse never gets through, and the ventricles develop their own rhythm independent of the atrial rhythm. *(first-degree heart block, second-degree heart block, complete heart block)*

4. _____ is a ventricular contraction that occurs early and independently in the cardiac cycle before the SA node initiates an electrical impulse. *(Premature ventricular contraction, Ventricular tachycardia, Ventricular fibrillation)*

5. _____ is the rhythm of a dying heart; the ventricles do not contract effectively, and there is no cardiac output. *(Premature ventricular contraction, Ventricular tachycardia, Ventricular fibrillation)*

6. An _____ is commonly located in public places such as worksites and locations where large numbers of people gather. The machine analyzes the heart's rhythm to determine whether an electric shock to the heart is indicated. *(automatic external defibrillator, automatic implanted cardioverter defibrillator, implanted pacemaker)*

7. A _____ provides an electrical stimulus to the heart muscle to treat an ineffective bradydysrhythmia. *(defibrillator, pacemaker, cardioversion)*

8. _____ is a procedure in which a heated catheter tip destroys dysrhythmia-producing tissue. *(Automatic external defibrillator, Radiofrequency catheter ablation, Elective electrical cardioversion)*

Activity B   *Write the correct term for each description.*

1. The usual cardiac rhythm. _____

2. The most common cause of dysrhythmias. _____

3. The use of drugs to eliminate dysrhythmia. _____

4. Refers to disorders in the conduction pathway that interfere with the transmission of impulses from the SA node through the AV node to the ventricles.

_____

5. If performed within the first 3 minutes of ventricular fibrillation or sudden cardiac arrest, the potential for survival is 74%; survival decreases 7% to 10% with every minute that this intervention is delayed. _____

6. A nonemergency procedure done by a physician to stop rapid, but not necessarily life-threatening, atrial dysrhythmias. _____

7. The only treatment for a life-threatening ventricular dysrhythmia; used when there is no functional ventricular contraction. _____

8. A totally implanted device used to manage a chronic bradydysrhythmia. _____

Activity C *Given in Column A are types of premature ventricular contractions (PVC). Match these with their descriptions given in Column B.*

Column A

_____ 1. Bigeminy

_____ 2. Couplets

_____ 3. A run of PVCs

_____ 4. Multifocal PVCs

_____ 5. R-on-T phenomenon

Column B

a. PVCs that originate from more than one location.

b. A PVC whose R wave falls on the T wave of the preceding complex.

c. Two PVCs in a row.

d. Every other beat is a PVC.

e. Three or more PVCs in a row.

Activity D *Use the following table to compare the dysrhythmias based on the given criteria.*

Dysrhythmia	Rhythm	Atrial Rate (beats per minute)	Ventricular Rate (beats per minute)	Treatment
Sinus bradycardia				
Sinus tachycardia				
Premature atrial contraction				
Supraventricular tachycardia				
Atrial flutter				
Atrial fibrillation				
First-degree AV block				
Second-degree AV block				
Complete heart block				
Ventricular tachycardia				
Ventricular fibrillation				

Activity E *Consider the following figure.*

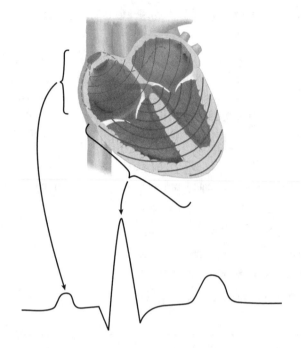

1. Name the first wave before the complex. What does this wave correlate with?

_____

_____

_____

2. Name the complex. What does the complex correlate with?

_____

_____

_____

3. Name the wave following the complex. What does this wave correlate with?

_____

_____

_____

Activity F *Briefly answer the following questions.*

1. Describe atrial flutter.

_____

_____

_____

2. How can atrial fibrillation result in the formation of blood clots? What is the treatment?

_____

_____

_____

3. What is the Maze procedure? What dysrhythmia is it used to treat?

_____

_____

_____

4. Identify common causes of occasional premature ventricular contractions that are usually harmless. What are the associated symptoms?

_____

_____

_____

5. What does electrical cardioversion do to the heart?

_____

_____

_____

6. What is the purpose of an electrophysiology study?

_____

_____

_____

SECTION 2: APPLYING YOUR KNOWLEDGE

Activity G *Give rationale for the following questions.*

1. Why can sinus bradycardia be dangerous for the client?

_____

_____

_____

2. Why is supraventricular tachycardia dangerous for the client?

_____

_____

_____

3. Why does atrial fibrillation result in an irregular ventricular heart rate?

_____

_____

_____

4. Why do clients with coronary artery disease and supraventricular tachycardia develop chest pain?

_____

_____

_____

5. Why do some clients with dysrhythmias not require anti-dysrhythmic drugs?

_____

_____

_____

6. Why are digitalis and diuretics withheld for 24 to 72 hours before cardioversion?

_____

_____

_____

Activity H *Answer the following questions related to caring for clients with cardiac dysrhythmias.*

1. Describe the origin and appearance of a premature atrial contraction. What are common causes of the dysrhythmia?

_____

_____

_____

2. Describe the characteristics of ventricular tachycardia.

_____

_____

_____

3. What are the assessment findings for a client with a dysrhythmia?

_____

_____

_____

4. What is an automatic implanted cardioverter defibrillator?

_____

_____

_____

5. What is the difference between demand (synchronous) mode pacemakers and fixed-rate (asynchronous) mode pacemakers?

_____

_____

_____

6. What is the difference between the following temporary pacemakers: transcutaneous, transvenous, and transthoracic?

_____

_____

_____

Activity I   *Think over the following questions. Discuss them with your instructor or peers.*

1. You are preparing a client for an elective electrical cardioversion. What are the nursing assessments and interventions indicated pre- and postprocedure?

_____

_____

_____

2. Your client is symptomatic with a heart rate of 42 beats/minute and unresponsive to medication. What nursing assessments and interventions are indicated with the use of a transcutaneous pacemaker?

_____

_____

_____

3. Your client goes into ventricular fibrillation. What actions will you take?

_____

_____

_____

SECTION 3:   GETTING READY FOR NCLEX

Activity J   *Answer the following questions.*

1. Which of the following is evidence to the nurse that the clients heart rhythm is providing a consistently adequate cardiac output? Select all that apply.
   1. The client is alert when awake.
   2. The client's capillary refill is greater than 3 seconds.
   3. The client's heart rate is 72 beats per minute.
   4. The client is oriented to person, place, and time.
   5. The client sleeps throughout the night.
   6. The client's urine output is over 100 mL/hr.

2. Which of the following should suggest to a nurse that a client is experiencing a cardiac dysrhythmia?
   1. The client's pulse is strong.
   2. The client's pulse feels irregular.
   3. The client's pulse is difficult to palpate.
   4. The client's pulse feels full.

3. The nurse is most accurate in identifying the location where the most lethal dysrhythmias originate as which of the following?
   1. Atria
   2. Atrioventricular node
   3. Bundle of His
   4. Ventricles

4. Which of the following is the nurse correct in identifying as a potential precursor of lethal dysrhythmias?
   1. Premature atrial contractions (PACs)
   2. Suprarventricular tachycardia (SVT)
   3. First degree AV heart block
   4. Premature ventricular contractions (PVCs)

5. When a nurse uses an automatic electronic defibrillator (AED) to resuscitate a pulseless person, where should the lower paddle be placed?
   1. To right of the sternum below the clavicle
   2. To the left of the sternum below the clavicle
   3. To the left of the nipple in the midaxillary line
   4. To the right of the nipple in the midaxillary line

6. Before shocking the heart with an automatic electronic defibrillator, which of the following nursing actions is essential?
   1. Notify the local police department.
   2. Ensure every one is positioned clear of the victim.
   3. Determine the identity of the victim.
   4. Ask if anyone knows cardiopulmonary resuscitation

7. At what rate should the nurse administer cardiac compressions to a child during a resuscitation attempt?
   1. 100/minute
   2. 90/minute
   3. 80/minute
   4. 70/minute

8. If all of the following drugs are ordered for a client who is scheduled for an elective cardioversion, the nurse is correct in consulting the physician about withholding which one?
   1. Digoxin (Lanoxin)
   2. Dexamethasone (Decadron)
   3. Levothyroxine (Synthroid)
   4. Loratidine (Claritin)

9. When teaching a client with a permanent implanted pacemaker, what should the nurse tell the client to do first if he or she experiences dizziness?
   1. Lie down and elevate your feet to avoid injury.
   2. Change the pacemaker battery as soon as possible.
   3. Have someone call an ambulance immediately.
   4. Move to another location and check your pulse.

10. Calculate the number of tablets per dose a nurse should administer to a client for whom the physician has written the following medical order: verapamil 480 mg/daily p.o. in three equally divided doses. Verapamil comes supplied in 80 mg tablets.

27 Caring for Clients With Hypertension

LEARNING OBJECTIVES

1. Identify the two physiologic components that create blood pressure.
2. List factors that influence blood pressure.
3. List three structures that physiologically control arterial pressure.
4. Explain systolic and diastolic arterial pressure.
5. Discuss the potential value in assessing central aortic systolic pressure.
6. Define hypertension and identify groups at risk for it.
7. Differentiate essential and secondary hypertension.
8. Identify causes of secondary hypertension.
9. List consequences of chronic hypertension.
10. Discuss the assessment findings in hypertension.
11. Discuss the medical and nursing management of the client with hypertension.
12. Differentiate between accelerated and malignant hypertension.
13. Identify potential complications of uncontrolled malignant hypertension.
14. Discuss the medical and nursing management of the client with malignant hypertension.

SECTION 1: ASSESSING YOUR UNDERSTANDING

Activity A *Fill in the blanks by choosing the correct word from the options given in parentheses.*

1. _____ is the force produced by the volume of blood in arterial walls. *(Stroke volume, Cardiac output, Blood pressure)*

2. _____ is determined by the force and volume of blood that the left ventricle ejects and the ability of the arterial system to distend at the time of ventricular contraction. *(Systolic blood pressure, Diastolic blood pressure, Hypertensive disease)*

3. _____ is a systolic blood pressure of 120 to 139 mm Hg or a diastolic blood pressure between 80 and 89 mm Hg. *(Normal blood pressure, Prehypertension, Stage 1 hypertension)*

4. _____ may cause a persistent cough until the medication is discontinued. *(Thiazide diuretics, ACE inhibitors, Beta-blockers)*

5. _____ describes markedly elevated BP accompanied by hemorrhages and exudates in the eyes. *(Stage 1 hypertension, Stage 2 hypertension, Accelerated hypertension)*

Activity B *Write the correct term for each description.*

1. Reflects arterial pressure during ventricular relaxation. _____

2. The ethnic group at highest risk for development of hypertension. _____

3. Vascular changes in the eyes, retinal hemorrhages, or edema of the optic nerves associated with hypertension. _____

4. A possible adverse effect with all antihypertensive drugs. _____

5. Describes dangerously elevated BP accompanied by papilledema. _____

Activity C *Match the various terms given in Column A to their associated definitions or effects given in Column B.*

Column A

_____ 1. Essential hypertension

_____ 2. Secondary hypertension

_____ 3. White-coat hypertension

Column B

a. A term describing elevated BP that develops during evaluation by medical personnel.

b. Sustained elevated BP with no known cause.

c. Elevated BP that results from or is secondary to some other disorder.

Activity D *Briefly answer the following questions.*

1. What does the measured BP reflect?

_____

_____

_____

2. What factors affect blood pressure?

_____

_____

_____

3. What causes an increase in peripheral vascular resistance, which in turn increases systolic blood pressure?

_____

_____

_____

4. Describe the difference between hypertensive heart disease, hypertensive vascular disease, and hypertensive cardiovascular disease.

_____

_____

_____

_____

5. How is medication usually prescribed for the hypertensive client?

_____

_____

_____

6. What types of clients develop accelerated or malignant hypertension?

_____

_____

_____

7. How is accelerated and malignant hypertension medically managed?

_____

_____

_____

SECTION 2: APPLYING YOUR KNOWLEDGE

Activity E *Provide rationale for the following questions.*

1. Why does blood pressure tend to increase with age?

_____

_____

_____

2. How can hypertension lead to heart failure?

_____

_____

_____

3. How can hypertension lead to angina?

_____

_____

_____

4. Why is caffeine intake reduced or eliminated in clients with hypertension?

_____

_____

_____

5. Why is the client who is on antihypertensive medication advised to rise slowly from a sitting or lying position?

_____

_____

_____

6. Why is malignant hypertension fatal unless BP is quickly reduced?

_____

_____

_____

Activity F   *Answer the following questions related to caring for clients with hypertension.*

1. What predisposing conditions may cause secondary hypertension?

_____

_____

_____

2. What changes to the arterial vascular system and serious complications may occur as a result of hypertension?

_____

_____

_____

3. What are risk factors for the development of hypertension?

_____

_____

_____

4. What are the signs and symptoms of hypertension?

_____

_____

_____

5. What nonpharmacologic interventions are used for clients with prehypertension?

_____

_____

_____

6. How is the client with hypertension assessed?

_____

_____

_____

7. Describe the signs and symptoms associated with accelerated and malignant hypertension.

_____

_____

_____

Activity G *Think over the following questions. Discuss them with your instructor or peers.*

1. Your client is admitted with malignant hypertension. What are the indicated nursing assessments and interventions to care for this client?

_____

_____

_____

2. Your client requires education on the DASH diet. What information would you provide?

_____

_____

_____

3. Your client is diagnosed with prehypertension. The client asks how he can reduce his blood pressure without the use of medications. What information will you provide?

_____

_____

_____

Activity H *Read the following case study. Use critical thinking skills to discuss and answer the questions that follow it.*

A client is admitted to the emergency room (ER) presenting with signs and symptoms of congestive heart failure (CHF), dizziness, edema, and fluid overload. The client's medical history indicates non-insulin-dependent (NID) diabetes, obesity, coronary artery disease (CAD), and newly diagnosed essential hypertension. The client's current BP is 98/60 mm Hg, well below his normal blood pressure range of 140 to 158 systolic over 90 to 98 diastolic. The ER nurse reviews the client's current medications, which are Micronase 2.5 mg twice a day, Procardia XL 30 mg daily, ASA 81 mg daily, and one multivitamin daily.

1. What is the relationship between the client's presenting symptoms and his current blood pressure medication?

_____

_____

_____

2. What stage of hypertensive disease does this client have?

_____

_____

_____

3. What effects may this client's diagnosis of hypertension (HTN) have on his already at risk heart and health?

_____

_____

_____

4. Concept Map: Using the information from the given case study, identify the client's current risk factors for chronic health issues.

```
                    ┌──────────────┐
                    │ RISK FACTORS │
                    └──────────────┘
         ┌──────────┬────┴─────┬──────────┐
    ┌─────────┐┌─────────┐┌─────────┐┌─────────┐
    │         ││         ││         ││         │
    └─────────┘└─────────┘└─────────┘└─────────┘
```

SECTION 3: GETTING READY FOR NCLEX

Activity I *Answer the following questions.*

1. Which of the following is the best technique when a nurse initially assesses a client's blood pressure?
   1. Take the blood pressure with an adult size cuff.
   2. Take the blood pressure first before other asessments.
   3. Take the blood pressure while the client stands, sits, and lies down.
   4. Take the blood pressure using a doppler stethoscope.

2. What is the most accurate explanation of the nurse's use of the term of "white coat" hypertension?
   1. It is a consequence of anxiety.
   2. It occurs when the weather is cold.
   3. It is a result of not dressing warmly.
   4. It is a response to a white color.

3. The nurse would be correct in suspecting clients with secondary hypertension to include which of the following? Select all that apply.
   1. A client who is recovering after surgery.
   2. A client who has blood relatives with hypertension.
   3. A client who has chronic kidney disease.
   4. A client who is grossly obese.

4. Which of the following are likely to increase a client's blood pressure? Select all that apply.
   1. Salting food heavily.
   2. Drinking wine occasionally.
   3. Straining to pass feces.
   4. Smoking cigarettes.
   5. Dealing with stress.
   6. Eating meals irregularly.

5. Which of the following diets is best for the nurse to recommend for clients with hypertension under the physician's guidance?
   1. The MyPlate diet
   2. Life's Simple7 diet
   3. The South Beach diet
   4. The DASH diet

6. Which of the following serum electrolytes is most important for the nurse to monitor when a client has been prescribed a loop diuretic like furosemide (Lasix)?
   1. Calcium
   2. Magnesium
   3. Chloride
   4. Potassium

7. What teaching should the nurse provide to promote safety when a client has been prescribed an antihypertensive medication?
   1. Take your medication with a full glass of water.
   2. Rise slowly from sitting or lying positions.
   3. Weigh yourself each day at the same time.
   4. Take your medication when eating a meal.

8. When a client who has been prescribed an angiotensin converting enzyme (ACE) inhibitor reports all of the following to the nurse, which one is most likely a side effect from the medication?
   1. Persistent cough
   2. Decreased appetite
   3. Weight loss
   4. Nose bleeds

9. Which of the following is the nurse correct in identifying as a sexual side effect common among males who are prescribed various antihypertensives?
   1. Premature ejaculation
   2. Absence of orgasms
   3. Erectile dysfunction
   4. Painful intercourse

10. A critical care nurse caring for a client with accelerated hypertension has piggybacked an intravenous infusion of 250 mL of D5W containing 50 mg of nitroglycerin into a client's IV and asks the practical nurse to monitor the infusion. The order is to administer the nitroglycerin solution at a rate of 6 mcg/min. If an electronic infusion device is used, what is the rate of infusion in mL/hr?

28 Caring for Clients With Heart Failure

LEARNING OBJECTIVES

1. Discuss the pathophysiology and etiology of heart failure.
2. Distinguish between acute and chronic heart failure.
3. Identify differences between left-sided and right-sided heart failure.
4. Describe the symptoms, diagnosis, and treatment of left-sided and right-sided heart failure.
5. Discuss the nursing management of clients with heart failure.
6. Discuss the pathophysiology, etiology, symptoms, diagnosis, and treatment of pulmonary edema.
7. Discuss the nursing management of clients with pulmonary edema.

SECTION 1: ASSESSING YOUR UNDERSTANDING

Activity A *Fill in the blanks by choosing the correct word from the options given in parentheses.*

1. An estimate of the heart's efficiency as a pump is its _____, the percentage of blood the left ventricle ejects when it contracts. *(ejection fraction, preload, afterload)*

2. _____ is a sudden change in the heart's ability to contract. It can cause life-threatening symptoms and pulmonary edema. *(Acute heart failure, Chronic heart failure, Intermittent heart failure)*

3. _____ is the force that the ventricle must overcome to empty its diastolic volume; it may increase as a result of arterial hypertension, aortic stenosis, pulmonary hypertension, or excessive blood volume from renal failure. *(Preload, Afterload, Interload)*

4. _____ restores synchrony in the contractions of the right and left ventricles, which is achieved with a biventricular pacemaker. *(Intra-aortic balloon pump, Cardiac resynchronization therapy, Multiple gated acquisition scan)*

5. _____ may be used if cardiogenic shock accompanies acute left ventricular heart failure. *(An intra-aortic balloon pump, Cardiac resynchronization therapy, A multiple gated acquisition scan)*

Activity B *Write the correct term for each description.*

1. The inability of the heart to pump sufficient blood to meet the body's metabolic needs. _____

2. Occurs when the heart's ability to pump effectively is gradually compromised and its impaired contractility remains prolonged. _____

3. A reduction in the ventricular ejection volume because diastole is shortened as a result of a tachydysrhythmia. _____

4. The major cause of right-sided heart failure. _____

5. The most accurate noninvasive test that measures the left ventricle's ejection fraction during rest and activity. _____

6. An auxiliary heart pump that supplements the heart's ability to eject blood; used for some clients awaiting heart transplants. _____

Activity C *Match the medications in Column A with their mechanisms of action in Column B.*

Column A

_____ **1.** Cardiac glycosides

_____ **2.** Diuretics

_____ **3.** Vasodilators

_____ **4.** Nonglycoside inotropic agents

_____ **5.** ACE inhibitors

_____ **6.** hBNP

Column B

a. Promote sodium and water excretion, thus reducing circulating blood volume and decreasing the heart's workload.

b. Improve stroke volume by reducing afterload; reduce preload by dilating veins and arteries.

c. Block ACE from converting angiotensin I to angiotensin II (a potent vasoconstrictor); promote fluid and sodium loss and decrease peripheral vascular resistance.

d. Increase cardiac output by slowing heart rate and increasing force of contraction.

e. Peptide hormone that acts on the kidney to increase the excretions of sodium and water and reduce blood pressure.

f. Relieve cardiogenic shock by strengthening force of myocardial contraction and increasing cardiac output.

Activity D *Briefly answer the following questions.*

1. What two mechanisms can cause heart failure?

_____

_____

_____

2. How do chronic respiratory disorders affect the right side of the heart?

_____

_____

_____

3. What is the compensatory response of the renal system to a decrease in cardiac output?

_____

_____

_____

4. What is the compensatory response of the adrenal gland to the presence of angiotensin in response to a decrease in cardiac output?

_____

_____

_____

5. Describe a cardiomyoplasty.

_____

_____

_____

SECTION 2: APPLYING YOUR KNOWLEDGE

Activity E *Give rationale for the following questions.*

1. How does β-type natriuretic peptide decrease blood pressure?

_____

_____

_____

2. Why are small, frequent meals offered to clients with heart failure?

_____

_____

_____

3. Why are clients with heart failure instructed to avoid activities that engage the Valsalva maneuver, such as straining with bowel elimination or using the arms to pull and reposition oneself?

_____

_____

_____

4. Why is pulmonary edema a serious complication of left-sided heart failure?

_____

_____

_____

5. Why is morphine administered to clients with acute pulmonary edema?

_____

_____

_____

Activity F *Answer the following questions related to caring for clients with heart failure.*

1. Describe the compensatory response of the sympathetic nervous system to a decrease in cardiac output.

_____

_____

_____

2. What is the medical treatment for heart failure?

_____

_____

_____

3. What types of medications are used to manage heart failure?

_____

_____

4. What is ventricular restoration?

_____

_____

_____

5. What is an artificial heart?

_____

_____

_____

Activity G

Think over the following questions. Discuss them with your instructor or peers.

1. Your client has a new onset of heart failure and requires education. What information will you provide to assist the client in managing this disease process?

_____

_____

_____

2. What nursing assessments and interventions are indicated for the client with heart failure?

_____

_____

_____

Activity H

Read the following case study. Use critical thinking skills to discuss and answer the questions that follow it.

A client, hospitalized for left-sided heart failure, turns on his call light for the nurse. When the nurse arrives to check on the client, the client indicates he is suddenly short of breath and feels he can't breathe even with the head of the bed elevated. The client is wheezing and appears restless, cyanotic, and severely anxious. The client's cough is productive, expectorating pinkish sputum. The nurse listens to the client's lung sounds, which are moist throughout, and obtains a set of vital signs. The client's vital signs are as follows: temperature, 99.6° F; pulse rate, 124 beats/minute; respiratory rate, 44 breaths/min; and BP 100/54 mm Hg. Pulse oximeter is 85%. The nurse places supplemental oxygen on the client, while the RN administers 2 mg of morphine IVP (an as-needed order), and calls the physician. Stat ABGs show severe hypoxemia. A stat chest x-ray shows the lungs are filled with fluid. Client will be transferred to the intensive care unit.

1. Given the client's left-sided heart failure, what is the likely cause of the client's sudden change in condition and rationale?

_____

_____

_____

2. What rationale would the nurse have for administering IV morphine?

_____

_____

_____

3. If the client does not respond to traditional medication therapy, what alternative measures might be used?

_____

_____

_____

4. Concept Map: Using the information from the given case study, identify at least two nursing diagnoses with "related to" and "as evidenced by" statements.

| Diagnosis: | Reason for seeking healthcare:

Left-Sided Heart Failure | Diagnosis: |

SECTION 3: GETTING READY FOR NCLEX

Activity I   *Answer the following questions.*

1. A client with a suspected left-sided heart failure is scheduled to undergo a multiple gated acquisition (MUGA) scan. Which nursing action is required before the test?
   1. Diuretics are administered.
   2. Client is medicated to relieve coughing.
   3. Fluids are restricted for 6 hours.
   4. An analgesic is administered.

2. The nurse should instruct a client who has been pre-scribed a potassium wasting diuretic to consume which of the following to compensate for its loss? Select all that apply.
   1. Bananas
   2. Potatoes
   3. Green beans
   4. Orange juice

3. When a client asks for clarification of information the dietitian provided about restricting dietary sodium, what are correct examples for the nurse to identify? Select all that apply.
   1. Soy sauce
   2. Bouillon powder
   3. Lemon juice
   4. Table salt
   5. Onion powder
   6. Baking soda

4. When caring for a client with heart disease, which of the following is the earliest sign or symptom of heart failure that a nurse is likely to note during an assessment?
   1. Urinary frequency
   2. Swollen joints
   3. Dyspnea on exertion
   4. Nausea after eating

5. When administering digoxin (Lanoxin) to a client in heart failure, which of the following is an indication to the nurse that the medication should be temporarily withheld?
   1. The client's respiratory rate is 28/min.
   2. The client's BP is 168/92 while supine.
   3. The client's apical pulse rate is 54/min.
   4. The client's oral temperature is 97.4 degrees F

6. Which of the following is an assessment finding the nurse is most likely to observe when caring for a client with right-sided heart failure?
   1. Dependent edema
   2. Exertional dyspnea
   3. Orthopnea
   4. Hemoptysis

7. A physician plans to digitalize a client in heart failure. The medical order is to administer 0.5 mg p.o. stat followed by 0.25 mg q 6h for a total of 5 doses. If the supplied dose is 125 mcg per tablet, calculate the number of tablets the nurse should administer for the first dose.

   _____

8. If a client receiving digoxin (Lanoxin) reported all of the following to the nurse, which one is most sugges-tive of digitalis toxicity?
   1. Seeing yellow halos around lights
   2. Hearing loud sounds that echo
   3. Having a metallic taste in the mouth
   4. Feeling a tingling skin sensation

9. Which electrolyte is most important for the nurse to monitor to detect a client's potential for developing digitalis toxicity?
   1. Sodium
   2. Potassium
   3. Calcium
   4. Magnesium

10. Which nursing assessment is most important determin-ing the amount of fluid that the client is retaining or losing?
   1. Heart sounds
   2. Peripheral pulses
   3. Daily weights
   4. Peripheral edema

29 Caring for Clients Undergoing Cardiovascular Surgery

LEARNING OBJECTIVES

1. Describe the purpose of cardiopulmonary bypass and its disadvantages.
2. Name indications for cardiac surgery.
3. Describe how coronary artery blood flow is surgically restored.
4. Name four surgical procedures for revascularizing the myocardium.
5. Identify techniques to correct valvular disorders.
6. Describe two methods for controlling bleeding from heart trauma.
7. List five problems associated with heart transplantation.
8. List three types of surgery performed on central or peripheral blood vessels.
9. Discuss the nursing management of clients undergoing cardiovascular surgery.

SECTION 1: ASSESSING YOUR UNDERSTANDING

Activity A *Fill in the blanks by choosing the correct word from the options given in parentheses.*

1. _____ refers to surgical techniques that improve the delivery of oxygenated blood to the myocardium for clients who have coronary artery disease. *(Myocardial revascularization, Cardiopulmonary bypass, Extracorporeal circulation)*

2. _____ uses a balloon catheter to stretch the stenosed valve. *(A commissurotomy, A valvuloplasty, An annuloplasty)*

3. When a donor heart becomes available, it must be removed from the donor and transplanted within _____ hours of being harvested. *(3, 6, 10)*

4. _____ is the resection and removal of the lining of an artery. It is performed to remove obstructive atherosclerotic plaques from the aortic, carotid, femoral, or popliteal arteries. *(A thrombectomy, An embolectomy, An endarterectomy)*

Activity B *Write the correct term for each description related to cardiovascular surgery.*

1. This type of surgery improves myocardial oxygenation by bypassing or detouring around the occluded portion of one or more coronary arteries with a relocated blood vessel. _____

2. This procedure is performed by means of a thoracotomy. The surgeon places a purse-string suture in the wall of the heart, makes an incision, and inserts his or her finger or a metal dilator into the narrowed valve, stretching its opening. _____

3. To prevent and manage tissue rejection following a heart transplant, recipients are given this type of medication. As a result of taking this medication, clients are at risk for infection. _____

4. Body surface area is obtained from this chart based on height and weight. _____

Activity C

Match the types of heart valves given in Column A with their corresponding disadvantages given in Column B.

Column A

_____ **1.** Hemodynamic monitoring

_____ **2.** Direct blood pressure monitoring

_____ **3.** Central venous pressure

_____ **4.** Pulmonary artery pressure monitoring

_____ **5.** Pulmonary capillary wedge pressure

_____ **6.** Cardiac index

Column B

a. Reflects the cardiac output in relation to the particular client's body size.

b. A monitor continuously displays the waveform and indicates the client's systolic, diastolic, and mean arterial pressures.

c. Methods include direct BP monitoring, central venous pressure (CVP) monitoring, and pulmonary artery pressure monitoring.

d. Intracardiac pressures and cardiac output can be measured to assess left ventricular function.

e. The retrograde pressure from the fluid on the left side of the heart at the end of left ventricular diastole.

f. The pressure produced by venous blood in the right atrium.

Activity D

Compare the types of surgical myocardial revascularization listed in the table based on the following criteria.

Surgery	Description	Procedure
Conventional coronary artery bypass graft (CABG)		
Off-pump coronary artery bypass graft (OPCAB)		
Minimally invasive direct coronary artery bypass (MIDCAB)		
Port access coronary artery bypass (PACAB)		

Activity E

Briefly answer the following questions.

1. How are heart tumors surgically managed?

2. When is a heart transplant indicated in adults, newborns, and infants?

3. When is a coronary artery bypass performed?

4. In regard to clients who have undergone cardiovascular surgery, where are they cared for postoperatively?

5. What problems are associated with heart transplants?

SECTION 2:   APPLYING YOUR KNOWLEDGE

Activity F   *Give rationale for the following questions.*

1. Why is antibiotic therapy given for 1 to 2 months following a prosthetic heart valve replacement?

_____

_____

_____

2. Why does a transplanted heart beat faster than the client's natural heart? Why do transplant recipients not experience angina?

_____

_____

_____

3. Why can a thrombectomy or embolectomy be an emergency surgical procedure? How is it performed?

_____

_____

_____

4. Why does the nurse hyperoxygenate with 100% oxygen before suctioning and suction for no longer than 10 to 15 seconds?

_____

_____

_____

5. Why does the nurse provide preoperative instruction for coughing, deep breathing, leg exercises, and splinting?

_____

_____

_____

Activity G   *Answer the following questions related to caring for clients undergoing cardiovascular surgery.*

1. What is the most lethal complication among clients who survive the acute stage of a myocardial infarction? What is the treatment?

_____

_____

_____

2. How are penetrating and nonpenetrating heart trauma injuries medically and surgically managed?

_____

_____

_____

3. How are central and peripheral graft procedures performed?

_____

_____

_____

4. What nursing assessments and interventions will the nurse implement to monitor for postoperative hemorrhage?

_____

_____

_____

Activity H *Think over the following questions. Discuss them with your instructor or peers.*

1. Your client has undergone an aortic graft. What nursing assessments and interventions are indicated?

_____

_____

_____

2. You client has undergone a myocardial revascularization. What nursing assessments and interventions are indicated?

_____

_____

_____

3. You client has undergone a heart transplant. What signs and symptoms are indicative of organ rejection?

_____

_____

_____

SECTION 3: GETTING READY FOR NCLEX

Activity I *Answer the following questions.*

1. When a nurse cares for a client following a heart transplant, which of the following is a sign of organ rejection?
   1. Low white blood cell count
   2. Fever over 100.4° F (38° C)
   3. Weight loss of 2 lb for 2 days in a row
   4. Decreased blood pressure

2. When a client asks the nurse which blood vessels are used when a coronary artery bypass is performed, the most correct answer would include which of the following? Select all that apply.
   1. The basilic and cephalic veins in the arm
   2. The internal mammary and internal thoracic arteries in the chest
   3. The saphenous vein in the leg
   4. The radial artery in the arm
   5. The femoral artery in the groin
   6. The subclavian vein in the chest

3. Which nursing intervention is appropriate to include on the care plan of a client who has had cardiac surgery to prevent ineffective peripheral tissue perfusion?
   1. Restrict oral fluid intake to 1500 mL/day.
   2. Caution the client to avoid prolonged sitting.
   3. Keep the lower extremities below heart level.
   4. Perform leg exercises once per shift.

4. Which of the following should a nurse include in the discharge teaching plan for a client after cardiac surgery?
   1. Avoid taking showers and take tub baths until all incisions are healed.
   2. Notify the physician if a painless lump is felt at the top of the chest incision.
   3. Continue to wear support hose or elastic stockings during the night and remove them during the day.
   4. Sexual relations typically can be resumed in 2 to 4 weeks depending on tolerance for activity.

5. When a client asks the nurse how heart transplant rejection is determined, which of the following is the most accurate answer?
   1. A biopsy of heart tissue is obtained.
   2. A cardiac catheterization is performed.
   3. An electrocardiogram provides specific evidence.
   4. Abnormal heart sounds are heard with a stethoscope.

6. When a client returns from cardiac surgery in which the saphenous vein was harvested, what nursing assessment indicates that circulation is compromised?
   1. The client has pain at the wound site.
   2. The pedal pulse is weak when palpated.
   3. The client resists doing leg exercises.
   4. There is evidence of bleeding on the dressing.

7. When the client who has a chest incision is required to deep breathe and cough, what nursing instruction is most appropriate?
   1. Breathe in and out with a paper bag.
   2. Blow into a bedside spirometer.
   3. Purse your lips during expiration.
   4. Splint your chest with a pillow.

8. Following the repair of an abdominal aortic aneurysm, the nurse notes that the client's bowel sounds are hypoactive and the abdomen is distended. Which one of the following prescribed medications is most likely the cause?
   1. morphine sulfate
   2. enoxaparin (Lovenox)
   3. clopidogrel (Plavix)
   4. furosemide (Lasix)

9. When a nurse caring for a client following cardiac surgery who has water-seal chest tube drainage, which assessment finding is most indicative that the distal end of the chest tube has been displaced?
   1. There is a sudden increase in bloody drainage in the collection chamber.
   2. The fluid in the water seal chamber moves up and down with each breath.
   3. There is crackling in the skin around the tube insertion site.
   4. There is air bubbling in the suction chamber.

10. Following cardiac surgery, a client requires a blood transfusion. To avoid over-hydrating the client, which of the following can the nurse expect the physician will order?
    1. Whole blood
    2. Packed red blood cells
    3. Fresh frozen plasma
    4. Platelets

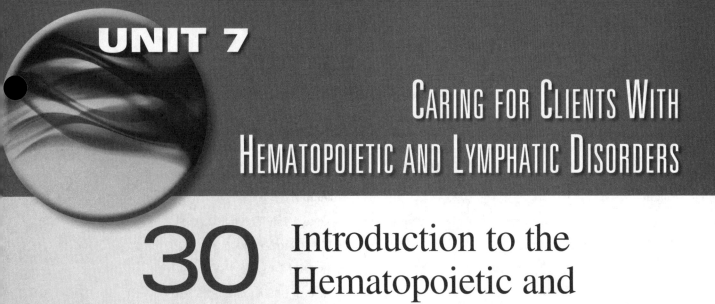

30 Introduction to the Hematopoietic and Lymphatic Systems

LEARNING OBJECTIVES

1. Define hematopoiesis.
2. Name the major structures in the hematopoietic system.
3. Name three types of blood cells produced by bone marrow, and discuss the function of each.
4. List at least five components of plasma.
5. Name three plasma proteins and explain the function of each.
6. Identify the four blood groups and discuss the importance of transfusing compatible types.
7. Explain the components and function of the lymphatic system and its role in hematopoiesis.
8. Describe the pertinent assessments of the hematopoietic and lymphatic systems when obtaining a health history and conducting a physical examination.
9. Name laboratory and diagnostic tests for disorders of the hematopoietic and lymphatic systems.
10. Discuss the nursing management of clients with hematopoietic or lymphatic disorders.

SECTION 1: ASSESSING YOUR UNDERSTANDING

Activity A *Fill in the blanks by choosing the correct word from the options given in parentheses.*

1. The _____ manufactures blood cells and hemoglobin. *(red marrow, yellow marrow, white marrow)*

2. _____ require iron, B_{12}, B_6, and folate to mature properly. *(Leukocytes, Thrombocytes, Erythrocytes)*

3. The red color of blood is caused by _____, an iron-containing pigment attached to erythrocytes. *(hemoglobin, red marrow, yellow marrow)*

4. Approximately _____ of the thrombocytes remain in the spleen unless needed in cases of significant bleeding. *(1/3, 1/2, 2/3)*

5. Blood cells are suspended in a fluid called plasma, which consists of 90% water and 10% _____. *(marrow, lymphokine, protein)*

Activity B *Write the correct term for each description given in parentheses.*

1. The manufacture and development of blood cells. _____

2. The soft tissue that fills spaces in the interior of the long bones and spongy bones of the skeleton. _____

3. The type of marrow that consists primarily of fat cells and connective tissue. _____

4. This hormone, released by the kidneys, regulates the rate of erythrocyte production. _____

5. The most abundant protein in the plasma formed in the liver. _____

Activity C *Match the cell type in Column A with the normal range in Column B.*

Column A

_____ **1.** Normal amount of hemoglobin in an adult

_____ **2.** Normal leukocyte count

_____ **3.** Normal thrombocyte count

_____ **4.** Normal erythrocyte count

Column B

a. 3.6 to 5.4 million/mm^3

b. 150,000 to 350,000/mm^3

c. 12.0 to 17.4 g/dL

d. 5000 to 10,000/mm^3

Activity D *Compare the types of blood cells based on the given criteria.*

Type of Blood Cell	Function
Leukocytes	
Neutrophils	
Basophils	
Eosinophils	
B Lymphocytes	
T Lymphocytes	
Monocytes	
Erythrocytes	
Thrombocytes	

Activity E *Briefly answer the following questions.*

1. Where is red marrow primarily found?

_____

_____

_____

2. How do red blood cells deliver oxygen to the cells of the body?

_____

_____

_____

3. What happens to red blood cells when they are removed from circulation by the body?

_____

_____

_____

4. What is a Schilling test? How is it performed?

_____

_____

_____

SECTION 2:   APPLYING YOUR KNOWLEDGE

Activity F   *Give rationale for the following questions.*

1. Why are leukocytes in constant demand by the body?

_____

_____

_____

2. Why is a bone marrow aspiration performed?

_____

_____

_____

3. Why is vitamin C important in hematopoiesis?

_____

_____

_____

4. Why are older adults susceptible to infections and malignancies?

_____

_____

_____

_____

Activity G   *Answer the following questions related to caring for clients with hematopoietic and lymphatic disorders.*

1. What is the role of proteins in the hematopoietic and lymphatic systems?

_____

_____

_____

2. Explain the relationship between blood type and antigen/antibodies.

_____

_____

_____

3. Describe the lymphatic system and its function.

_____

_____

_____

4. What assessment data is significant to the hematopoietic and lymphatic systems?

_____

_____

_____

5. Some medications affect the hematopoietic system, causing a decrease in various blood components. What signs and symptoms should be monitored?

_____

_____

_____

6. When obtaining a history, the nurse asks about foreign travel. How is this related to the hematopoietic and lymphatic systems?

_____

_____

_____

Activity H *Think over the following questions. Discuss them with your instructor or peers.*

1. Your client is advised that she needs to change her dietary habits to improve red blood cell formation. How will you instruct her?

2. Your client is scheduled for a bone marrow aspiration. What is your role in this procedure?

_____

_____

_____

SECTION 3: GETTING READY FOR NCLEX

Activity I *Answer the following questions.*

1. When providing nursing care for an older adult, which of the following is the most likely consequence of reduced leukocytes?
   1. Tendency to bleed
   2. Potential for infection
   3. Chronic fatigue
   4. Prediposition for allergies

2. The nurse is correct in identifying which of the following as an indication that donor and recipient blood are compatible?
   1. There is no change in the blood color when both samples are mixed
   2. There are blood clots when both samples are mixed
   3. There is no clumping or hemolysis when both samples are mixed
   4. A blood drop floats when dropped in water after both samples are mixed

3. What is the most important reason that the nurse should obtain a dietary history when assessing a client with a disorder of the hematopoietic or lymphatic system?
   1. Compromised nutrition interferes with the production of blood cells and hemoglobin.
   2. A high fat diet interferes with the production of blood cells and hemoglobin.
   3. Inconsistent dieting interferes with the production of blood cells and hemoglobin.
   4. An excess intake of iron and protein interferes with the production of blood cells and hemoglobin.

4. Which of the following should the nurse monitor to detect as a sign or symptom of medications that reduce the formation of thrombocytes?
   1. Sore throat
   2. Unusual bleeding
   3. Feeling chilled
   4. Swollen glands

5. The nurse is correct in identifying which of the following as someone who has an increased susceptibility to infections?
   1. A client who has had a splenectomy
   2. A client who has had an appendectomy
   3. A client who has had a cholecystecomy
   4. A client who has had a nephrectomy

6. Which of the following clients should the nurse expect will have a potential for developing anemia?
   1. Client A who has chronic pulmonary disease
   2. Client B who has an autoimmune disorder
   3. Client C who has chronic renal failure
   4. Client D who has irritable bowel syndrome

7. When a nurse assists with a bone marrow aspiration, which of the following infection control precautions are required?
   1. Contact precautions
   2. Airborn precautions
   3. Droplet precautions
   4. Standard precautions

8. When conscious sedation is used while obtaining a bone marrow specimen, which of the following is best for monitoring the client's oxygenation?
   1. Request an arterial blood gas analysis
   2. Check the client's hemoglobin level
   3. Attach a pulse oximeter to a finger
   4. Review the client's last prothrombin time

9. A nurse is preparing to administer epoietin alfa (Epogen) to increase the client's red blood cell count. The medical order is to give 50 Units/kg subcutaneously once a month. The client weighs 158 lbs. The medication is supplied in a vial that contains 4000 Units/mL. When converting the client's weight to kilograms, round to the nearest whole number. Calculate the volume of epoietin alfa the nurse should administer per dose.

   _____

10. If a nurse cares for a client with a low albumin level, which of the following signs is the most likely manifestation?
    1. Generalized edema
    2. Tarry black stools
    3. Light amber urine
    4. Enlarged spleen

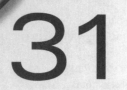

31 Caring for Clients With Disorders of the Hematopoietic System

LEARNING OBJECTIVES

1. List seven types of anemia, including examples of inherited types.
2. Identify nutritional deficiencies that can lead to anemia.
3. Discuss clinical problems that clients with any type of anemia experience.
4. Discuss factors that cause sickling of erythrocytes and related adverse effects.
5. List activities a person with sickle cell disease can do to reduce the potential for a sickle cell crisis.
6. Explain the term *erythrocytosis*, give one example of a characteristic disease, and list possible complications.
7. Explain how forms of leukemia are classified.
8. List clinical problems or nursing diagnoses common among clients with leukemia.
9. Explain how the bone marrow dysfunction of multiple myeloma has an effect on the skeletal system.
10. Differentiate agranulocytosis from leukopenia.
11. Explain the term *pancytopenia* and give an example of a disorder that represents this condition.
12. Discuss the meaning of *coagulopathy* and name two coagulopathies.
13. Discuss nursing responsibilities when managing the care of clients with coagulopathies.

SECTION 1:   ASSESSING YOUR UNDERSTANDING

Activity A   *Fill in the blanks by choosing the correct word from the options given in parentheses.*

1. _____ are abnormalities in the numbers and types of blood cells. (*Blood dyscrasias, Coagulopathies, Thalassemias*)

2. _____ are found in people from Southeast Asia and Africa. (*Alpha-thalassemias, Beta-thalassemias, Gamma-thalassemias*)

3. _____ is an increase in circulating erythrocytes. (*Erythrocytosis, Leukocytosis, Leukemia*)

4. _____ refers to any malignant blood disorder in which proliferation of leukocytes, usually in an immature form, is unregulated. There often is an accompanying decrease in production of erythrocytes and platelets. (*Erythrocytosis, Leukocytosis, Leukemia*)

5. _____ is a malignancy involving plasma cells, which are B-lymphocyte cells in bone marrow. (*Leukemia, Multiple myeloma, Agranulocytosis*)

6. _____ is a decreased production of granulocytes, which places the client at risk for infection. (*Aplastic anemia, Agranulocytosis, Multiple myeloma*)

7. _____ is a consequence of inadequate stem cell production in the bone marrow. (*Aplastic anemia, Multiple myeloma, Coagulopathy*)

8. _____ refers to conditions in which a component that is necessary to control bleeding is missing or inadequate. (*Aplastic anemia, Agranulocytosis, Coagulopathy*)

Activity B   *Write the correct term for each description.*

1. Bleeding disorders that involve platelets or clotting factors. _____

2. Hereditary hemolytic anemias. _____

3. A severe form of beta-thalassemia; clients exhibit symptoms of severe anemia and a bronzing of the skin caused by hemolysis of erythrocytes. _____

4. Characterized by a greater-than-normal number of erythrocytes, leukocytes, and platelets. _____

5. An increased number of leukocytes above normal limits. _____

6. A general reduction in all white blood cells (WBCs). _____

7. Insufficient numbers of erythrocytes, leukocytes, and platelets. _____

8. A lower-than-normal number of thrombocytes. _____

9. A genetically inherited disorder involving an absence or reduction of a clotting factor. _____

Activity C   *Given in Column A are different types of anemia. Match these with their associated signs and symptoms given in Column B.*

Column A

_____ 1. Hypovolemic anemia

_____ 2. Iron deficiency anemia

_____ 3. Sickle cell disease

_____ 4. Hemolytic anemia

_____ 5. Pernicious anemia

_____ 6. Folic acid deficiency anemia

Column B

a. Symptoms are similar to those associated with hypovolemic anemia. In more severe forms, the client is jaundiced and the spleen is enlarged.

b. Erythrocytes become crescent-shaped when oxygen supply in the blood is inadequate.

c. Severe fatigue, a sore and beefy red tongue, dyspnea, nausea, anorexia, headaches, weakness, and light-headedness occur.

d. Pallor, fatigue, chills, postural hypotension; rapid heart and respiratory rates occur.

e. Some clients develop stomatitis and glossitis, digestive disturbances, and diarrhea.

f. Clients have reduced energy, feel cold all the time, and experience fatigue and dyspnea with minor physical exertion. The heart rate usually is rapid even at rest.

Activity D   *Briefly answer the following questions.*

1. What are possible reasons a client may develop iron deficiency anemia?

_____

_____

_____

2. Which ethnic groups are affected by sickle cell disease? How does sickle cell disease differ from carrying the sickle cell trait?

_____

_____

_____

3. Which clients are at risk for developing pernicious anemia?

_____

_____

_____

4. What types of clients are at risk for developing folic acid anemia?

_____

_____

_____

5. What are the symptoms of polycythemia vera?

_____

_____

_____

6. How are leukemias classified? What are the four types?

_____

_____

_____

7. What are the signs and symptoms of agranulocytosis?

_____

_____

_____

8. What is the medical management of aplastic anemia?

_____

_____

_____

9. Describe the pathophysiology and etiology of thrombocytopenia.

_____

_____

_____

10. What is the medical treatment for hemophilia?

_____

_____

_____

SECTION 2: APPLYING YOUR KNOWLEDGE

Activity E *Give rationale for the following questions.*

1. Why is iron deficiency anemia unusual in older adults?

_____

_____

_____

2. Why are older adults more susceptible to hemolytic anemia?

_____

_____

_____

3. There are many leukocytes present with leukemia, so why is the client at risk for infection? Why are clients at risk for anemia and bleeding?

_____

_____

_____

4. Why do clients with multiple myeloma experience hypercalcemia, pathologic fractures, and significant pain?

_____

_____

_____

5. How does multiple myeloma cause renal failure and interfere with the immune response?

_____

_____

_____

Activity F   *Answer the following questions related to caring for clients with disorders of the hematopoietic system.*

1. What problems do clients with sickle cell disease have?

_____

_____

_____

2. What is the pathophysiology of polycythemia vera?

_____

_____

_____

3. What is the treatment for polycythemia vera?

_____

_____

_____

4. How is leukemia medically managed?

_____

_____

_____

5. What are the signs and symptoms of multiple myeloma?

_____

_____

_____

6. What is the medical treatment for multiple myeloma?

_____

_____

_____

7. What are the signs and symptoms of aplastic anemia?

_____

_____

_____

8. What is the medical treatment for thrombocytopenia?

_____

_____

_____

Activity G   *Think over the following questions. Discuss them with your instructor or peers.*

1. Your client is diagnosed with sickle cell disease. What educational information will you provide to this client?

_____

_____

_____

2. Your client is diagnosed with acute lymphocytic leukemia. His absolute neutrophil count indicates that he is at high risk for infection. You place the client in neutropenic precautions. What guidelines will you follow?

_____

_____

_____

3. What general nursing assessments and interventions will you provide to all clients diagnosed with anemia?

_____

_____

_____

4. What nursing assessments and interventions will you provide to clients that are specific to each type of the seven anemias?

_____

_____

_____

Activity H *Read the following case study. Use critical thinking skills to discuss and answer the questions that follow.*

A client presents to the local emergency room with signs and symptoms of an infection. The client complains of a sore throat, fatigue, fever, chills, and a headache. During the nurse's assessment, the client's medical history and current medications are obtained. The client informs the nurse that he is being treated for multiple myeloma and is receiving a combination of antineoplastics: vincristine (Oncovin), doxorubicin (Adriamycin), and a steroid dexamethasone (Decadron). The physician orders a white blood cell (WBC) count with differential and electrolytes. The WBC results indicate low granulocyte counts (neutrophils, basophils, and eosinophils). The blood chemistry panel an elevated blood sugar level.

1. Given the client's symptoms, history, and current medications, what is the likely cause of the client's illness?

_____

_____

_____

2. Why is the client's blood sugar elevated in the blood chemistry panel results?

_____

_____

_____

3. Upon admission, what type of nursing care would you provide for this client?

_____

_____

_____

4. What advantages does using this combination of drugs—vincristine (Oncovin), doxorubicin (Adriamycin), and dexamethasone (Decadron)—provide for the client as treatment for his multiple myeloma?

_____

_____

_____

SECTION 3: GETTING READY FOR NCLEX

Activity I *Answer the following questions.*

1. When caring for a client with decreasing blood pressure and tachycardia, the nurse is accurate in indentifying which of the following as an underlying etiology?
1. Vasoconstriction
2. Hypoxemia
3. Anemia
4. Hypovolemia

2. When the nurse cares for all of the following clients, which one has the highest iron requirement?
1. Client A who is pregnant
2. Client B who is a newborn
3. Client C who is an older adult
4. Client D who is a male teen

3. In a client with suspected sickle cell disease, which assessment finding should alert the nurse that the client is experiencing an accelerated rate of erythrocyte destruction?
1. Bleeding
2. Edema
3. Jaundice
4. Bradycardia

4. Which of the following sexual effects of sickle cell disease is the nurse most accurate as affecting males?
1. Erectile dysfunction
2. Low sperm count
3. Undescended testicle
4. Prolonged erection

5. Following dental surgery on a client with hemophilia, the physician orders aminocaproic acid (Amicar) 5 g p.o. immediately postoperatively. Aminocaproic acid is supplied in a syrup that is labeled 1.25 g per 5 mL. Calculate the volume the nurse should administer.

_____

6. For a client with polycythemia vera, how can the nurse help the client decrease the risk for thrombus formation?
   1. Tell the client to walk 15 min/day.
   2. Advise wearing thromboembolic stockings during waking hours.
   3. Recommend reducing oral fluids to 1 L/day drinking 3 quarts (L) of fluid per day.
   4. Instruct the client to rest if chest pain develops.

7. Which of the following is best for the nurse to recommend to increase the absorption of dietary iron?
   1. Sources of vitamin C
   2. Sources of vitamin D
   3. Sources of calcium
   4. Sources of magnesium

8. When caring for a client with leukemia on neutropenic precautions, which of the following nursing actions is appropriate? Select all that apply.
   1. Assign the client to a private room.
   2. Schedule blood draws hours apart.
   3. Eliminate consumption of fresh fruit.
   4. Limit bathing to every 3 days.
   5. Remove cut flowers from the room.

9. When a client is admitted in sickle cell crisis, which of the following assessment findings will the nurse most likely detect?
   1. Fever
   2. Lethargy
   3. Oliguria
   4. Pain

10. When caring for a client with a bleeding disorder, which of the following are appropriate nursing actions? Select all that apply.
    1. Modify oral hygiene with foam mouth swabs.
    2. Request a soft diet from nutritional services.
    3. Apply prolonged pressure to injection sites.
    4. Take the client's temperature rectally.

32 Caring for Clients With Disorders of the Lymphatic System

LEARNING OBJECTIVES

1. Explain the cause and characteristics of lymphedema.
2. Discuss the role of the nurse when managing the care of clients with lymphedema.
3. Describe nursing interventions that promote the resolution of lymphangitis and lymphadenitis.
4. Explain the nature and transmission of infectious mononucleosis.
5. List suggestions the nurse can offer to individuals who acquire infectious mononucleosis.
6. Define the term *lymphoma* and name two types.
7. Name the type of malignant cell diagnostic of Hodgkin's disease.
8. List three forms of treatment used to cure or promote remission of lymphomas.
9. Name at least four problems that nurses address when caring for clients with Hodgkin's disease and non-Hodgkin's lymphoma.

SECTION 1:   ASSESSING YOUR UNDERSTANDING

Activity A   *Fill in the blanks by choosing the correct word from the options given in parentheses.*

1. The tonsils, thymus gland, and spleen are _____ lymphatic structures. *(specialized, accessory, primary)*

2. _____ is a condition that results from impaired lymph circulation. *(Lymphedema, Lymphangitis, Lymphadenitis)*

3. _____ refers to a group of cancers that affect the lymphatic system. *(Infectious mononucleosis, Lymphangitis, Lymphoma)*

4. Symptoms of _____ include fatigue, fever, sore throat, headache, and cervical lymph node enlargement. The tonsils ooze white or greenish-gray exudates. *(infectious mononucleosis, lymphoma, lymphedema)*

5. Monoclonal antibody therapy is a form of _____. *(radiation, chemotherapy, immunotherapy)*

Activity B   *Write the correct term for each description.*

1. Clusters of bean-sized structures located primarily in the neck, axilla, chest, abdomen, pelvis, and groin. _____

2. Lymphatic disorder caused by a parasitic worm transmitted by mosquitoes. _____

3. Inflammation of lymphatic vessels. _____

4. A viral disease that affects lymphoid tissues such as the tonsils and spleen, caused by the Epstein-Barr virus. _____

5. This form of treatment for lymphoma requires marrow from a human donor. _____

Activity C
Match the type of complex decongestive physiotherapy treatment for lymphedema given in Column A with the description given in Column B.

Column A

_____ 1. Distal-to-proximal massage

_____ 2. Compression dressings

_____ 3. Active exercise

_____ 4. Mechanical pulsating compression device

Column B

a. Relieves edema by reducing the excess volume of fluid in the interstitial space.

b. The alternating filling and emptying "milks" the lymph toward the duct, leading to venous drainage.

c. Facilitates lymphatic drainage into collateral vessels.

d. Promotes lymphatic circulation and maintains functional use of the limb.

Activity D
Compare the two types of lymphomas based on the given criteria.

Type of Lymphoma	Description	Cause
Hodgkin's disease		
Non-Hodgkin's lymphomas		

Activity E
Briefly answer the following questions.

1. How is lymphatic fluid circulated?

_____

_____

_____

2. What are the assessment findings with lymphangitis and lymphadenitis?

_____

_____

_____

3. How is infectious mononucleosis spread? Whom does it most commonly affect?

_____

_____

_____

4. What is monoclonal antibody therapy? How is it performed?

_____

_____

_____

5. How is an autologous bone marrow transplant performed?

_____

_____

_____

6. What are the advantages of an allogenic bone marrow transplant?

_____

_____

_____

SECTION 2: APPLYING YOUR KNOWLEDGE

Activity F *Give rationale for the following questions.*

1. Why are antibiotics not prescribed for uncomplicated infectious mononucleosis?

_____

_____

_____

2. Why is the risk of lymphoma increased in older adults?

_____

_____

_____

3. Why do clients with Hodgkin's disease develop pain, fever, and itching?

_____

_____

_____

4. Why are staging and subclassification an important part of medical care for Hodgkin's disease?

_____

_____

_____

5. Why would an endotracheal tube, laryngoscope, and bag-valve mask be placed at the bedside for a client with Hodgkin's disease?

_____

_____

_____

Activity G *Answer the following questions related to caring for clients with disorders of the lymphatic system.*

1. Describe the pathophysiology of lymphedema.

_____

_____

_____

2. What are Reed-Sternberg cells? How are the cells identified?

_____

_____

_____

3. What are the signs and symptoms of Hodgkin's disease?

_____

_____

_____

4. What is the medical treatment for Hodgkin's disease?

_____

_____

_____

5. A client with Hodgkin's disease is at risk for infection related to immunosuppression, secondary to impaired lymphocytes and drug or radiation therapy. What precautions would be taken?

_____

_____

_____

6. What is the pathophysiology of non-Hodgkin's lymphoma? How is the disease classified?

_____

_____

_____

Activity H *Think over the following questions. Discuss them with your instructor or peers.*

1. Your client is diagnosed with lymphedema. What nursing assessments and interventions are indicated?

_____

_____

_____

2. Your client is diagnosed with Hodgkin's disease. What are your priority nursing diagnoses? What is your rationale for these diagnoses? What nursing assessments and interventions are indicated?

_____

_____

_____

SECTION 3: GETTING READY FOR NCLEX

Activity I *Answer the following questions.*

1. A female client with lymphedema expresses her anxiety about the abnormal enlargement of an arm. Which of the following suggestions can a nurse give to support the client's self-image?
   1. Place the arm in a commercial sling.
   2. Provide examples of concealing clothes.
   3. Assist with cold soaks to the affected arm.
   4. Apply a compression garment to the arm.

2. Under which of the following situations should a nurse notify the physician when caring for a client with lymphangitis?
   1. Affected area appears to enlarge.
   2. Lymph nodes are palpable.
   3. Red streaks extend up the limb.
   4. Liver and spleen become enlarged.

3. When a client with Hodgkin's disease experiences itching, which of the following nursing measures are appropriate? Select all that apply.
   1. Use an antibacterial soap for bathing.
   2. Pat to dry the skin after bathing.
   3. Trim the fingernails to a short length.
   4. Consult with the physician about an analgesic.

4. What is the best criterion that indicates the nurse should implement supplemental oxygen therapy for a client with Hodgkin's disease involving cervical lymph nodes?
   1. The client's respiratory rate is 24 bpm.
   2. The client prefers a Fowler's position.
   3. The client's SpO2 is 86% on room air.
   4. The client's apical heart rate is 90 per min.

5. Which of the following nursing instructions is best for a client with non-Hodgkin's lymphoma who is being treated with radiation and chemotherapy?
   1. Increase oral fluid intake.
   2. Eat soft, bland foods.
   3. Restrict calories from dietary fat.
   4. Take a supplement of vitamin C.

6. For which of the following clients, should the nurse monitor most for the development of lymphedema?
   1. Client A who has had a radical mastectomy.
   2. Client B who has a severe case of tonsillitis.
   3. Client C who has had a ruptured spleen removed.
   4. Client D who is undergoing cancer chemotherapy.

7. What infection control measure is most appropriate to recommend when the nurse cares for a client with infectious mononucleosis?
   1. Wear a mask when interacting with others.
   2. Remain at home until symptoms are gone.
   3. Avoid exposing others to your saliva.
   4. Never donate blood in the future.

8. When a client with infectious mononucleosis experiences inflammation of the oral and pharyngeal mucosa, which nursing suggestions are best? Select all that apply.
   1 Eat frequent high calorie meals.
   2. Gargle frequently with warm salt water.
   3. Drink cold or iced beverages.
   4. Avoid eating food with rough textures

9. A client with multiple myeloma is to receive thalido-mide (Thalmid) 200 mg p.o. daily in combination with dexamethasone (Decadron). If the thalidomid is supplied in 50 mg capsules, calculate the number of capsules the nurse should administer.

_____

10. When caring for a client who has just undergone a bone marrow transplant, for which potential complication is it most important for the nurse to monitor to detect?
1. Renal failure
2. Infection
3. Hair loss
4. Dysrhythmias

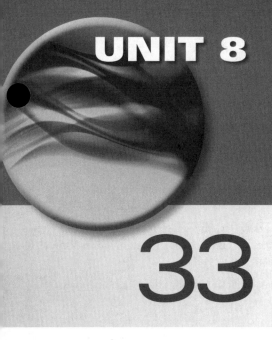
33 Introduction to the Immune System

LEARNING OBJECTIVES

1. Explain the meaning of an immune response.
2. List two general components of the immune system.
3. Discuss the role of T-cell and B-cell lymphocytes.
4. Differentiate between an antigen and an antibody.
5. Name examples of lymphoid tissue.
6. List some cells and chemicals that enhance the function of the immune system.
7. Name three types of immunity, describing how each develops.
8. Discuss techniques for detecting immune disorders.
9. Describe the role of the nurse when caring for a client with an immune disorder.

SECTION 1: ASSESSING YOUR UNDERSTANDING

Activity A   *Fill in the blanks by choosing the correct word from the options given in parentheses.*

1. Primary targets of the _____ are infectious, foreign, or cancerous cells. *(immune system, colony-stimulating factor, tumor necrosis factor)*

2. Formation of antibodies is called a _____ response. *(cell-mediated, humoral, cytotoxic)*

3. _____ are chemical messengers released by lymphocytes, monocytes, and macrophages. There are many subgroups including interleukins, interferons,

tumor necrosis factor, and colony-stimulating factors. *(Immunoglobulins, Nonantibody proteins, Cytokines)*

4. _____ results from the administration of a killed or weakened microorganism or toxoid. *(Naturally acquired active immunity, Artificially acquired active immunity, Passive immunity)*

5. _____ is the inability to mount an immune response. *(Anergy, Inergy, Energy)*

Activity B   *Write the correct term for each description.*

1. Mechanism that enables the immune system to differentiate self from nonself. _____

2. Occurs when T cells survey proteins in the body, actively analyze the surface features, and respond to those that differ from the host by directly attacking the invading antigen. _____

3. The process of engulfing and digesting bacteria and foreign material. _____

4. These tissues filter bacteria from tissue fluid. Because they are exposed to pathogens in the oral and nasal passages, they can become infected and locally inflamed. _____

5. Lymphocyte-like cells that circulate throughout the body looking for virus-infected cells and cancer cells. _____

Activity C   *Match the cytokines in Column A with their functions in Column B.*

Column A

_____ **1.** Interleukins

_____ **2.** Interferons

_____ **3.** Tumor necrosis factor

_____ **4.** Colony-stimulating factors

Column B

a. Chemicals that primarily protect cells from viral invasion; they enable cells to resist viral infection and slow viral replication.

b. Helps in cellular repair when administered in small doses; excess amounts destroy healthy tissue.

c. Carry messages between leukocytes and tissues that form blood cells; some enhance the immune response, whereas others suppress it.

d. Regulate the production, maturation, and function of blood cells.

Activity D   *Compare the specialized white blood cells based on the given criteria.*

Type of Cells	Function
Neutrophils (microphages)	
Monocytes (macrophages)	
Regulator T cells *Helper T cells* (also called T4 or CD4 cells) *Suppressor T cells*	
Effector T cells *Cytotoxic T cells* (also called T8 or CD8 cells)	
B-cell lymphocytes *Plasma cells* *Memory cells*	

Activity E   *Briefly answer the following questions.*

1. What are the types of lymphocytes? What is their function?

_____

_____

_____

2. What are the functions of the thymus gland?

_____

_____

_____

3. What is the function of the spleen?

_____

_____

_____

4. Explain the process of artificially acquired active immunity.

_____

_____

_____

5. How does the complement system assist in the immune response?

_____

_____

_____

SECTION 2: APPLYING YOUR KNOWLEDGE

Activity F *Give rationale for the following questions.*

1. Why are immunosuppressive drugs prescribed following an organ transplant?

_____

_____

_____

2. Why are viral vaccines less effective in older adults?

_____

_____

_____

3. Why are natural killer cells unable to destroy cancer cells?

_____

_____

_____

4. Why is the older client at increased risk for problems related to immunity?

_____

_____

_____

Activity G *Answer the following questions related to the immune system.*

1. Where is lymphoid tissue found?

_____

_____

2. What are the components of the lymphatic system and the functions it performs?

_____

_____

_____

3. How do antibodies destroy invading cells? What is another name for antibodies?

_____

_____

_____

4. What information will the nurse explain and what interventions will the nurse take when a client undergoes immune-related tests?

_____

_____

_____

5. What are examples of interleukin activity?

_____

_____

_____

Activity H *Think over the following questions. Discuss them with your instructor or peers.*

1. What dietary modifications can clients make to boost their immune system?

_____

_____

2. A client states that he has heard that high levels of vitamins and minerals can provide assistance to the immune system. What would you tell him?

_____

_____

_____

3. A mother states she does not want her child immunized. Her rationale is that her child was born with natural immunities and immunizations are not required. What information would you provide?

_____

_____

_____

SECTION 3: GETTING READY FOR NCLEX

Activity I   *Answer the following NCLEX-style questions.*

1. What can the nurse tell the mother of a school age who received a rubellla (measles) vaccine as an infant, but was recently exposed to someone with the infectious disease?
1. The child needs to be revaccinated.
2. The earlier vaccination protects the child.
3. The child may develop a milder case.
4. Confine the child to avoid exposing others.

2. A client is suspected of an immune system disorder. Which of the following is the most important information for the nurse to assess?
1. The client's diet history
2. The client's drug history
3. The client's history of immunizations
4. The client's family history of chronic diseases

3. The nurse is correct in identifying which one of the following as the major factor for older clients having increased susceptibility to immune system disorders?
1. Age-related changes
2. Minimally adequate diet
3. Multiple prescribed drugs
4. Reduced activity levels

4. What is the best nursing response when a pregnant woman asks if she can obtain an injection of influenza vaccine?
1. Wait until after your baby is born to avoid fetal harm.
2. You are protected if you recently had the flu.
3. An injected influenza vaccine is safe during pregnancy.
4. An injection of gamma globulin is better.

5. A client who is undergoing cancer chemotherapy has a low white blood cell count that could interrupt drug therapy. The nurse is correct to anticipate that the physician will order a drug from which category to increase the client's white blood cell count?
1. Interferons
2. Tumor necrosis factor inhibitors
3. Colony stimulating factors
3. Interleukins

6. When the nurse cares for the following clients, which one is at highest risk for an infectious disorder due to immune suppression?
1. Client A with rheumatoid arthritis being treated with steroid therapy
2. Client B with a thombus being treated with anticoagulants
3. Client C with gastritis being treated with a proton pump inhibitor
4. Client D with hypertension being treated with a loop diuretic

7. Prior to undergoing therapy with a tumor necrosis factor (TNF) inhibitor, such as etanercept (Enbrel), the nurse is correct in knowing the client should be tested for which infectious disease?
1. Chickenpox
2. Mumps
3. Hepatitis
4. Tuberculosis

8. When a nurse reviews the hematology laboratory results of a client, which one of the following is most indicative of an increased risk for infections?
1. Low neutrophil count
2. Low eosinophil count
3. Low basophil count
4. Low reticulocyte count

9. When a nurse explains various types of immunity, which client is an example of one who has acquired passive immunity?
   1. An older adult with a history of many infectious disease
   2. A school age child who is exposed to many infectious pathogens
   3. A toddler who is undergoing scheduled immunizations
   4. A newborn who was delivered three days ago

10. Calculate the volume the nurse should administer when the physician orders adalimumab (Humira) 35 mg SC every other week. Adalimumab is supplied in a pre-filled pen that contains 40 mg in 0.8 mL.

_____

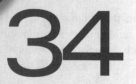

34 Caring for Clients With Immune-Mediated Disorders

LEARNING OBJECTIVES

1. Describe an allergic disorder.
2. List five examples of allergic signs and symptoms.
3. Name four categories of allergens, and give an example of each.
4. Give four examples of allergic reactions, including two that are potentially life threatening.
5. Describe diagnostic skin testing.
6. Name three methods for treating allergies.
7. Discuss the nursing management of a client with an allergic disorder.
8. Explain the meaning of autoimmune disorder, and give at least three examples of related diseases.
9. Discuss theories that explain the development of an autoimmune disorder.
10. Name three categories of drugs used in the treatment of autoimmune disorders.
11. Discuss the nursing management of a client with an autoimmune disorder.
12. Give two explanations for how chronic fatigue syndrome develops.
13. List common symptoms experienced by people with chronic fatigue syndrome.
14. Name common nursing diagnoses, desired outcomes, and related nursing interventions for clients who have chronic fatigue syndrome.

SECTION 1: ASSESSING YOUR UNDERSTANDING

Activity A *Fill in the blanks by choosing the correct word from the options given in parentheses.*

1. An _____ is characterized by a hyperimmune response to weak antigens that usually are harmless. *(allergic disorder, allergen, anaphylaxis response)*

2. _____ is the process by which cellular and chemical events occur after a second or subsequent exposure to an allergen. *(Anaphylaxis, Chemotaxis, Sensitization)*

3. Immediate hypersensitivity response type _____ is mediated by immunoglobulin E (IgE) antibodies. IgE antibodies attach to basophils or mast cells; the response occurs within minutes. *(I, II, III)*

4. In an _____, killer T cells and autoantibodies attack or destroy natural cells—those cells that are "self." *(allergic disorder, autoimmune disorder, anaphylaxis response)*

5. Autoimmune disorders sometimes have inflammatory symptoms that are episodic. Periods of acute flare-ups are called _____. *(exacerbations, remissions, alloimmunity)*

6. _____ is a complex of symptoms primarily characterized by profound fatigue with no identifiable cause. *(An autoimmune disorder, Chronic fatigue syndrome, An allergic disorder)*

7. A(n) _____ is a test in which the client lies horizontally on a table whose incline is elevated to approximately 70° for 45 minutes. *(tilt-table test, flat-table test, elevated-table test)*

Activity B *Write the correct term for each description.*

1. The antigens that can cause an allergic response. _____

2. This type of immediate hypersensitivity response is mediated by IgG antibodies, and its responses reach a peak within 6 hours after exposure. _____

3. A process of attracting migratory cells to a particular area in the body. _____

4. Acute swelling of the face, neck, lips, larynx, hands, feet, genitals, and internal organs. _____

5. Cells that are targeted by autoantibodies and whose antigens match the individual's own genetic code. _____

6. Period during which clients with autoimmune disorders are asymptomatic. _____

7. Pain in fibrous tissues of the body such as muscles, ligaments, and tendons. _____

Activity C *Match the medications in Column A with their mechanisms of action in Column B.*

Column A

_____ **1.** Antihistamines

_____ **2.** Oral corticosteroids

_____ **3.** Oral decongestant agents

_____ **4.** Bronchodilators

_____ **5.** Oral or parenteral sympathomimetic agents

_____ **6.** Leukotriene antagonists

Column B

a. Block receptors for leukotrienes.

b. Block histamine (H_1) receptors.

c. Act on alpha and beta receptors.

d. Dilate airways by stimulating adrenergic receptors located throughout the lungs.

e. Regulate immune response, control inflammatory response.

f. Vasoconstrict nasal membranes.

Activity D *Briefly answer the following questions.*

1. Describe the pattern of allergies.

_____

_____

_____

2. Which organs and structures are primarily involved in allergic reactions?

_____

_____

_____

3. Describe a delayed hypersensitivity response: type IV.

_____

_____

_____

4. What happens to the client during anaphylaxis?

_____

_____

_____

5. What is a patch test?

_____

_____

_____

6. What are complications of inhalant allergies?

_____

_____

_____

7. What types of tests are used to detect autoimmune disorders?

_____

_____

_____

SECTION 2: APPLYING YOUR KNOWLEDGE

Activity E *Give rationale for the following questions.*

1. When testing for food allergies with an elimination diet, why may clients experience symptoms based on their expectations, not from a true allergy?

_____

_____

_____

2. Why does the nurse instruct clients who are scheduled for diagnostic skin testing to avoid taking prescribed or over-the-counter antihistamines or cold preparations for at least 48 to 72 hours before testing?

_____

_____

_____

3. Why are older adults more susceptible to autoimmune disorders?

_____

_____

_____

4. Why does drug therapy for autoimmune disorders cause the client to be at increased risk for infection?

_____

_____

_____

5. Why do some believe that chronic fatigue syndrome should be called "chronic viral reactivation syndrome"?

_____

_____

_____

Activity F *Answer the following questions.*

1. How does the body suppress the allergic response via the eosinophil chemotactic factor?

_____

_____

2. What signs and symptoms can occur with anaphylaxis?

_____

_____

_____

3. What is a scratch (prick) test?

_____

_____

_____

4. What is desensitization?

_____

_____

_____

5. How is an autoimmune disorder medically managed?

_____

_____

_____

6. What is included in the nursing assessment of a client with an autoimmune disorder?

_____

_____

7. Explain the theory of the HPA axis as it relates to chronic fatigue syndrome.

_____

_____

_____

8. What are signs and symptoms of chronic fatigue syndrome?

_____

_____

_____

Activity G *Think over the following questions. Discuss them with your instructor or peers.*

1. What educational information would you provide to a client diagnosed with an autoimmune disorder?

_____

_____

_____

2. What educational information would you provide to a client diagnosed with an allergic disorder?

_____

_____

_____

3. What would be your priority nursing diagnoses for a client with chronic fatigue syndrome? Why? What nursing assessments and interventions are indicated?

_____

_____

_____

Activity H *Read the following case study. Use critical thinking skills to discuss and answer the questions that follow it.*

A 56-year-old female meets with the nurse practitioner in her primary care physician's office. The client is complaining of unrelenting fatigue, malaise, joint pain, muscle pain, and a headache. The client tells the nurse that even after periods of rest, she continues to feel fatigued. During the nurse's review of the client's history, it is discovered that the client was treated 7 months ago for an upper respiratory infection. The nurse continues with her assessment, noting that the client has been experiencing these symptoms for 6 months and has had difficulty with forgetfulness and concentration. The client reports that activity seems to make the fatigue worse, and after standing for just a short period, she becomes light-headed and has to sit down. The client has had to quit her part-time job due to the symptoms she is experiencing. The nurse suspects the client may have chronic fatigue syndrome (CFS) and is experiencing neurally mediated hypotension (NMH).

1. What is NMH and how does it relate to chronic fatigue syndrome?

_____

_____

_____

2. Upon being diagnosed, the client is placed on ENADA. What is ENADA and what client education about its administration does the nurse need to provide?

_____

_____

_____

3. How can nutritional therapy aid in the holistic treatment of CFS?

_____

_____

_____

4. When looking for alternative therapeutic approaches to CFS, what is important for clients to keep in mind?

_____

_____

_____

5. The client in the case study is seeking support to help cope with her CFS. What educational assistance can the nurse provide?

_____

_____

_____

SECTION 3: GETTING READY FOR NCLEX

Activity I _Answer the following questions._

1. What is the role of a nurse during the scratch test to detect allergies?
1. Applying the liquid test antigen
2. Measuring the raised wheal
3. Determining the type of allergy
4. Documenting the findings

2. Which of the following is the most severe complication the nurse can expect among clients with allergies, regardless of type?
1. Bronchitis
2. Cardiac arrest
3. Anaphylaxis
4. Asthma

3. What is the best nursing response when a client asks for the reason he or she must avoid taking antihistamine or cold preparations for at least 24 to 72 hours before undergoing a diagnostic skin test?
1. They may sensitize the skin.
2. They may aggravate the allergic reaction.
3. They may cause false-negative test results.
4. They may alter vital signs.

4. A client is experiencing itching and redness of the eyes. Which of the following would be the best nursing recommendation?
1. Consult an ophthalmologist for evaluation.
2. Instill over-the-counter eye preparations.
3. Stay indoors temporarily on windy days.
4. Avoid close contact with others.

5. What is the most appropriate information for the nurse to give a client with an autoimmune disorder who is taking a corticosteroid such as prednisone (Medicorten)?
1. Do not stop taking the drug suddenly.
2. Increase sources of dietary sodium.
3. Monitor for significant weight loss.
4. Report if you observe bloody urine.

6. When a client is diagnosed with an autoimmune disorder, which of the following statements by the nurse is accurate?
1. These disorders may have remissions.
2. These disorders are always fatal.
3. These disorders can lead to malignancies.
4. These disorders can be cured.

7. A physican who is treating a client with rheumatoid arthritis orders methotrexate (Rheumatrex) 2.5 mg p.o. q 12 h for 3 days. The drug is supplied in 5 mg tablets. Calculate the total number of tablets the nurse will need to implement the medical order.

_____

8. Which of the following is the most important nursing action in the management of a client with CFS?
1. Teaching the client how changes in weather aggravate the disease
2. Informing the client about side effects of prescribed drugs drug therapy
3. Advising the client to include daily aerobic exercise
4. Educating the client about the disease and its limitations

9. What is the best nursing explanation for why antihistamines are used cautiously in older men with prostatic hypertrophy?
   1. They may experience increased drowsiness
   2. They may experience difficulty voiding
   3. They face a greater risk of cardiac arrest
   4. They have a weakened immune response

10. What data does the nurse monitor during a tilt-table test?
    1. Respiratory rate
    2. Temperature and pulse
    3. Pulse and blood pressure
    4. Level of consciousness

35 Caring for Clients With HIV/AIDS

LEARNING OBJECTIVES

1. Explain the term *acquired immunodeficiency syndrome* (AIDS).
2. Identify the virus that causes AIDS.
3. Discuss the characteristics of a retrovirus.
4. Explain how human immunodeficiency virus (HIV) is transmitted.
5. Name at least four methods for preventing transmission of HIV.
6. List three criteria for diagnosing AIDS.
7. Discuss the pathophysiologic process of AIDS.
8. List at least five manifestations characteristic of acute retroviral syndrome.
9. Name two laboratory tests used to screen for HIV antibodies and one that confirms a diagnosis of AIDS.
10. Name two laboratory tests used to measure viral load, and give two purposes for their use.
11. Identify categories of drugs that are used to treat individuals infected with HIV, and give an example of a specific drug in each category.
12. Give the criterion for successful drug therapy for HIV/AIDS.
13. Discuss the nursing management of a client with AIDS, including client teaching.
14. Describe techniques for preventing HIV infection among healthcare workers who care for infected clients.
15. Discuss two ethical issues that affect healthcare workers in relation to clients with HIV infection.

SECTION 1: ASSESSING YOUR UNDERSTANDING

Activity A *Fill in the blanks by choosing the correct word from the options given in parentheses.*

1. _____ is an infectious and eventually fatal disorder that profoundly weakens the immune system. (*Acquired immunodeficiency syndrome, Opportunistic infection, Human immunodeficiency virus*)

2. At the time of primary HIV infection, one third to more than one half of those infected develop _____, which often is mistaken for "flu" or some other common illness. (*acute retroviral syndrome, Kaposi's sarcoma, pneumocystis pneumonia*)

3. _____ is an ineffective response to a prescribed drug because of the survival and replication of exceptionally virulent mutations and noncompliance with drug therapy regimens. (*Drug resistance, Drug dominance, Drug cross-resistance*)

4. When _____ is done, the blood is examined for genetic changes in circulating HIV particles. (*genotype testing, ELISA testing, phenotype testing*)

5. _____ inhibits an enzyme that functions in DNA synthesis. When combined with antiretrovirals, this drug interferes with viral replication, increasing anti-HIV effects. (*Interferon, Interleukin-2, Hydroxyurea*)

6. _____ is an opportunistic infection that affects immunosuppressed people such as clients with AIDS. It can infect the choroid and retinal layers of the eye, leading to blindness. (*Cryptosporidium, Cytomegalovirus, Candidiasis*)

7. Immunosuppressed clients may develop serious diarrhea as a result of infection with a protozoan called _____. (*Cryptosporidium, Cytomegalovirus, Candidiasis*)

Activity B *Write the correct names for the following conditions and treatments of clients with AIDS.*

1. A disease infecting large numbers of people throughout the world; HIV/AIDS is an example. _____

2. A double layer of lipid material surrounding the incomplete HIV. _____

3. A type of connective tissue cancer common among those with AIDS. _____

4. Diminished drug response to similar HIV drugs. _____

5. Sequences of DNA on HIV genes where mutations occur. _____

6. In this type of testing, a measured amount of antiviral drug is mixed with the virus until there is a quantity that prevents the virus from reproducing. _____

7. Activates the cell's own defenses against viruses and is believed to increase blood levels of antiretroviral drugs. _____

8. This yeast infection may develop in the oral, pharyngeal, esophageal, or vaginal cavities or in folds of the skin. _____

Activity C *Match diagnostic tests in Column A with the descriptions given in Column B.*

Column A

_____ 1. Enzyme-linked immunosorbent assay (ELISA) test

_____ 2. Western blot

_____ 3. A total T-cell count

_____ 4. p24 antigen test and polymerase chain reaction test

_____ 5. Papanicolaou cervical test

Column B

a. A positive test result confirms the diagnosis; however, false-positive and false-negative results are possible.

b. This type of cancer screening recommended for women infected with HIV.

c. An initial HIV screening test; results are positive when there are sufficient HIV antibodies or antibodies from other infectious diseases. The test is repeated if results are positive.

d. Measure viral loads; used as a guide for drug therapy and to follow the progression of the disease.

e. Determines the status of T lymphocytes.

Activity D *Compare the following antiretroviral medications based on the given criteria.*

Classification	Mechanism of Action

Reverse transcriptase inhibitors
    Nucleoside reverse transcriptase inhibitors (NRTIs)
    Non-nucleoside reverse transcriptase inhibitors (NNRTIs)
    Nucleotide analogues	

Protease inhibitors	
Entry inhibitors (fusion inhibitors)	
Integrase inhibitors	

Activity E   *Briefly answer the following questions.*

1. What factors have contributed to the statistical decline and actual decline in mortality from AIDS?

_____

_____

_____

2. How did HIV originate?

_____

_____

_____

3. How does the capsid insert its contents into the helper T cell?

_____

_____

_____

4. How is HIV transmitted?

_____

_____

_____

5. What events mark the conversion from HIV to AIDS?

_____

_____

_____

6. What determines the rate of progression from HIV to AIDS?

_____

_____

_____

7. What are the benefits of highly active antiretroviral therapy (HAART)?

_____

_____

_____

SECTION 2:   APPLYING YOUR KNOWLEDGE

Activity F   *Give rationale for the following questions.*

1. Why is AIDS a major public health problem in the United States, especially among African Americans?

_____

_____

_____

2. How can a person with HIV donate blood and the virus not be detected?

_____

_____

_____

3. Why must nurses immediately report any needlestick or sharp injury to a supervisor?

_____

_____

_____

4. Why should a client take antiretroviral medications exactly as prescribed?

_____

_____

_____

5. Most people infected with HIV die of their disease; a few are long-term survivors. Why do some individuals have long-term survival?

_____

_____

_____

6. Why do some physicians feel that delaying drug therapy is justified?

_____

_____

_____

7. Why is it difficult to diagnose distal sensory polyneuropathy?

_____

_____

_____

8. What is AIDS dementia complex? What are the symptoms?

_____

_____

_____

Activity G _Answer the following questions related to caring for the clients with HIV/AIDS._

1. What are the characteristics of HIV-1 and HIV-2?

_____

_____

_____

2. How does HIV replicate?

_____

_____

_____

3. What prevention strategies can reduce or eliminate the transmission of HIV?

_____

_____

_____

4. How does immunodeficiency develop?

_____

_____

_____

5. What are symptoms of acute retroviral syndrome?

_____

_____

_____

6. What are current guidelines for initiation of drug therapy?

_____

_____

_____

7. What is the approximate cost of drug therapy? What are options for funding?

_____

_____

_____

Activity H *Think over the following questions. Discuss them with your instructor or peers.*

1. When providing education to the clients with HIV/AIDS, what information would you provide related to diet?

_____

_____

_____

2. When caring for the clients with HIV/AIDS on an outpatient basis, what educational information would you provide?

_____

_____

_____

3. What steps will you take to ensure safe handling of needles and sharp instruments as a healthcare provider?

_____

_____

_____

SECTION 3: GETTING READY FOR NCLEX

Activity I *Answer the following questions.*

1. When a nurse leads a discussion about HIV transmission, what substances will the nurse correctly identify as body fluids that are potentially infectious? Select all that apply.
   1. Saliva
   2. Blood
   3. Semen
   4. Tears
   5. Vaginal secretions
   6. Breast milk

2. When a nurse assesses a client who is HIV positive, which of the follow findings suggests that the client has developed AIDS-related distal sensory polyneuropathy (DSP)?
   1. Staggering gait and muscle incoordination
   2. Abnormal sensations such as burning and numbness
   3. Delusional thinking
   4. Stress incontinence

3. Which of the following precautions must a nurse take while caring for clients with HIV/AIDS to reduce occupational risks?
   1. Transport specimens of body fluids in leak-proof containers.
   2. Seek prescription for a fusion inhibitor to reduce risk of infection.
   3. Request an order for oral rather than parenteral medications. Avoid administering.
   4. Avoid cleaning items that contain urine, stool, or emesis.

4. Which are appropriate nursing interventions when caring for a client with AIDS who develops pneumocystis pneumonia? Select all that apply.
   1. Encourage forced coughing
   2. Restrict caffeinated beverages
   3. Perform chest percussion
   4. Request blenderized food
   5. Suction the client's airway
   6. Attach a pulse oximeter

5. A client with HIV has been prescribed antiviral medications. What instructions related to administration of medications should the nurse give such a client?
   1. Comply with the timing of antiviral medications.
   2. Avoid all nonprescription medications after taking the medication.
   3. Take the medications with plenty of fruit juice.
   4. Take an increased dose of the medications if the symptoms worsen.

6. A client asks the nurse what evidence suggests that antiretroviral drug therapy is successful. Which of the following are accurate responses? Select all that apply.
   1. The CD4 cell count increases.
   2. No opportunistic infections occur.
   3. The viral load is nondetectable.
   4. HIV is no longer drug dependent.
   5. Treatment is reduced to one drug.

7. What dietary advice is best for the nurse to reinforce when caring for clients with HIV/AIDS?
   1. Encourage multivitamin and mineral supplements.
   2. Suggest limiting food intake to control diarrhea.
   3. Increase food sources rich in iron and zinc.
   4. Avoid food items with gravies, sauces, and broth.

8. Which nursing explanation is accurate for why older clients with AIDS need more care than their younger counterparts?
   1. Older clients lack in balanced diet and activity.
   2. Older clients lack knowledge about disorders.
   3. Older clients have a faster progression of disease.
   4. Older clients do not generally adhere to a therapy.

9. An HIV infected client develops oral candidiasis for which the physician prescribes nystatin (Mycostatin) oral suspension 400,00 Units qid. Calculate the volume the nurse should administer when the pharmacy sends a 60 mL that contains a total of 6,000,000 Units of nystatin oral suspension.

_____

10. What nursing instruction is most appropriate for a client to whom the nurse administers nystatin (Mycostatin) oral suspension.
    1. Swish then swallow the solution.
    2. Gargle then swallow the solution.
    3. Swallow the solution and rinse with water.
    4. Swallow the solution and brush your teeth.

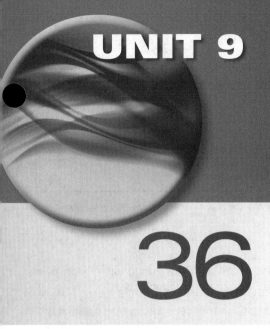

36 Introduction to the Nervous System

LEARNING OBJECTIVES

1. Name the two anatomic divisions of the nervous system.
2. Name the three parts of the brain.
3. List the four lobes of the cerebrum.
4. Give two functions of the spinal cord.
5. Name and describe the function of the two parts of the autonomic nervous system.
6. Describe methods used to assess motor and sensory function.
7. List six diagnostic procedures performed to detect neurologic disorders.
8. Discuss the nursing management of the client undergoing neurologic diagnostic testing.

SECTION 1:   ASSESSING YOUR UNDERSTANDING

Activity A   *Fill in the blanks by choosing the correct word from the options given in parentheses.*

1. The basic structure of the nervous system is the _____. *(neuron, dendrite, axon)*

2. _____ transmit(s) impulses from the CNS. *(Sensory neurons, Myelin, Motor neurons)*

3. The _____ is the surface of the cerebrum. *(corpus callosum, cerebral cortex, midbrain)*

4. The two main functions of the _____ are to provide centers for reflex action and to serve as a pathway for impulses to and from the brain. *(spinal cord, meninges, vertebrae)*

5. _____ allergies suggest an allergy to iodine. *(Dairy, Peanut, Seafood)*

Activity B   *Write the correct term for each description.*

1. The part of the nervous system that consists of all the sensory and motor nerves outside the central nervous system (CNS); it includes the cranial, spinal, and sympathetic and parasympathetic nerves of the autonomic nervous system. _____

2. The type of neurons that transmit impulses to the CNS. _____

3. These substances accomplish the transmission of an impulse from one neuron to the next; they can either excite or inhibit neurons. _____

4. The cerebrum consists of two hemispheres; each hemisphere has four lobes: _____, _____, _____, and _____.

5. The part of the brain, located behind and below the cerebrum, that controls and coordinates muscle movement. _____

6. Within the brain are four hollow structures called the ventricles, which manufacture and absorb this fluid. _____.

Activity C   *Match the levels of consciousness (LOC) given in Column A with their corresponding characteristics given in Column B.*

Column A

_____ **1.** Conscious

_____ **2.** Somnolent or lethargic

_____ **3.** Stuporous

_____ **4.** Semicomatose

_____ **5.** Comatose

Column B

a. The client is aroused only by vigorous and repetitive physical, auditory, or visual stimulation.

b. Spontaneous motion is uncommon, but the client may groan or mutter.

c. There is no spontaneous movement, and the respiratory rate is irregular.

d. The client responds immediately, fully, and appropriately to visual, auditory, and other stimulation.

e. The client is drowsy or sleepy at inappropriate times but can be aroused, only to fall asleep again.

Activity D   *Identify the following postures in the illustration.*

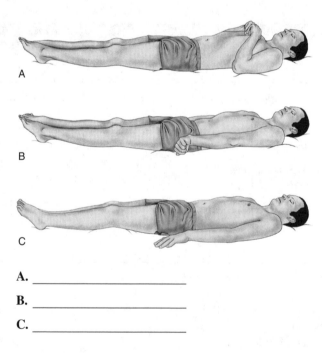

A. _____

B. _____

C. _____

Activity E   *Match the cranial nerve in Column A to its corresponding function in Column B.*

Column A

_____ **1.** Olfactory nerve

_____ **2.** Optic nerve

_____ **3.** Oculomotor nerve

_____ **4.** Trochlear nerve

_____ **5.** Trigeminal nerve

_____ **6.** Abducens nerve

_____ **7.** Facial nerve

_____ **8.** Vestibulocochlear (or auditory) nerve

_____ **9.** Glossopharyngeal nerve

_____ **10.** Vagus nerve

_____ **11.** Accessory (or spinal accessory) nerve

_____ **12.** Hypoglossal nerve

Column B

a. Facial expression, taste, secretions of salivary and lacrimal glands

b. Head and shoulder movement

c. Eye movement

d. Taste, sensory fibers of pharynx and tongue, swallowing, secretions of parotid gland

e. Eye movement

f. Contraction of iris and eye muscles

g. Sense of smell

h. Movement of the tongue

i. Sensory nerve to face, chewing

j. Hearing, balance

k. Sight

l. Production of digestive enzymes regulates, heart rate controls, muscles of speech, gastrointestinal motility, respiration, swallowing, coughing, vomiting reflex

Activity F   *Identify the method, purpose, and precautions for the diagnostic tests related to the nervous system that are listed in the following table.*

Diagnostic test	Method	Purpose	Precautions
Computed tomography			
Magnetic resonance imaging			
Positron emission tomography			
Single-photon emission computed tomography			
Lumbar puncture			
Vascular contrast studies			
Electroencephalogram			
Brain scan			
Electromyography			
Nerve conduction studies			
Echoencephalogram			

Activity G *Give rationale for the following questions.*

1. What pharmacologic considerations should be noted when performing a neurologic assessment?

_____

_____

_____

2. How are intellectual and speech patterns assessed?

_____

_____

_____

3. What assessments will the nurse make if the client has sustained head trauma?

_____

_____

_____

4. How is motor response evaluated in the comatose or unconscious client?

_____

_____

_____

5. What are the three parts of the Glasgow Coma Scale?

_____

_____

_____

SECTION 2: APPLYING YOUR KNOWLEDGE

Activity H *Give rationale for the following questions.*

1. Why does the nurse stand close to the client when performing the Romberg test?

_____

_____

2. Why can assessment of the older adult be difficult?

_____

_____

3. Why do some rehabilitation centers prefer the Rancho Los Amigos Scale over the Glasgow Coma Scale?

_____

_____

4. Why is it important to monitor temperature with a CNS disorder?

_____

_____

Activity I   *Answer the following questions related to the nervous system.*

1. Describe the function of the spinal nerves.

_____

_____

_____

2. What information is essential to gather when obtaining a history from a client with a possible neurologic diagnosis?

_____

_____

_____

3. Describe the assessment of motor function during a neurologic examination.

_____

_____

_____

4. Describe the assessment of sensory function during a neurologic examination.

_____

_____

_____

5. When assessing the client's pupils, what information should be reported to the physician immediately?

_____

_____

_____

Activity J   *Think over the following questions. Discuss them with your instructor or peers.*

1. Calculate the client's Glasgow Coma Scale based on the following findings: eye opening response: to pain; best verbal response: incomprehensible sounds; and best motor response: withdraws (pain). What is the client's total score? What high-priority nursing diagnoses would be pertinent? What nursing interventions would you provide?

_____

_____

_____

2. You are assessing an older client's pupillary response and note pupil response is sluggish. What further information will you need to obtain?

_____

_____

_____

3. You are preparing a client for a lumbar puncture. The client is fearful about the procedure. How will you explain the procedure? What educational information will you provide? What nursing interventions will you use to reduce the client's fears?

_____

_____

_____

SECTION 3: GETTING READY FOR NCLEX

Activity K *Answer the following questions.*

1. What nursing intervention is most appropriate for preventing a headache following a lumbar puncture?
   1. Position the client flat for the time specified by the physician.
   2. Play some soothing music the client enjoys.
   3. Help the client perform a light leg exercises.
   4. Provide some reading material that appeals to the client's interests.

2. What is the best explanation for the nurse to keep a client awake from midnight until an EEG the next morning?
   1. Excess sleep may interfere with client cooperation.
   2. Minimal sleep helps regulate the breathing patterns during the EEG.
   3. Wakefulness helps the client to fall asleep naturally during the EEG.
   4. Sleep deprivation reduces the chances of getting a postprocedural headache.

3. During the physical examination of a client for a possible neurologic disorder, what is the best technique the nurse can use to examine the client for stiffness and rigidity of the neck?
   1. Position the client flat on the bed for at least 3 hours
   2. Move the head and chin of the client toward the chest
   3. Ask the client to pick up objects on the floor
   4. Apply a painful stimulus to the client's neck

4. When a nurse notes a sudden change in the vital signs a client with a neurologic disorder, what is the first action the nurse should take? Which of the following steps should the nurse take immediately?
   1. Report the trend in vital signs to the physician.
   2. Transfer the client to a private room.
   3. Withhold the client's intake of food and fluids.
   4. Restrict the client's activity to bathroom privileges.

5. Which assessment technique is most appropriate for determining a client's motor function during a neurologic examination?
   1. Check the client's sensitivity to heat, cold, touch, and pain.
   2. Have the client push his or her palm against the nurse's palm.
   3. Ask questions that require cognition and logic.
   4. Tell the client to throw a ball to the nurse.

6. Which of the following is the nurse accurate in correlating with the actions involving the sympathetic nervous system? Select all that apply.
   1. Rapid heart rate
   2. Increased peristalsis
   3. Increased perspiration
   4. Decreased blood pressure
   5. Dilated pupils

7. Prior to a magnetic resonance imaging (MRI) test, which nursing instruction is accurate?
   1. Wash your hair.
   2. Remove your watch.
   3. Do not drink coffee.
   4. Remove your underwear.

8. When assessing the pupils of a client who is unconscious, which of the following findings are abnormal responses? Select all that apply.
   1. Each pupil constricts upon light stimulation.
   2. Pupils are unequal.
   3. Pupils are dilated upon light stimulation.
   4. The unstimulated pupil constricts when stimulated pupil constricts.

9. A client who has difficulty swallowing pills and capsules requests sedation prior to an MRI. The physician orders liquid diphenhydramine (Benadry) 50 mg po. 1 hr before the MRI. The supplied dose of liquid diphenhydramine is 12.5 mg per 5 mL. Calculate the amount the nurse should administer.

   _____

10. Which of the following side effects of diphenhydramine (Benadryl) can the nurse expect the client will most likely experience?
    1. Oliguria
    2. Seizure
    3. Drowsiness
    4. Hypertension

37 Caring for Clients With Central and Peripheral Nervous System Disorders

LEARNING OBJECTIVES

1. Discuss at least four signs and symptoms and nursing care of the client with increased intracranial pressure.
2. Name four infectious or inflammatory diseases that affect the central or peripheral nervous system.
3. Discuss three neuromuscular disorders, common related problems, and nursing management.
4. Discuss the nursing management of clients with a cranial nerve disorder.
5. List the signs and symptoms of Parkinson's disease.
6. Discuss the purpose of drug therapy and drugs commonly prescribed for Parkinson's disease.
7. Describe signs and symptoms of Huntington's disease and related nursing management.
8. Discuss the pathophysiology of seizure disorders and different types of seizures.
9. Discuss the nursing management of clients with seizure disorders.
10. Discuss the nursing management of clients with brain tumors.

SECTION 1: ASSESSING YOUR UNDERSTANDING

Activity A   *Fill in the blanks by choosing the correct word from the options given in parentheses.*

1. Shallow, rapid breathing followed by periods of apnea is known as _____. *(Cushing's triad, Cheyne-Stokes respirations, papilledema)*

2. Normal intracranial pressure (ICP) in the ventricles is _____ mm Hg. *(0 to 5, 1 to 15, 5 to 20)*

3. Although the ICP varies, a rise of _____ mm Hg from a previous measurement is cause for concern. *(2, 4, 6)*

4. _____ is a disorder that occurs from inflammation around one of the paired facial nerves, blocking motor impulses to muscles on one side of the face. *(Bell's palsy, Trigeminal neuralgia, Parkinson's disease)*

5. _____ is an extrapyramidal disorder that is transmitted genetically and inherited by people of both genders. *(Parkinson's disease, Trigeminal neuralgia, Huntington's chorea)*

6. A _____ is a growth of abnormal cells within the cranium. *(brain abscess, brain tumor, brain lesion)*

Activity B   *Write the correct term for each of the following descriptions that relate to nervous system disorders or conditions.*

1. An increase in systolic BP and decrease in diastolic BP (widened pulse pressure), bradycardia, and irregular respirations. _____

2. The client's head is maintained in this position to promote venous drainage of blood and cerebrospinal fluid (CSF). _____

3. An inflammation of the meninges caused by various infectious microorganisms, such as bacteria, viruses, fungi, or parasites. _____

4. This treatment for Guillain-Barré syndrome involves removal of plasma from the blood and reinfusion of the cellular components with saline. _____

5. A collection of purulent material in the brain. If untreated, it can be fatal. _____

6. A surgical procedure that destroys a part of the globus pallidus to eliminate or reduce tremor, stooped posture, shuffling gait, and stiff movement. _____

Activity C *Match the neurologic disorders in Column A with their signs and symptoms in Column B.*

Column A

_____ **1.** Bell's palsy

_____ **2.** Huntington's disease

_____ **3.** Trigeminal neuralgia

_____ **4.** Parkinson's disease

Column B

a. Early signs include stiffness (referred to as rigidity) and tremors of one or both hands (described as pill rolling). Bradykinesia develops; clients have a masklike expression, stooped posture, hypophonia, and difficulty swallowing saliva and food. Weight loss occurs, a shuffling gait is apparent, and the client has difficulty turning or redirecting forward motion.

b. The client describes the pain as sudden, severe, and burning. The pain ends as quickly as it begins, usually lasting a few seconds to several minutes. The cycle repeats many times each day. During a spasm, the face twitches and the eyes tear.

c. Symptoms develop slowly and include mental apathy and emotional disturbances, choreiform movements, grimacing, difficulty chewing and swallowing, speech difficulty, intellectual decline, and loss of bowel and bladder control. Severe depression is common and can lead to suicide.

d. Involves the seventh cranial nerve, which supplies the muscles for facial movement. Symptoms develop in a few hours or over 1 to 2 days. Facial pain, pain behind the ear, numbness, diminished blink reflex, ptosis of the eyelid, and tearing on the affected side occur. Speaking and chewing become difficult.

Activity D *Compare and contrast the early and late signs of increased ICP.*

1. Early signs: _____

2. Late signs: _____

Activity E *Briefly answer the following questions.*

1. Why are isotonic intravenous solutions and supplemental oxygen or mechanical ventilation significant to the medical care of the client with increased ICP?

_____

_____

_____

2. Why would medications such as anticonvulsants and benzodiazepines be used in the treatment of increased ICP?

_____

_____

_____

3. Describe the treatment for bacterial meningitis.

_____

_____

_____

4. What is encephalitis? What are common causes?

_____

_____

_____

5. Surgical division of the sensory root of the trigeminal nerve may be performed as treatment for trigeminal neuralgia. What problems may result from this procedure?

_____

_____

_____

6. What are the signs and symptoms of a brain tumor?

_____

_____

_____

SECTION 2:   APPLYING YOUR KNOWLEDGE

Activity F   *Give rationale for the following questions.*

1. Why are hypotonic intravenous solutions and solutions containing glucose not administered to clients with increased ICP?

_____

_____

_____

2. Why are narcotics withheld from clients with increased ICP unless absolutely necessary?

_____

_____

_____

3. Why are respiratory status, nutrition, and immobility priority concerns for a nurse caring for a client with Guillain-Barré?

_____

_____

_____

4. Why are CT scans, MRIs, and skull radiographs safer techniques than a lumbar puncture for diagnosing and locating a brain abscess?

_____

_____

_____

5. Why can an absence seizure go unnoticed?

_____

_____

_____

6. Why should anticonvulsant medications be withdrawn slowly when used in the symptomatic treatment of acute neurologic disorders?

_____

_____

_____

Activity G   *Answer the following questions related to central and peripheral nervous system disorders.*

1. Describe the signs and symptoms of meningitis.

_____

_____

_____

2. What are signs and symptoms of encephalitis?

_____

_____

_____

3. Describe the pathophysiology of Guillain-Barré syndrome and the usual course of the disorder.

_____

_____

_____

4. List the category of drugs used to treat Parkinson's disease, an example of a drug in the category, and its mechanism of action.

_____

_____

_____

5. Describe the difference between a partial elementary seizure with motor symptoms, a partial elementary seizure with sensory symptoms, and a partial seizure with complex symptoms.

_____

_____

_____

6. Describe the difference between these generalized seizures: a myoclonic seizure and a tonic-clonic seizure.

_____

_____

_____

Activity H   *Think over the following questions. Discuss them with your instructor or peers.*

1. What priority nursing diagnoses and interventions would you identify for clients with increased ICP?

_____

_____

_____

2. What priority nursing diagnoses and interventions would you identify for clients with neurologic infectious or inflammatory disorders?

_____

_____

_____

3. What priority nursing diagnoses and interventions would you identify for clients with neuromuscular disorders?

_____

_____

_____

4. What educational information would you provide to a client diagnosed with a seizure disorder?

_____

_____

_____

Activity I   *Read the following case study. Use critical thinking skills to discuss and answer the questions that follow.*

A client diagnosed with Parkinson's disease is being cared for at home by his spouse. The client exhibits hand tremors, bradykinesia, masklike expression, stooped posture, a shuffling gait, hypophonia, and difficulty swallowing. The home health nurse visits to monitor the client's current status and assist with any problems the client or spouse may be experiencing. The nurse asks how the client is responding with his current medication, levodopa (Sinemet). The spouse states that the client is currently having a few "off episodes" of decreased response. The nurse also takes the client's vital signs and weight. The nurse identifies that the client has lost 5 lb since the last visit. The spouse reports that the client doesn't have much of an appetite and that his swallowing difficulty only adds to the problem. The spouse questions the nurse about adding a multivitamin to make sure the client is getting the nutrients he needs. The nurse informs the spouse that the multivitamin is fine as long as it doesn't contain pyridoxine. The spouse appears stressed, and the nurse inquires about the health and well-being of the spouse as caregiver.

1. Why should the client taking levodopa (Sinemet) avoid taking multivitamins with pyridoxine?

_____

_____

_____

2. What strategies can the nurse teach the client and spouse to prevent unintentional weight loss?

_____

_____

_____

3. What dietary precaution should the nurse inform the spouse and client who takes levodopa (Sinemet)?

_____

_____

_____

4. What are some nursing challenges when managing the drug therapy caring for clients with Parkinson's disease?

_____

_____

_____

5. Concept Map: Using the information from the given case study, identify five nursing diagnoses for this client.

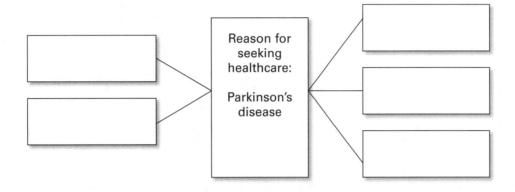

Reason for seeking healthcare:

Parkinson's disease

SECTION 3: GETTING READY FOR NCLEX

Activity J _Answer the following questions._

1. What advice is most appropriate to avoid neurologic disorders transmitted via insect bites?
1. Stay indoors when vacationing in wooded areas.
2. Apply insect repellant to clothing and exposed skin.
3. Wear thick woolen clothing to cover the skin while outdoors.
4. Take a shower with highly scented soap.

2. When caring for a client with a seizure disorder, which of the following nursing measures are appropriate? Select all that apply.
1. Pad the side rails of the bed with soft material.
2. Suction the client's mouth after the seizure.
3. Give supplemental oxygen following the seizure.
4. Raise the client's head during the seizure.
5. Keep a bite guard in the client's mouth at all times.
6. Keep the client awake after the seizure is over.

3. Which nursing interventions are best when caring for a client with impaired swallowing? Select all that apply.
1. Relax while feeding the client.
2. Help the client sit upright.
3. Request thin watery foods.
4. Lower the client's chin when swallowing.

4. Which one of the following is a classic assessment finding when the nurse cares for a client with suspected meningitis?
1. Arching of the back and hyperextension of the head.
2. Drooping of an eyelid, cheek, and lip on one side of the face.
3. Flexing of the arms, clenched fists, and extended legs.
4. Having seizures, muscle weakness, and lethargy.

5. When caring for a client with a neuromuscular disorder at risk for impaired skin integrity, which of the following is best for preventing skin breakdown?
1. Assist with range of motion exercises.
2. Use devices that reduce pressure.
3. Keep the client in a high Fowler's position.
4. Bathe the client with a liquid cleanser. Avoid giving daily baths with soap.

6. Which of the following nursing measures can help clients with neuromuscular disorders cope with feelings of helplessness? Select all that apply.
1. Suggest joining a support group.
2. Allow the client to make choices.
3. Refer the client to a clergy person.
4. Encourage diversional activities.
5. Limit social contacts to close friends.
6. Urge the client to discuss feelings.

7. What is the first sign or symptom a nurse may detect when assessing a client with increased intracranial pressure?
1. Decrease in level of consciousness (LOC)
2. Decreased response to painful stimuli
3. Periods of apnea
4. Elevated systolic blood pressure

8. What is the best method the nurse can use to evaluate the effectiveness of a histamine antagonist like famotidine (Pepcid) used to prevent stress ulcers in clients with increased intracranial pressure?
1. Assess gastric pH.
2. Insert a nasogastric tube.
3. Monitor for vomiting.
4. Auscultate bowel sounds.

9. The physician orders neostigmine (Prostigmin) 0.5 mg IM stat for a client in myasthenic crisis. Calculate the volume the nurse should give when the supplied dose is a 1:2000 solution.

10. A client with Parkinson's disease is considering treatment with deep brain stimulation. What is the nurse most accurate in identifying as a potential outcome of this procedure?
1. Relief of stooped posture
2. Relief of shuffling gait
3. Relief of masklike expression
4. Relief of hand tremors

38 Caring for Clients With Cerebrovascular Disorders

LEARNING OBJECTIVES

1. Identify three common types of headaches and their characteristics.
2. List nursing techniques that supplement drug therapy in reducing or relieving headaches.
3. Explain the cause and significance of a transient ischemic attack.
4. Discuss medical and surgical techniques used to reduce the potential for a cerebrovascular accident.
5. Differentiate between ischemic and hemorrhagic strokes.
6. Identify five manifestations of a cerebrovascular accident; discuss those that are unique to right-sided and left-sided infarctions.
7. Identify at least five nursing diagnoses common to the care of a client with a cerebrovascular accident and interventions for them.
8. Describe a cerebral aneurysm and the danger it presents.
9. Discuss appropriate nursing interventions when caring for a client with a cerebral aneurysm.

SECTION 1:   ASSESSING YOUR UNDERSTANDING

Activity A   *Fill in the blanks by choosing the correct word from the options given in parentheses.*

1. _____, the most common of the three types of headaches, occur when a person contracts the neck and facial muscles for a prolonged period of time. *(Tension headaches, Migraine headaches, Cluster headaches)*

2. Prophylactic drug therapy may be necessary if _____ occur several times a month and produce severe impairment, or if acute attacks are not adequately relieved. *(tension headaches, migraine headaches, cluster headaches)*

3. A _____ is a sudden, brief episode of neurologic impairment caused by a temporary interruption in cerebral blood flow. *(cerebrovascular accident [CVA], cerebral aneurysms, transient ischemic attack [TIA])*

4. _____ is the antidote for oral anticoagulants. *(Vitamin A, Vitamin E, Vitamin K)*

5. _____ develop at a weakened area in the blood vessel wall. The defect is congenital or secondary to hypertension and atherosclerosis. *(TIAs, CVAs, Aneurysms)*

Activity B   *Write the correct term for each description.*

1. These types of headaches may be a variant of migraine headaches; they are episodic, reoccurring over 6 to 8 weeks, with only brief periods of recovery between multiple daily attacks. _____

2. These types of headaches are usually relieved by rest, a mild analgesic, and stress management techniques such as relaxation or imaging. _____

3. A warning that a cerebrovascular accident can occur in the near future; one third of people who experience this develop a stroke. _____

4. An abnormal sound caused by blood flowing over the rough surface of one or both carotid arteries. _____

5. This type of medication has been found to limit neurologic deficits when given within 3 hours after the onset of an ischemic CVA. _____

Activity C *Match the nursing intervention listed in Column A with the rationale in Column B.*

Column A

_____ 1. Eliminate environmental factors that intensify pain, such as bright light and noise.

_____ 2. Administer prescribed medications as early as possible and note their effects.

_____ 3. Offer a back massage to promote muscle relaxation.

_____ 4. Apply warm (or cool) cloths to the forehead or back of the neck.

_____ 5. Provide distraction with soft, soothing music, or suggest using an audio CD that provides relaxation or guided imagery.

Column B

a. Relaxes tense muscles, causes local dilation of blood vessels, and relieves headache; this approach is not likely to help a client with a migraine or cluster headache.

b. Reduced anxiety can relieve a tension headache; clients with migraine or cluster headaches are not receptive to this approach.

c. Sensory stimuli decrease pain tolerance.

d. Treatment can abort symptoms. If ineffective, collaborate with the physician to modify symptom management.

e. Warmth promotes vasodilation; cool applications stimuli reduce blood flow.

Activity D *Compare and contrast the symptoms of right-sided hemiplegia (stroke on left side of brain) and left-sided hemiplegia (stroke on right side of brain).*

_____

_____

_____

Activity E *Briefly answer the following.*

1. A client who has "classic" migraines may experience an "aura." What is an aura? What other symptoms do clients often experience with a "common" migraine?

_____

_____

_____

2. What are the symptoms of a transient ischemic attack (TIA)?

_____

_____

_____

3. What procedures may be performed on the carotid arteries to increase blood flow to the brain?

_____

_____

_____

4. Define hemiplegia, expressive aphasia, receptive aphasia, and hemianopia.

_____

_____

_____

5. What are the clinical manifestations following a cerebral hemorrhage?

_____

_____

_____

6. What are the symptoms of a cerebral aneurysm?

_____

_____

_____

SECTION 2:   APPLYING YOUR KNOWLEDGE

Activity F   *Give rationale for the following questions.*

1. Why might an older adult ignore symptoms of a TIA?

_____

_____

_____

2. Why are clients who are at risk for a TIA given aspirin prophylactically?

_____

_____

_____

3. Why may an older adult, who is diagnosed with hypertension and given a prescription for medication to treat the disorder, still be at risk for a CVA?

_____

_____

_____

4. Why is it essential to monitor a client's cardiac rhythm following carotid artery surgery?

_____

_____

_____

5. Why is surgery not always an option for treatment of an aneurysm?

_____

_____

_____

Activity G   *Answer the following questions related to caring for clients with cerebrovascular disorders.*

1. Describe the pathophysiology of a TIA.

_____

_____

_____

2. Describe the basic events and effects that occur as a result of a CVA.

_____

_____

_____

3. What are the signs of an impending CVA?

_____

_____

_____

4. How are clients who are at risk for a TIA or CVA medically managed?

_____

_____

_____

5. What assessment data should the nurse obtain when caring for a client with a cerebrovascular disorder?

_____

_____

_____

6. How are clients with an aneurysm medically managed?

_____

_____

_____

Activity H *Think over the following questions. Discuss them with your instructor or peers.*

1. What educational information should the nurse provide to clients about controllable risk factors to prevent a TIA or CVA?

_____

_____

_____

2. What are high priority nursing diagnoses and nursing interventions for the client experiencing a CVA? What educational information should the nurse provide?

_____

_____

_____

3. What nursing interventions are appropriate when caring for the client with an aneurysm?

_____

_____

_____

SECTION 3: GETTING READY FOR NCLEX

Activity I *Answer the following questions.*

1. When a nurse assesses a client, which of the following suggests that the cause of the client's discomfort is a tension headache?
   1. A heavy feeling over the frontal region and sensitivity to light
   2. Pressure or steady constriction on both sides of the head
   3. Occipital discomfort and temporary unilateral paralysis
   4. Throbbing sensation in the periorbital area

2. What should the nurse teach an older client with TIA?
   1. Do not worry about the symptoms because they are only temporary.
   2. Seek care in a nursing home for the time being for observation.
   3. Comply with the medication regimen prescribed by the physician.
   4. Report heart palpitations or fluttering in the chest.

3. Which of the following is the best nursing explanation for why clients who take warfarin (Coumadin) should limit consumption of green, leafy vegetables?
   1. They contain vitamin K, which counteracts the drug's action.
   2. They contain vitamin B6 that controls homocystine levels.
   3. They increase erythrocyte production.
   4. They increase the potential for anemia.

4. When caring for a client after a balloon angioplasty of the carotid artery, which of the following assessment findings requires immediate attention?
   1. Dyspnea
   2. Hyperglycemia
   3. Oliguria
   4. Drowsiness

5. When caring for a client who receives warfarin (Coumadin) which nursing action is appropriate if the client's international normalized ratio (INR) result is a value of 2?
   1. Withhold the medication and consult the physician.
   2. Prepare to give protamine sulfate as an antidote.
   3. Give the medication in the prescribed dose for the day.
   4. Request that the laboratory repeat the test again.

6. When the nurse collects data from a client who is exhibiting signs of having had a recent stroke, which of the following would exclude the use of a thrombolytic agent?
   1. The client will be 68 years old next month.
   2. The onset of symptoms was 2 hours ago.
   3. The client had a heart valve replaced 10 days ago.
   4. The client's apical heart rate is 92 per minute.

7. When the nurse prepares the dietary tray for a client who has had a recent stroke, which of the following items should the nurse remove?
   1. Cooked oatmeal
   2. Stewed prunes
   3. Whole wheat toast
   4. Soft boiled egg

8. When a nurse discusses stroke prevention with a group of adults, which of the following represent controllable risk factors. Select all that apply.
   1. Smoking
   2. Obesity
   3. Racial origin
   4. Hypertension
   5. Aging
   6. Diabetes

9. The physician orders heparin sodium 4000 Units SC q6h as stroke prevention for a client with atrial fibrillation. Calculate the volume the nurse should administer from a vial with a supplied dose of 5000 Units/mL.

   _____

10. Which is the preferred site for the nurse to administer a subcutaneous injection of heparin?
    1. Deltoid
    2. Abdomen
    3. Rectus femoris
    4. Vastus lateralis

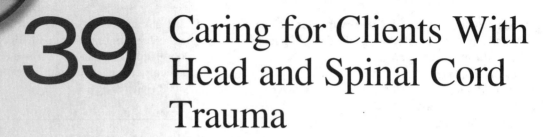

39 Caring for Clients With Head and Spinal Cord Trauma

LEARNING OBJECTIVES

1. Differentiate a concussion from a contusion.
2. Explain the cause and effects of chronic traumatic encephalopathy.
3. Identify differences between epidural, subdural, and intracerebral hematomas.
4. Discuss the nursing management of a client with a head injury.
5. Discuss the nursing management of a client undergoing intracranial surgery.
6. Explain spinal shock, listing four symptoms.
7. Discuss autonomic dysreflexia and at least five manifestations.
8. List possible long-term complications of spinal cord injury.
9. Describe the nursing management of a client with a spinal cord injury.
10. Identify the anatomic difference between intramedullary and extramedullary spinal nerve root compression.

SECTION 1: ASSESSING YOUR UNDERSTANDING

Activity A *Fill in the blanks by choosing the correct word from the options given in parentheses.*

1. When the head is struck, dual bruising can result if the force is strong enough to send the brain ricocheting to the opposite side of the skull. This is called a _____. (*coup injury, contrecoup injury, skull fracture*)

2. A _____ is a surgical opening of the skull. (*craniotomy, craniectomy, cranioplasty*)

3. To detect any cerebrospinal fluid (CSF) drainage, the nurse looks for a _____, which is a bloodstain surrounded by a clear or yellowish stain. (*Battle's sign, periorbital ecchymosis, halo sign*)

4. _____ refers to weakness, paralysis, and sensory impairment of all extremities and the trunk; this occurs when there is a spinal injury at or above the first thoracic (T1) vertebrae. (*Tetraplegia, Paraplegia, Hemiplegia*)

5. _____ is a neuroprotective drug that blocks the neurotoxic effects of glutamate. (*Rilutek, Cetherin, Gabapentin*)

6. A(n) _____ lesion is a type of spinal nerve root compression that involves the spinal cord. (*extramedullary, laminectomy, intramedullary*)

Activity B *Write the correct term for each description.*

1. A contusion caused when the head is struck directly. _____

2. Removal of part of the cranial bone. _____

3. A break in the continuity of the cranium. _____

4. Weakness or paralysis and compromised sensory functions of both legs and the lower pelvis, which occurs with spinal injuries below the T1 level. _____

5. May be used to activate paralyzed muscles and prevent muscle atrophy. _____

6. A type of spinal nerve root compression that involves the tissues surrounding the spinal cord. _____

Activity C *Match the type of cerebral hematoma given in Column A with the corresponding description given in Column B.*

Column A

_____ **1.** Epidural hematoma

_____ **2.** Subdural hematoma

_____ **3.** Acute subdural hematoma

_____ **4.** Subacute and chronic subdural hematomas

_____ **5.** Intracerebral hematoma

Column B

a. Results from venous bleeding, with blood gradually accumulating in the space below the dura.

b. Symptoms progressively worsen within the first 24 hours of the head injury.

c. Bleeding within the brain that results from an open or closed head injury or from a cerebrovascular condition such as a ruptured cerebral aneurysm.

d. Stems from arterial bleeding, usually from the middle meningeal artery, and blood accumulation above the dura. It is characterized by rapidly progressive neurologic deterioration.

e. Clients become symptomatic after 24 hours and up to 1 week later.

Activity D *Provide the description/causes and manifestations of complications associated with spinal cord injury.*

Complication	Description /Causes	Manifestations
Respiratory failure		
Spinal shock		
Autonomic dysreflexia		
Pressure ulcers		
Respiratory infections		
Urinary impairment		
Fecal impairment		
Spasticity and contractures		
Weight change		
Calcium depletion		
Urinary calculi		
Sexual dysfunction: male		
Sexual dysfunction: female		
Pain		

Activity E *Briefly answer the following questions.*

1. When a client is discharged following a concussion, what changes would the family be instructed to watch for as common signs of increased ICP?

_____

_____

_____

2. The rapidity and severity of neurologic changes caused by a cerebral hematoma depend on which factors?

_____

_____

_____

3. What is the purpose of burr holes?

_____

_____

_____

4. What are the common sites and causes of spinal cord injuries?

_____

_____

_____

5. What is the purpose of treadmill training? Is it appropriate for all clients with spinal cord injuries?

_____

_____

_____

6. What types of clients may benefit from tendon transfer surgery?

_____

_____

_____

7. Describe the usual symptoms of a spinal nerve root compression.

_____

_____

_____

SECTION 2:   APPLYING YOUR KNOWLEDGE

Activity F   *Give rationale for the following questions.*

1. Why do epidural hematomas require prompt intervention?

_____

_____

_____

2. Why would mannitol be used following intracranial surgery?

_____

_____

_____

3. Why are fluids restricted before intracranial surgery?

_____

_____

_____

4. Why is it important to monitor temperature following intracranial surgery?

_____

_____

_____

5. Why are open head injuries more likely to create a risk for infection but less likely to result in increased ICP?

_____

_____

_____

6. Why are basilar skull fractures especially dangerous?

_____

_____

_____

Activity G   *Answer the following questions related to caring for the clients with head and spinal cord trauma.*

1. To reduce the potential for both minor and life-threatening head injuries, the nurse should stress the importance of which activities?

_____

_____

_____

2. What types of signs and symptoms can a basilar skull fracture produce?

_____

_____

_____

3. Describe the medical and surgical treatment for a skull fracture.

_____

_____

_____

4. Describe how trauma, edema, and bleeding can cause damage to the spinal cord.

_____

_____

_____

5. Describe how immobilization and traction are used with a spinal cord injury.

_____

_____

_____

6. Describe the benefits of functional electrical stimulation.

_____

_____

_____

7. What is the medical and surgical treatment involved with a spinal nerve root compression?

_____

_____

_____

Activity H   *Think over the following questions. Discuss them with your instructor or peers.*

1. What nursing care would you provide for a client returning to your unit after intracranial surgery?

_____

_____

_____

2. A client who has suffered a traumatic spinal cord injury is being transferred to your unit following the acute care phase. What will be your priority nursing diagnoses and interventions for the physiologic needs of the client? What will be your priority nursing diagnoses and interventions for the psychosocial needs of the client? What educational information will you need to provide to the client and family?

_____

_____

_____

3. What are the ethical considerations related to spinal cord injuries and embryonic stem cell transplantation?

_____

_____

_____

SECTION 3: GETTING READY FOR NCLEX

Activity I *Answer the following questions.*

1. When the nurse assesses a client with a basilar skull fracture, which of the following is likely to be present?
   1. Raccoon eyes
   2. Halo sign
   3. Amnesia
   4. Paresthesia

2. Which of the following is the most correct rationale the nurse can identify for administering phenytoin (Dilantin) to a client before intracranial surgery?
   1. Phenytoin reduces the potential for seizures.
   2. Phenytoin avoids intraoperative inflammation.
   3. Phenytoin reduces intracranial pressure.
   4. Phenytoin prevents postoperative vomiting.

3. When teaching a client who has had a spinal cord injury, which iinstruction is best for preventing renal calculi?
   1. Eat foods high in natural fiber.
   2. Increase protein consumption.
   3. Drink a large volume of fluid.
   4. Take a calcium supplement.

4. A client with spinal cord injury at the level of T3 complains of a sudden severe headache and nasal congestion. The nurse observes that the client has a flushed skin with goosebumps. Which of the following actions should the nurse take first?
   1. Raise the client's head.
   2. Place the client on a firm mattress.
   3. Call the physician immediately.
   4. Administer an analgesic.

5. Which of the following nursing interventions is taken as a precautionary measure if shock develops when a client with spinal cord injury is hospitalized?
   1. Ensure that IV line is inserted.
   2. Immobilize the client's head.
   3. Apply weights to cervical traction.
   4. Transfer the client to a turning frame.

6. When a nurse cares for all of the following clients, which one is at greatest risk for devloping a cerebral hematoma?
   1. A client who has a relative with hemophilia.
   2. A client with neutropenia from chemotherapy.
   3. A client with anemia taking an iron supplement.
   4. A client with atrial fibrillation on warfarin.

7. The nurse provides discharge teaching to a client who has halo vest traction. Which of the following instructions are appropriate? Select all that apply.
   1. Drive a car with an automatic transmission.
   2. Inspect the pin sites for signs of drainage.
   3. Adjust the vest if it becomes tight or loose.
   4. Wear supportive shoes with flat heels.

8. The nurse administers phentolamine (Regitine) intramuscularly to a client experiencing autonomic dysreflexia. What assessment finding is the best indication that the client is experiencing a therapeutic effect?
   1. The client's blood pressure is reduced.
   2. The client's urine output is increased.
   3. The client's nausea has been relieved.
   4. The client's vision is greatly improved.

9. The physician prescribes lioresal (Baclofen) 60 mg p.o. in 4 equally divided doses. Calculate the number of tablets the nurse should administer per dose from the medication that is supplied in 10 mg scored tablets.

10. Which of the following are appropriate nursing measures when caring for a client immediately following a lumbar laminectomy and spinal fusion?
   1. Log roll the client when changing bed positions.
   2. Help the client to sit in an overstuffed chair.
   3. Advise the client to bend from the waist.
   4. Encourage the client to turn by him- herself.

40 Caring for Clients With Neurologic Deficits

LEARNING OBJECTIVES

1. Define neurologic deficit.
2. Describe the three phases of a neurologic deficit.
3. Give the primary aims of medical treatment of a neurologic deficit.
4. Name six members of the healthcare team involved with the management of a client with a neurologic deficit.
5. Describe nursing management of a client with a neurologic deficit.

SECTION 1: ASSESSING YOUR UNDERSTANDING

Activity A *Fill in the blanks by choosing the correct word from the options given in parentheses.*

1. A _____ position facilitates functional use of the limbs. *(flexed, neutral, hyperextended)*

2. The urge to void occurs when the bladder contains _____ of urine. *(50 to 100 mL, 150 to 300 mL, 350 to 500 mL)*

3. _____ is a normal response to loss. *(Grief, Despair, Hopelessness)*

Activity B *Write the correct term for each description.*

1. A condition in which one or more functions of the central and peripheral nervous systems are decreased, impaired, or absent. _____

2. Increases fecal bulk and pulls water in to the feces to promote regular bowel elimination. _____

3. Exercises that should be performed slowly and smoothly, with a momentary pause when spasticity causes resistance. _____

Activity C *Given in Column A are some measures used in the treatment of clients with neurologic deficits. Match these with the corresponding benefits given in Column B.*

Column A

_____ 1. Flotation mattress

_____ 2. Footboard

_____ 3. Disposable, porous pad

_____ 4. Mechanical lift

Column B

a. Positions the foot and ankle in such a way as to prevent plantar flexion.

b. Used for safe transfer of the client.

c. Keeps urine away from skin and keeps bedding dry.

d. Relieves pressure when the client is lying and sitting.

Activity D *Provide information in the three columns that correspond with the phases of clients with neurologic deficits.*

Phase	Time Frame	Client's Condition	Focus of Treatment
Acute phase			
Recovery phase			
Chronic phase			

Activity E *Briefly answer the following questions.*

1. What are examples of a neurologic deficit?

_____

_____

_____

2. What is the purpose of occupational and recreational therapy?

_____

_____

_____

3. Who are the members of the healthcare team involved in the care of the client with a neurologic deficit?

_____

_____

_____

SECTION 2: APPLYING YOUR KNOWLEDGE

Activity F *Give rationale for the following questions.*

1. Why are social services and other agencies involved in the care of clients with neurologic deficits following discharge?

_____

_____

_____

2. Why is it important for the family to discuss medication administration with the physician when the client has impaired swallowing?

_____

_____

_____

3. What is the advantage of positioning a client with paraplegia or tetraplegia in an upright posture?

_____

_____

_____

4. Why should caution be used when moving and lifting clients who have been chronically immobile?

_____

_____

_____

Activity G *Answer the following questions related to caring for clients with neurologic deficits.*

1. What types of psychosocial issues may the client and family have as a result of the change in the client's condition?

_____

_____

_____

2. How can the nurse assist the client in coping with his disability?

_____

_____

_____

3. How can the nurse facilitate positive family processes in coping with altered lifestyles, strained financial resources, conflicts, and the new responsibilities people must accept?

_____

_____

_____

4. What elements are included in the assessment of a client with a neurologic deficit?

_____

_____

_____

Activity H *Think over the following questions. Discuss them with your instructor or peers.*

1. A client you are caring for is in the chronic phase after recovering from an accident that left him a paraplegic. What will be your priority nursing diagnoses and interventions for the physiologic needs of the client? What will be your priority nursing diagnoses and interventions for the psychosocial needs of the client?

_____

_____

_____

_____

2. What information about sexuality and reproduction will you need to provide if the client is male? If the client is female?

_____

_____

_____

SECTION 3: GETTING READY FOR NCLEX

Activity I *Answer the following questions.*

1. Which of the following is best for the nurse to perform to monitor for dehydration in a client with a neurologic deficit?
1. Measure intake and output.
2. Review electrolyte lab results.
3. Weigh the client every other day.
4. Assess vital signs each day.

2. Which nursing assessment finding correlates with urinary retention experienced by older adults with a neurologic deficit?
1. Increased thirst
2. Hypotension
3. Hypertension
4. Behavioral change

3. Which of the following nursing measures are appropriate when implementing bladder retraining? Select all that apply.
   1. Withhold fluids following supper; resume in AM.
   2. Record the voiding pattern for several weeks.
   3. Help the client to the toilet q 30 min to 2 hrs.
   4. Run water in the sink when toileting the client.

4. What nursing measures are appropriate for managing the care of a client with chronic constipation? Select all that apply.
   1. Toilet the client frequently.
   2. Increase oral fluid intake.
   3. Include more fresh fruits.
   4. Add bran to the client's diet.
   5. Promote more activity.

5. Which of the following actions should the nurse perform before a client with impaired physical mobility gets up? Select all that apply.
   1. Use a mechanical lift.
   2. Apply elastic stockings.
   3. Dangle the client.
   4. Obtain crutches.

6. Which of the following nursing interventions may reduce hemostasis and decrease the potential for thrombophlebitis for a client with a neurologic disorder?
   1. Remove and reapply elastic stockings.
   2. Change the client's position.
   3. Keep extremities in neutral position.
   4. Use a flotation mattress.

7. Which of the following are correctly identified by a nurse in reference to males following a spinal cord injury that results in tetraplegia? Select all that apply.
   1. A spermatocele can develop.
   2. Impotence can be expected.
   3. The scrotum will be smaller.
   4. Infertility is a potential problem.
   5. Ejaculate will be minimal to none.

8. When a nurse cares for a male client with a neurologic deficit who has an external condom catheter to manage urinary incontinence, which of the following is correct?
   1. Change the catheter once a week.
   2. Leave a space below the meatus.
   3. Unclamp the drainage tube q 2h.
   4. Lubricate the penis before applying.

9. Which of the following activity-related strategies is most important for the nurse to stress to a client who has a neurologic deficit prior to a home discharge?
   1. Avoid fatigue and take frequent rest periods.
   2. Enroll in a yoga class for relaxation.
   3. Try walking in a gym or shopping mall.
   4. Work out on a treadmill once a day.

10. What nursing measure is most important when caring for a client who takes powdered psyllium (Metamucil) to prevent constipation?
    1. Restrict consuming dietary fat.
    2. Give the drug at a mealtime.
    3. Ensure a large fluid intake.
    4. Use honey to sweeten the taste.

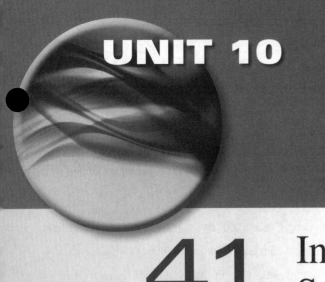
41 Introduction to the Sensory System

LEARNING OBJECTIVES

1. Describe the anatomy and physiology of the eyes.
2. Discuss tests that are used for visual screening.
3. Identify questions to ask during an eye assessment.
4. Describe diagnostic studies for eye function.
5. Explain the anatomy and physiology of the ears.
6. Describe methods for assessing the ear and hearing acuity.
7. Describe specific diagnostic tests for ear function.

SECTION 1: ASSESSING YOUR UNDERSTANDING

Activity A   *Fill in the blanks by choosing the correct word from the options given in parentheses.*

1. The superior and inferior rectus muscles permit eye movement _____. *(up and down, toward the nose and the temple, left and right)*

2. The eyelids, eyelashes, and tears _____ the anterior or exposed surface of the eye. *(maintain placement of, protect, nourish)*

3. The process of _____ occurs when the ciliary muscles contract or relax, changing the shape of the lens, which allows the person to clearly see distant or near objects. *(refraction, near point, accommodation)*

4. The _____ is used to evaluate near vision. *(Snellen eye chart, Rosenbaum Pocket Vision Screener, Ishihara polychromatic plates)*

5. The _____ equalizes air pressure in the middle ear. *(eustachian tube, labyrinth, external acoustic meatus)*

6. A _____ is used to measure gross auditory acuity. *(Weber test, Romberg test, whisper test)*

Activity B   *Write the correct term for each description.*

1. These innervate the eye, ocular muscles, and lacrimal apparatus. They include the optic, oculomotor, trochlear, trigeminal, abducens, and facial nerves. _____

2. The closest point at which a person can clearly focus on an object. _____

3. A simple screening tool for determining visual acuity, defined as the ability to see far images clearly. _____

4. This part of the ear helps maintain balance. _____

5. An examination that involves inspecting the external acoustic canal and tympanic membrane. _____

6. A more precise method for evaluating vestibular function, the mechanisms that facilitate maintaining balance. It is performed in conjunction with caloric stimulation. _____

Activity C *Match the structures of the eye given in Column A with their related descriptions given in Column B.*

Column A

_____ **1.** Sclera

_____ **2.** Uvea

_____ **3.** Iris

_____ **4.** Pupil

_____ **5.** Ciliary process

_____ **6.** Ciliary muscle

_____ **7.** Aqueous humor

_____ **8.** Vitreous humor

_____ **9.** Retina

_____ **10.** Macula

_____ **11.** Cornea

Column B

a. An opening that dilates and constricts in response to light.

b. A nutrient-rich liquid that nourishes eye structures.

c. Commonly referred to as the "white of the eye"; it is composed of tough connective tissue, which protects structures in the eye.

d. Produces aqueous humor.

e. The vascular coat of the eye; this structure includes the choroid, which prevents light from scattering inside the eye.

f. Helps change the shape of the lens when adjusting to near or far vision.

g. Contains nerve cells called rods and cones; rods function in night (or dim) light and assist in distinguishing black and white. Cones function in bright light and are sensitive to color.

h. The highly vascular, pigmented portion of the eye.

i. Provides central vision, defined as the ability to discriminate letters, words, and the details of any image.

j. A thick, gelatinous material that maintains the spherical shape of the eyeball and maintains the placement of the retina.

k. The transparent domelike structure that covers most of the anterior portion of the eyeball.

Activity D *Differentiate the following eye tests based on the given criteria.*

Test	Purpose
Ophthalmoscopy	
Retinoscopy	
Tonometry	
Visual field examination	
Color vision testing	
Amsler grid	
Slit-lamp examination	
Retinal angiography	
Ultrasonography	
Retinal imaging	

Activity E *Briefly answer the following questions.*

1. Name the bones that form the walls of the orbit. What protects the posterior, superior, inferior, and lateral aspects of each eyeball?

_____

_____

_____

2. What conditions minimize glare for the older adult experiencing age-associated lens changes?

_____

_____

_____

3. What is the purpose of the corneal light reflex test? How is it performed?

_____

_____

_____

4. Identify common medications that are potentially ototoxic.

_____

_____

_____

5. Identify the structures and function of the outer ear.

_____

_____

_____

6. What is the difference between conductive and sensorineural hearing loss?

_____

_____

_____

SECTION 2: APPLYING YOUR KNOWLEDGE

Activity F *Give rationale for the following questions.*

1. Why does aging often result in the need for reading glasses for near vision?

_____

_____

2. Why is a positions test performed?

_____

_____

3. Why should the examiner remain close to the client when performing the Romberg test?

_____

_____

4. Why is it important to carefully document conduction times assessed using the Rinne and Weber tests?

_____

_____

Activity G   *Answer the following questions related to the sensory system.*

1. Describe how the eyes convert light energy into nerve signals that are transmitted and interpreted in the cerebral cortex.

_____

_____

_____

2. What information is obtained in the nursing assessment of ocular health?

_____

_____

_____

3. What questions would the nurse ask during an eye examination?

_____

_____

_____

4. Describe the sequence of events that makes sound perception possible.

_____

_____

_____

5. What is the purpose of the Rinne test and Weber test? How are they performed?

_____

_____

_____

Activity H   *Think over the following questions. Discuss them with your instructor or peers.*

1. Which high-priority nursing diagnoses and interventions would you implement for the client with diminished vision in the acute care setting? In the home care setting?

_____

_____

_____

2. Which high-priority nursing diagnoses and interventions would you implement for the client with diminished hearing?

_____

_____

_____

SECTION 3:   GETTING READY FOR NCLEX

Activity I   *Answer the following questions.*

1. During an ophthalmic assessment, which of the following is the nurse expected to observe carefully?
1. Level of central vision
2. Internal eye condition
3. Pupil responses
4. Rate of blinking

2. A nurse is reviewing monometer measurements on four clients. The nurse correctly identifies which of the following as normal intraocular pressure (IOP)?
1. 8 mm Hg
2. 11 mm Hg
3. 25 mm Hg
4. 28 mm Hg

3. A client has undergone the Snellen eye chart and has 20/40 vision. The correctly interprets this as which of the following descriptions?
   1. The client sees letters at 20 feet that others can read at 40 feet.
   2. The client sees letters at 40 feet that others can read at 20 feet.
   3. The client sees colors at 20 feet that others can see at 40 feet.
   4. The client sees colors at 40 feet that others can see at 20 feet.

4. When the client reports first perceiving sound at _____ dB, the nurse determines that the client's hearing acuity is normal.
   1. 10
   2. 20
   3. 30
   4. 40

5. A client has a Romberg test done. Which of the following results should the nurse recognize as abnormal?
   1. Hypotension
   2. Sneezing and wheezing
   3. Swaying, losing balance, or arm drifting
   4. Excessive cerumen in the outer ear

6. Which of the following nursing actions is helpful for older clients who are experiencing lens changes associated with aging?
   1. Offer teaching aids with large-sized letters
   2. Advise reduced visual activity, such as reading or watching television
   3. Recommend the use of eye drops for comfort
   4. Suggest the use of glasses or contact lenses

7. A 24-year-old client asks the nurse when is the best time to have an eye exam. There is not any personal history of eye problems, or any family history of eye disease. What is the nurse's best recommendation?
   1. Have an annual exam after the age of 30.
   2. Have the first complete eye exam in your 20s.
   3. Have a thorough eye exam when you turn 40.
   4. Have yearly eye exams after the age of 50.

8. A nurse is performing a health history on a client and determines that the client has some hearing loss. When reviewing medications the client has taken, which ones might have contributed to the hearing loss?
   1. Salicylates
   2. Penicillin
   3. Spironolactone
   4. Ceclor

9. The nurse is checking a client's color vision. Which of the following charts does the nurse use to check this?
   1. Ishihara polychromatic plates
   2. Rosenbaum Pocket Vision Screener
   3. Snellen eye chart
   4. Jaeger chart

10. Which of the following tests would a nurse use to test whether air conduction or bone conduction is greater in a client with hearing loss?
   1. Romberg test
   2. Rinne Test
   3. Weber test
   4. Otoscopic examination

11. A client is seen in an eye clinic complaining of burning and irritation after being struck in the eye by a pine branch. The nurse anticipates the client will need which of the following eye examinations?
   1. Retinoscopy
   2. Slit-lamp examination
   3. Tonometry
   4. Visual field examination

12. At an annual check-up a client complains of persistent itching in the right eye. What questions does the nurse need to include as part of the assessment? Select all that apply.
   1. Has this happened before?
   2. How long have you had this problem?
   3. Is the other eye ever itchy?
   4. Is there any drainage?
   5. Do any family members have eye conditions?

42 Caring for Clients With Eye Disorders

LEARNING OBJECTIVES

1. Explain the different types of refractive errors.
2. Differentiate the terms *blindness* and *visually impaired.*
3. Identify appropriate nursing interventions for a blind client.
4. Discuss the nursing management of clients with eye trauma.
5. Describe the technique for instilling ophthalmic medications.
6. Explain how different infectious and inflammatory eye disorders are acquired.
7. Specify the visual changes that result from delayed or unsuccessful treatment of macular degeneration.
8. Differentiate between open-angle and angle-closure glaucoma.
9. Distinguish categories and mechanisms of actions of medications used to control intraocular pressure.
10. Identify a category of drugs contraindicated in clients with glaucoma.
11. Name activities clients with glaucoma should avoid because they elevate intraocular pressure.
12. Describe methods for improving vision after a cataract is removed.
13. Discuss postoperative measures that help prevent complications after a cataract extraction.
14. Give classic symptoms associated with a retinal detachment.
15. Discuss the care and cleaning of an eye prosthesis.

SECTION 1: ASSESSING YOUR UNDERSTANDING

Activity A *Fill in the blanks by choosing the correct word from the options given in parentheses.*

1. In _____, vision is impaired because light rays are not sharply focused on the retina. *(refractive errors, infectious eye disorders, eye trauma)*

2. Untreated _____, especially when caused by *Neisseria gonorrhoeae* and *Chlamydia trachomatis,* can lead to blindness. *(conjunctivitis, uveitis, blepharitis)*

3. _____ seals the serous leak and destroys the encroachment of blood vessels in the area. It must be performed early to prevent progression of macular degeneration. *(Photodynamic therapy, Macular translocation, Laser photocoagulation)*

4. Carbonic anhydrase inhibitors used to treat glaucoma _____. *(constrict the pupil, decrease the flow rate of aqueous humor into the eye, slow the production of aqueous fluid)*

5. A diet with cold-water fish, green leafy vegetables, and supplements including zinc, lutein, and zeaxanthin may be effective for slowing the progression of _____. *(glaucoma, age-related macular degeneration, cataracts)*

6. A _____ occurs when the sensory layer becomes separated from the pigmented layer of the retina. *(cataract, retinal detachment, age-related macular degeneration)*

Activity B *Write the correct term for each description.*

1. Treatment includes oral and topical corticosteroids, mydriatic (dilating) eyedrops such as atropine, and antibiotic eyedrops. Analgesics are prescribed for pain. Sunglasses reduce the discomfort of photophobia. _____

2. An inflammation of the cornea; treatment is begun promptly to avoid permanent loss of vision. _____

3. This procedure uses an intravenous injection of a photosensitizing drug and a nonthermal laser application to reduce proliferation of abnormal blood vessels. This helps eliminate the risk to the retina for clients with macular degeneration. _____

4. The purpose of eyedrops used to treat glaucoma. _____

5. Signs and symptoms include gaps in vision or blind spots, a sensation of a curtain being drawn over the field of vision, flashes of light, and seeing spots or moving particles called floaters. Complete loss of vision may occur in the affected eye. This condition is not painful. _____

6. An alternative method of medication administration for clients with glaucoma; it eliminates the need for frequent eyedrop instillation. _____

7. The surgical removal of an eye. _____

Activity C *Match the inflammatory and infectious eye disorders in Column A with their descriptions and symptoms in Column B.*

Column A

_____ **1.** Keratitis

_____ **2.** Chalazion

_____ **3.** Uveitis

_____ **4.** Corneal ulcer

_____ **5.** Hordeolum

_____ **6.** Conjunctivitis

_____ **7.** Blepharitis

Column B

a. Results from a bacterial, viral, or rickettsial infection; some forms are highly contagious. Symptoms include redness, excessive tearing, swelling, pain, burning or itching, and possible purulent drainage from one or both eyes.

b. The cause is unknown, but it definitely produces inflammatory changes. Pathogens seldom are identified. Although the disorder occurs randomly, it is detected with some frequency among clients with autoimmune disorders; it may be an atypical antigen–antibody phenomenon.

c. Causes include trauma to the cornea and infectious agents. Symptoms include localized pain or the sensation that a foreign body is present; blinking increases the discomfort.

d. An erosion of the corneal tissue. Once corneal scar tissue has formed, the only treatment is corneal transplantation.

e. One form is associated with hypersecretion from sebaceous glands, which causes greasy scales to form. Infectious agents such as staphylococci cause other cases. Some cases are combinations of both. The lid margins appear inflamed. Patchy flakes cling to the eyelashes and are readily visible about the lids. Eyelashes may be missing. Purulent drainage may be present.

f. An inflammation and infection of the Zeis or Moll gland, types of oil glands at the edge of the eyelid. *Staphylococcus aureus* is the most common causative pathogen. A sty appears as a tender, swollen, red pustule in the internal or external tissue of the eyelid.

g. A cyst of one or more meibomian glands, a type of sebaceous gland in the inner surface of the eyelid at the junction of the conjunctiva and lid margin. The swelling in the upper or lower eyelid is not tender, and as it matures, it feels hard.

Activity D

Compare and contrast the pathophysiology and signs and symptoms of macular degeneration, glaucoma, and cataracts.

Disorder	Pathophysiology	Signs and Symptoms
Dry macular degeneration		
Wet macular degeneration		
Open-angle glaucoma		
Angle-closure glaucoma		
Cataracts		

Activity E

Briefly answer the following questions.

1. Define the following refractive errors: emmetropia, myopia, hyperopia, presbyopia, and astigmatism.

_____

_____

_____

2. Differentiate between blindness and visual impairment.

_____

_____

_____

3. Identify potential causes of eye injuries.

_____

_____

_____

4. How are minute foreign objects detected in the eye?

_____

_____

_____

5. Describe why mydriatics (drugs that dilate the pupil) must never be administered to clients with glaucoma.

_____

_____

_____

6. Differentiate between phacoemulsification and extra-capsular extraction.

_____

_____

_____

_____

SECTION 2: APPLYING YOUR KNOWLEDGE

Activity F

Give rationale for the following questions.

1. Why should the nurse introduce himself or herself each time he or she enters the room when the client is visually impaired?

_____

_____

_____

2. Why should the nurse call the client by name during group conversations when the client is visually impaired?

_____

_____

_____

3. Why should a night light be used for older adults?

_____

_____

_____

4. Why do clients with blepharitis become discouraged?

_____

_____

_____

5. Why are sties common in clients with diabetes mellitus?

_____

_____

_____

6. Why is acute angle-closure glaucoma an emergency?

_____

_____

_____

Activity G   _Answer the following questions related to caring for clients with eye disorders._

1. What are common signs of a refractive error? How are refractive errors commonly detected? What treatments are available to correct vision?

_____

_____

_____

2. Many types of conjunctivitis are contagious. What instructions would be provided to the client to reduce the risk of infection to others?

_____

_____

_____

3. What general instructions should be provided to the client with glaucoma?

_____

_____

_____

4. What postoperative instructions will the nurse provide to the client who has undergone cataract surgery?

_____

_____

_____

5. Describe the nursing management for the client with a detached retina.

_____

_____

_____

6. Describe the procedure for teaching a client to clean a prosthetic eye.

_____

_____

_____

Activity H   _Think over the following questions. Discuss them with your instructor or peers._

1. Following cataract surgery, vision may be corrected using one of three methods: corrective eyeglasses, a contact lens, or an intraocular lens (IOL) implant. Identify the benefits and disadvantages of each method.

_____

_____

_____

2. What high-priority nursing diagnoses and interventions would you identify for a client who is losing her vision?

_____

_____

_____

3. A neighbor seeks assistance from you because his child has a foreign object in her eye. What instructions would you provide?

_____

_____

_____

4. You are at a friend's house when she suddenly announces that bleach has splashed in her eye. What actions would you take?

_____

_____

_____

SECTION 3:   GETTING READY FOR NCLEX

Activity I   _Answer the following questions._

1. Which of the following actions should the nurse first carry out in a client with a chemical splash in the eye?
1. Irrigate the eyes with tap water.
2. Instill an antibiotic.
3. Apply an eye pad.
4. Rub the eyes vigorously.

2. In addition to assessing the degree of the client's impairment, which of the following types of information should a nurse obtain from a client who has recently turned blind?
1. Ask about the client's diet
2. Ask about the client's allergy history
3. Ask about the client's family's medical history
4. Ask about how the client is coping with the visual problems

3. Which of the following statements by a nurse is correct in informing the client of how to manage a nonsevere sty?
1. "Apply a cold compress for 20 minutes every 6 hours."
2. "Use warm soaks every 4 hours for at least 30 minutes."
3. "Limit any sensory stimulation to rest the eye."
4. "You will need to schedule an incision and drainage of the sty."

4. The nurse in the clinic is aware that which of the following is the first symptom that a client with dry macular degeneration may report?
1. Blurred vision
2. Loss of eyelashes
3. Affected peripheral field
4. Distortion of direct vision

5. Which of the following instructions should the nurse give a client with glaucoma?
1. Avoid going outdoors in the daylight.
2. Avoid getting up too quickly.
3. Avoid heavy lifting.
4. Use cough syrups containing atropine.

6. Which of the following symptoms should the nurse closely monitor for and report immediately in a client who has just undergone cataract surgery?
1. Hypotension
2. Nausea and vomiting
3. Intense pain in the eye or near the brow
4. Increased urine output

7. A nurse is caring for a client just diagnosed with emmetropia. What is the nurse's best explanation for this disorder for the client?
1. "Emmetropia involves difficulty with near vision."
2. "Emmetropia causes issues with far vision."
3. "Emmetropia results from an irregularly shaped cornea."
4. "Emmetropia is a term used for normal vision."

8. A nurse hears the physician explain to the client that the surgical procedure involves removing the epithelial layer (top surface) of the cornea while a laser sculpts the cornea to correct refractive errors. The nurse recognizes that this procedure is which of the following?
1. Photorefractive keratectomy (PRK)
2. Intrastromal corneal ring segments (ICRSs)
3. Laser-assisted in situ keratomileusis (LASIK)
4. Conductive keratoplasty (CK)

9. A nurse is giving a lecture to a group of nursing students on blindness. Which of the following best defines a client's blindness in terms of the best corrected visual acuity (BCVA)?
1. Less than 20/200 even with correction
2. Between 20/70 and 20/200 in the better eye with glasses
3. 20/400 or greater with no light perception
4. 20/40 in at least one eye with correction

10. A client is visually impaired and is admitted to the hospital. Which of the following interventions can help the visually impaired client to achieve independence?
1. Keep personal care items in a different location each day.
2. Ask client's preference for where to store hygiene articles and other objects needed for self-care.
3. At mealtimes, ask the client to feel where food is on the plate.
4. Place meal tray on overbed tray and leave the room.

11. The nurse is providing teaching for a client with blepharitis. Which of the following would the nurse be most likely to recommend?
1. Avoid outdoor activities.
2. Frequently wash the face and hair.
3. Avoid use of soap on the face.
4. Use dark glasses at all times.

12. A client has glaucoma that has not been treated. Which of the following symptoms caused by chronic progression of the disease is the client most likely to report to the nurse?
1. Bulging eyes
2. Double vision
3. Tunnel vision
4. Bloodshot eyes

43 Caring for Clients With Ear Disorders

LEARNING OBJECTIVES

1. List types of hearing impairment and the acuity levels for each.
2. Name techniques that clients with impaired hearing use to communicate with others.
3. Give examples of support services available for the hearing impaired.
4. Discuss the role of the nurse in caring for clients with a hearing loss.
5. Name conditions that involve the external ear.
6. Explain the technique for straightening the ear canal of adults to facilitate inspection and the administration of medication.
7. Discuss methods for preventing or treating disorders of the external ear.
8. Name conditions that affect the middle ear.
9. Describe nursing interventions appropriate for managing the care of a client with ear surgery.
10. Discuss the nursing management for clients experiencing vertigo.
11. Explain the symptoms clients have when diagnosed with Ménière's disease.

SECTION 1: ASSESSING YOUR UNDERSTANDING

Activity A *Fill in the blanks by choosing the correct word from the options given in parentheses.*

1. Hearing impairment is described as mild, moderate, severe, or profound, depending on the _____ of sound required for a person to hear it. *(quality, intensity, vibration)*

2. Diminished _____ results from conductive loss, sensorineural loss, mixed hearing loss, or central hearing loss. *(hearing, ototoxicity, otosclerosis)*

3. Clients with a _____ hearing loss benefit more from the use of a hearing aid because the structures that convert sound into energy (and facilitate perception of sound in the brain) continue to function. *(sensorineural, dual, conductive)*

4. _____ is an acute inflammation or infection in the middle ear. *(Otitis externa, Ototoxicity, Otitis media)*

5. _____ is the result of a bony overgrowth of the stapes and a common cause of hearing impairment among adults. Fixation of the stapes occurs gradually over many years. *(Mastoiditis, Labyrinthitis, Otosclerosis)*

6. For clients with otosclerosis, the best outcomes are achieved by using hearing aids when the hearing loss is _____. *(conductive, sensorineural, both)*

7. Generally, physicians attribute _____ to viral infections of the inner ear, a head injury, hereditary factors, or allergic reactions. More recent theories center on autoimmune factors. *(Ménière's disease, ototoxicity, acoustic neuromas)*

Activity B *Write the correct term for each description.*

1. The client hears buzzing, whistling, or ringing noises in one or both ears. _____

2. A battery-operated device that fits behind the ear, in the ear, or in the ear canal and amplifies sound. _____

3. A method for communication that uses a hand-spelled alphabet and word symbols. _____

4. To reduce the consequences of spontaneous rupture of the eardrum, subsequent scarring, and hearing loss, a physician may perform this procedure. The incised opening facilitates drainage of purulent material, eases pressure, and relieves throbbing pain. The incision heals readily, with little scarring. _____

5. A progressive, bilateral loss of hearing is the most characteristic symptom. Tinnitus appears as the loss of hearing progresses. The eardrum appears pinkish-orange from structural changes in the middle ear. _____

6. A disorder characterized by fluctuations in the fluid volume and pressure in the endolymphatic sac of the inner ear. _____

7. The detrimental effect of certain medications on the eighth cranial nerve or hearing structures. _____

Activity C   *Match the items in Column A with the alternate forms of use for the hearing impaired in Column B.*

Column A

_____ 1. Telephones

_____ 2. Television broadcasts

_____ 3. Light-activated equipment

_____ 4. Hearing dogs

_____ 5. Theaters

Column B

a. Use closed-caption inserts in which the dialogue is printed on the bottom of the screen or a person who simultaneously signs is displayed in a corner of the screen.

b. Provide headsets that amplify actors' voices for individual patrons.

c. Text-based telecommunications equipment.

d. These products allow the hearing impaired to perceive rather than hear sound.

e. Are specially trained to warn their owners when certain sounds occur.

Activity D   *Briefly answer the following questions.*

1. Describe how sound is transmitted with a cochlear implant.

_____

_____

_____

2. What signs would the nurse look for to identify a hearing impairment?

_____

_____

_____

3. What will influence the selection of a hearing aid?

_____

_____

_____

4. Describe the pathophysiology of otitis media.

_____

_____

_____

5. Describe the pathophysiology of otosclerosis.

_____

_____

_____

6. What are the symptoms of Ménière's disease?

_____

_____

_____

7. What are the symptoms of ototoxicity?

_____

_____

_____

SECTION 2: APPLYING YOUR KNOWLEDGE

Activity E *Give rationale for the following questions.*

1. Why might a client deny hearing loss and refuse to wear a hearing aid?

_____

_____

_____

2. Why has the overuse of antibiotics created a problem?

_____

_____

_____

3. Why can nystagmus occur with Ménière's disease?

_____

_____

_____

4. Why is smoking contraindicated with Ménière's disease? Why are clients placed on a low-sodium or sodium-free diet?

_____

_____

_____

5. Why does hearing loss occur with an acoustic neuroma?

_____

_____

_____

6. Why is surgical removal of an acoustic neuroma the preferred treatment?

_____

_____

_____

Activity F *Answer the following questions related to caring for clients with ear disorders.*

1. What considerations and interventions should be used when caring for a client with a hearing impairment?

_____

_____

_____

2. What complications can occur with otitis media?

_____

_____

_____

3. What is the etiology of otosclerosis?

_____

_____

_____

4. Describe the nursing management for the client undergoing ear surgery.

_____

_____

_____

_____

Activity G *Think over the following questions. Discuss them with your instructor or peers.*

1. A client smiles and nods yes to everything you say while you are explaining instructions related to her care. How would you confirm the client has heard the instructions?

_____

_____

_____

2. A client you are caring for has a severe hearing impairment. The client is from a foreign country and is unable to read or write in English. What methods could you use to communicate with the client? It is determined that the client requires surgery. What actions would you take to ensure that the client can provide informed consent?

_____

_____

_____

3. A client you are caring for has a hearing-impaired sibling who would like to visit. The sibling has a hearing dog. What would you tell your client about the hospital's policy on service dogs?

_____

_____

_____

Activity H *Read the following case study. Use critical thinking skills to discuss and answer the questions that follow it.*

A client is admitted to the local hospital by his primary care physician for diagnostic testing and evaluation. Over the past few months, the client has been experiencing a gradual hearing loss in the left ear accompanied by tinnitus, numbness, tingling, and impaired facial movement. The physician has ordered audiometric studies and an MRI with contrast to determine a diagnosis. The admitting nurse completes vital signs and begins her assessment and data collection.

1. Given the signs and symptoms the client has been experiencing and the tests the physician has ordered, what medical condition does this client most likely have?

_____

_____

_____

2. When managing care for this client, what specific information should the nurse include in her assessment?

_____

_____

_____

3. What potential surgical complications does the nurse need to consider when planning care for this client?

_____

_____

_____

4. If the client should opt for the nonsurgical, gamma-knife radiosurgery, what postoperative education should the nurse provide?

_____

_____

_____

SECTION 3: GETTING READY FOR NCLEX

Activity I   *Answer the following questions.*

1. Which of the following instructions should a nurse give a client who has been prescribed hearing aids and fears that wearing a hearing aid is a stigma?
   1. Purchase a hearing aid from a mail-order catalogue.
   2. Purchase a hearing aid from a company salesman.
   3. Use a hearing aid that fits almost unnoticeably in the ear.
   4. Avoid telling others about the use of a hearing aid.

2. When assessing a client for otitis media, what should the nurse expect for signs and symptoms?
   1. Signs of swelling and pus.
   2. Evidence of dried cerumen.
   3. Client complains of whistling noise.
   4. Client has an upper respiratory infection.

3. Which of the following should the nurse closely monitor in a client who has undergone surgery for otosclerosis?
   1. Hypotension
   2. Nausea and vomiting
   3. Decreased urine output
   4. Abnormal facial nerve function

4. The nurse correctly advises a client being treated for Meniere's disease that which of the following is contraindicated?
   1. Alcohol
   2. Smoking
   3. A high-protein diet
   4. Cough syrups and other CNS depressants

5. When a client with otitis media complains of tenderness behind the ear, the nurse is aware this may be a sign of which of the following conditions?
   1. Mastoiditis
   2. Tinnitus
   3. Labyrinthitis
   4. Septicemia

6. Which of the following strategies should the nurse encourage for older clients with hearing impairments to prevent disorientation?
   1. Use written notes and a walking cane for proper balance
   2. Refer client to a local support or self-help group
   3. Reorient the client frequently
   4. Avoid frequent outdoor activities

7. A nurse needs to irrigate a client's ear to remove wax. In which direction does the nurse hold the syringe when irrigating the ear?
   1. Toward the roof of the canal
   2. Toward the eardrum
   3. Toward the nasal cavity
   4. Toward the helix

8. Which of the following symptoms would a nurse suspect a client to have accompanied a medical diagnosis of acoustic neuroma?
   1. Altered facial sensation
   2. Vertigo only when standing
   3. Tinnitus in the unaffected ear
   4. Impaired facial movement when smiling

9. A nurse caring for a client with a sensorineural hearing loss is aware that this condition was most likely caused by which of the following?
   1. Otitis media
   2. Temporal bone fractures
   3. Otitis externa
   4. Vascular conditions

10. A client arrives at the emergency department after an insect has entered the ear. Which of the following solutions would the nurse instill into the client's ear to smother the insect?
    1. Carbamide peroxide
    2. Hot water
    3. Mineral oil
    4. Triethanolamine

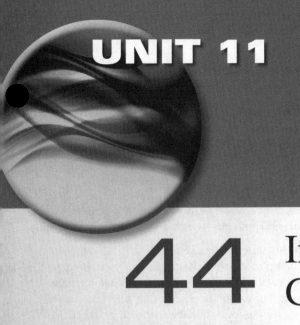
44 Introduction to the Gastrointestinal System and Accessory Structures

LEARNING OBJECTIVES

1. Identify major organs and structures of the gastrointestinal system.
2. Discuss important information to ascertain about gastrointestinal health.
3. Identify facts in the client's history that provide pertinent data about the present illness.
4. Discuss physical assessments that provide information about the functioning of the gastrointestinal tract and accessory organs.
5. Describe common diagnostic tests performed on clients with gastrointestinal disorders.
6. Describe nursing measures after liver biopsy.
7. Explain nursing management of clients undergoing diagnostic testing for a gastrointestinal disorder.

SECTION 1: ASSESSING YOUR UNDERSTANDING

Activity A *Fill in the blanks by choosing the correct word from the options given in parentheses.*

1. The _____ GI tract begins at the mouth and ends at the jejunum. *(upper, middle, lower)*

2. The client may receive up to three cleansing enemas prior to a _____ unless contraindicated in preparation for this test. *(radionuclide imaging, lower gastrointestinal series, cholangiography)*

3. A client must have _____ prior to a percutaneous liver biopsy, as bleeding is a major complication. *(coagulation studies, an ultrasound, CT scanning)*

4. _____ allows for the direct visual examination of the lumen of the GI tract. *(Gastrointestinal endoscopy, Radionuclide imaging, Lower gastrointestinal series)*

5. _____, a bacterium, is believed to be responsible for the majority of peptic ulcers. *(Salmonella, Shigella, Helicobacter pylori)*

Activity B *Write the correct term for each description.*

1. This portion of the GI tract begins at the ileum and ends at the anus. _____

2. In this test, to facilitate observation of the rectum, sigmoid colon, and descending colon fluoroscopically during filling, the examiner directs the client to make multiple position changes. _____

3. This test, contraindicated in pregnant women, requires women who are lactating to pump and discard their breast milk so that the nursing child remains safe from radioactivity. _____

4. Clients who are claustrophobic may need sedation before undergoing this test because it is imperative that they lie still and not panic during the test. _____

5. The physician obtains a small core of liver tissue by placing a needle through the client's lateral abdominal wall directly into the liver. _____

Activity C *Match the diagnostic tests in Column A to their corresponding purpose in Column B.*

Column A

_____ **1.** Cholangiography

_____ **2.** Upper gastrointestinal test

_____ **3.** Magnetic resonance imaging

_____ **4.** Radionuclide imaging

_____ **5.** Small bowel series

_____ **6.** Lower gastrointestinal series (barium enema)

_____ **7.** Computed tomography

_____ **8.** Magnetic resonance elastography

_____ **9.** Oral cholecystography (gallbladder series)

_____ **10.** Ultrasonography

_____ **11.** Enteroclysis

Column B

a. Used to visualize soft tissue structures; it is used to examine GI structures when CT scanning is inadequate.

b. Requires nasal or oral placement of a flexible feeding tube, the tip of which is positioned in the proximal jejunum; contrast media fill in and pass through the intestinal loops. The examiner observes the intestine continuously by fluoroscopy and takes periodic x-rays of the various sections of the small intestine.

c. Detects lesions of the liver or pancreas and assists in evaluating gastric emptying.

d. Used to identify polyps, tumors, inflammation, strictures, and other abnormalities of the colon; 1000 to 1500 mL of barium solution is instilled rectally. The rectum, sigmoid colon, and descending colon are observed fluoroscopically during filling.

e. Shows the size and location of organs and outlines structures and abnormalities; helps detect cholecystitis, cholelithiasis, pyloric stenosis, and some disorders of the biliary system.

f. This procedure involves a fluoroscopic study of the entire upper GI tract. It diagnoses structural abnormalities in the esophagus, such as tumors, strictures, varices, and hiatal hernia. Structural abnormalities below the esophagus include gastric tumors, peptic ulcers, and numerous gastric disorders.

g. May be performed to detect structural abnormalities of the GI tract. These tests help detect metastatic lesions that might not be apparent on regular GI x-rays.

h. Identifies stones in the gallbladder or common bile duct, tumors, or other obstructions. The test also determines the ability of the gallbladder to concentrate and store a dyelike, iodine-based, radiopaque contrast medium.

i. Determines the patency of the ducts from the liver and gallbladder.

j. Fluoroscopy of the small intestine after the ingestion of a contrast medium; it is used to identify tumors, inflammation, or obstruction in the jejunum or ileum.

k. The resulting images enable physicians to ascertain the firmness of the liver, thus allowing them to better predict clients who are at risk for developing fibrosis and eventually cirrhosis.

Activity D *Identify the following functions of the gastrointestinal system and accessory structures.*

Structure	Function
Mouth	
Esophagus	
Stomach	
Small intestine	
Large intestine	
Peritoneum	
Liver	
Gallbladder	
Pancreas	

Activity E *Briefly answer the following questions.*

1. What is the objective of gathering the client history related to the gastrointestinal system? What information is gathered?

2. How is family and work history significant to the gastrointestinal system and accessory structure assessment?

3. What are the precautions taken when a client undergoes an enteroclysis?

4. What are the therapeutic uses of a gastrointestinal endoscopy?

5. Following an endoscopy, the nurse monitors for signs of perforation. Which signs and symptoms indicate a perforation?

SECTION 2: APPLYING YOUR KNOWLEDGE

Activity F *Give rationale for the following questions.*

1. Why does disease of the large intestine, or surgical removal of any portion of the large intestine, place a client at risk for malabsorption, fluid and electrolyte imbalances, and skin breakdown?

2. Why may older adults have less control of the rectal sphincter?

3. Why does the nurse have the client lie supine, with the knees flexed slightly, for the abdominal examination?

_____

_____

_____

4. Why is abdominal auscultation completed before abdominal palpation during an examination?

_____

_____

_____

5. Why does the nurse examine the client's anus and stool?

_____

_____

_____

6. Why does the nurse discourage drinking through a straw, smoking, or chewing gum prior to ultrasonography?

_____

_____

_____

Activity G _Answer the following questions related to the gastrointestinal system and accessory structures._

1. What is the significance of a skin assessment in relationship to the gastrointestinal system and accessory structures?

_____

_____

_____

2. Describe the process and purpose of the nursing examination of the mouth.

_____

_____

_____

3. Describe the process of the nursing examination of the abdomen.

_____

_____

_____

4. Describe the preprocedure and postprocedure care for an upper gastrointestinal test.

_____

_____

_____

5. What is the purpose of stool analysis?

_____

_____

_____

Activity H _Think over the following questions. Discuss them with your instructor or peers._

1. Your client is at risk for fluid volume deficit following a gastrointestinal procedure. What actions will you take to ensure adequate intake and output?

_____

_____

_____

2. Which clients are at higher risk for fluid volume deficit when undergoing gastrointestinal procedures?

_____

_____

_____

3. What interventions would you implement to prevent constipation following a gastrointestinal procedure?

_____

_____

_____

4. What action will you take to decrease a client's anxiety related to a gastrointestinal procedure?

_____

_____

_____

SECTION 3: GETTING READY FOR NCLEX

Activity I   _Answer the following questions._

1. A client with a GI disorder has to undergo a barium swallow test. The nurse correctly states which of the following diet restrictions required for this client?
   1. "You need to be NPO 8 to 12 hours before the test."
   2. "You cannot have any solid food for 6 to 8 hours before the test."
   3. You can have normal fluid intake until 1 to 2 hours before the test."
   4. "You must avoid red meat for 3 days prior to the test."

2. A client has to undergo a barium enema for a suspected GI disorder. During the test, the client experiences a strong urge to defecate and seeks the nurse's advice. Which of the following should the nurse do?
   1. Advise the client to clear the bowel immediately.
   2. Assure the client that most people can resist the urge.
   3. Give the client analgesics to relieve the urge.
   4. Instruct the client to drink plenty of fluids.

3. What instruction should the nurse give to a client scheduled for a gallbladder series test?
   1. Remain on a low-residue diet 1 to 2 days before the test
   2. Take a laxative the evening before the test
   3. Do not eat or drink until the test is complete
   4. Take cleansing enemas the morning of the test

4. A client tells the nurse that the dye tablets needed to test the gallbladder cause the client to vomit. The nurse lets the client know that which of the following tests can be done as an alternative?
   1. Oral cholecystography
   2. Cholangiography
   3. Barium enema
   4. Barium swallow

5. The nurse is conducting an abdominal assessment on a client. After inspecting the skin of the abdomen, which assessment is done next?
   1. Listen for bowel sounds in all four quadrants.
   2. Observe the abdomen's contour for shape and distention.
   3. Palpate the abdomen for areas of tenderness or pain.
   4. Percuss the abdomen for to determine changes in sounds.

6. Which of the following pretest evaluation measures should the nurse ensure before a client undergoes the gallbladder series test?
   1. Determine the work environment of the client
   2. Determine whether the client has a family history of GI disorders
   3. Determine whether the client is pregnant
   4. Determine whether the client is allergic to iodine

7. What is most important for the nurse to assess for a client scheduled for a percutaneous liver biopsy?
   1. Coagulation studies
   2. Testing to determine allergy to iodine
   3. Assessment of family history for GI disorders
   4. Presence of radioactive material in the work environment

8. A client complained of a sore throat after an EGD. The nurse observed that the client's gag reflex has returned. What measure can the nurse take to relieve the client's discomfort?
   1. Provide the client with lots of fluids.
   2. Provide the client with ice chips.
   3. Provide the client with nourishment.
   4. Provide the client with medications.

9. A client scheduled for a colonoscopy has taken the oral preparations as ordered prior to the exam the next day. The client is now having liquid stools. What is the nurse's best action?
   1. Administer a cleansing enema.
   2. Explain that this is the expected response.
   3. Report these results to the physician.
   4. Start an intravenous infusion.

10. The client with epigastric pain is scheduled for an x-ray of the upper gastrointestinal tract. After the nurse explains the procedure, which statement best indicates that the client understands what the procedure involves?
   1. "A flexible tube will be inserted into my stomach."
   2. "Dye will be infused into my vein before the test."
   3. "I will have to swallow a large amount of barium."
   4. "My body will be placed within an imaging chamber."

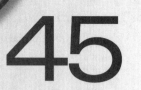

45 Caring for Clients With Disorders of the Upper Gastrointestinal Tract

LEARNING OBJECTIVES

1. Discuss assessment findings and treatment of eating disorders, esophageal disorders, and gastric disorders.

2. Describe the nursing management of a client with a nasogastric or gastrointestinal tube or gastrostomy.

3. Identify strategies for relieving upper gastrointestinal discomfort.

4. Discuss the nursing management of clients undergoing gastric surgery.

SECTION 1: ASSESSING YOUR UNDERSTANDING

Activity A *Fill in the blanks by choosing the correct word from the options given in parentheses.*

1. _____ feedings are not administered through gastric tubes placed below the pylorus, because abdominal cramping and diarrhea can occur. *(Bolus, Intermittent, Cyclic)*

2. _____ is a common disorder that develops when gastric contents flow upward into the esophagus. *(Esophageal diverticulum, Hiatal hernia, Gastroesophageal reflux disease)*

3. Administer _____ of water before and after medications and feedings and every 4 to 6 hours with continuous feedings to maintain tube patency. *(5 to 10 mL, 15 to 30 mL, 40 to 60 mL)*

4. The gastrointestinal tube used to relieve abdominal distention caused by problems after surgery, episodes of acute upper GI bleeding, or symptoms associated with intestinal obstruction, or for diagnostic purposes is _____ the one used for tube feeding. *(smaller than, larger than, the same size as)*

5. Signs and symptoms of _____ include foul breath and difficulty or pain when swallowing, belching, regurgitating, or coughing. Auscultation of the middle to upper chest may reveal gurgling sounds. *(gastroesophageal reflux, esophageal diverticula, peptic ulcer disease)*

6. _____ occurs when the normal balance between factors that promote mucosal injury and factors that protect the mucosa is disrupted. The single greatest risk factor for the development of this disease is infection with the gram-negative bacterium *H. pylori. (Gastroesophageal reflux, Esophageal diverticula, Peptic ulcer disease)*

7. Clients with _____ are at greater risk for diabetes, heart disease, hypertension, stroke, osteoarthritis, gallbladder disease, and some forms of cancer, most notably colorectal and kidney cancer. *(esophageal cancer, cancer of the stomach, extreme obesity)*

Activity B *Write the correct term for each description.*

1. A lack of appetite, which is a common symptom of many diseases. _____

2. A transabdominal opening into the stomach that provides long-term access for administering fluids and liquid nourishment. _____

3. The most common symptoms are epigastric pain or discomfort (dyspepsia), burning sensation in the esophagus (pyrosis), and regurgitation. _____

4. Never crush and administer this type of medication through any type of enteral feeding tube. _____

5. A protrusion of part of the stomach into the lower portion of the thorax. _____

6. Clients usually do not experience symptoms until the disease has progressed to interfere with swallowing and passage of food, leading to weight loss. _____

7. Most common among natives of Japan as well as in African Americans and Latinos. _____

8. Defined as a body mass index (BMI) of 40 or higher or a body weight of more than 20% over ideal. _____

Activity C *Match the gastric tubes in Column A with their corresponding description in Column B.*

Column A

_____ **1.** Nasogastric intubation

_____ **2.** Orogastric intubation

_____ **3.** Nasoenteric intubation

_____ **4.** Gastrostomy

_____ **5.** Jejunostomy

Column B

a. The tube passes through the nose, esophagus, and stomach to the small intestine.

b. The tube enters the stomach through a surgically created opening into the abdominal wall.

c. The tube enters the jejunum or small intestine through a surgically created opening into the abdominal wall.

d. The tube passes through the nose into the stomach via the esophagus.

e. The tube passes through the mouth into the stomach.

Activity D *Briefly answer the following questions.*

1. What types of issues can affect appetite?

_____

_____

_____

2. What serious signs and symptoms can occur as a result of nausea and vomiting?

_____

_____

_____

3. What is the focus of care for clients diagnosed with oral cancer?

_____

_____

_____

4. What equipment is kept at the client's bedside following oral surgery?

_____

_____

_____

5. Identify the functions of gastrointestinal intubation.

_____

_____

6. Identify the causes of gastritis.

_____

_____

_____

7. What are the long-term goals of gastric bypass surgery?

_____

_____

_____

SECTION 2: APPLYING YOUR KNOWLEDGE

Activity E *Give the rationale for the following questions.*

1. Why are older adults at increased risk for anorexia?

_____

_____

_____

2. Why would the use of a gastric sump tube be preferred to a nonvented tube?

_____

_____

_____

3. Why are intermittent, cyclic, or continuous feedings preferred to bolus feedings?

_____

_____

_____

4. Why is it essential to readminister the gastric contents after checking for residual?

_____

_____

_____

5. Why must the client be placed in semi-Fowler's position during (and 30 to 60 minutes after) an intermittent feeding and at all times for a continuous feeding?

_____

_____

_____

_____

Activity F *Answer the following questions related to caring for clients with disorders of the upper gastrointestinal tract.*

1. Identify the signs and symptoms of anorexia.

_____

_____

_____

2. How are nausea and vomiting medically managed?

_____

_____

_____

3. What are appropriate nursing assessments and goals when caring for a client with gastrointestinal intubation?

_____

_____

_____

4. How is a gastrostomy tube stabilized? What are the advantages and disadvantages of each method?

_____

_____

_____

5. Describe the postoperative care following a gastrostomy.

_____

_____

_____

6. What interventions will the nurse use to prevent infection when caring for a client with tube feeding?

_____

_____

_____

7. Describe the treatment options for esophageal cancer.

_____

_____

_____

8. What dietary guidelines will the nurse provide after Roux-en-Y gastric bypass surgery?

_____

_____

_____

Activity G _Think over the following questions. Discuss them with your instructor or peers._

1. What high-priority nursing diagnoses and interventions would you identify for clients diagnosed with anorexia?

_____

_____

_____

2. What high-priority nursing diagnoses and interventions would you identify for clients diagnosed with nausea and vomiting?

_____

_____

_____

3. What high-priority nursing diagnoses and interventions would you identify for a client following oral surgery?

_____

_____

_____

4. What educational information about nutrition would you provide to a client diagnosed with esophageal cancer?

_____

_____

_____

Activity H _Read the following case study. Use critical thinking skills to discuss and answer the questions that follow it._

A 42-year-old client is admitted to the emergency room with complaints of abdominal pain and black, tarry stools. The client describes the pain as burning and that it occurs a few hours after eating. The client states, "It wakes me up and I can't sleep." After completing a focused assessment of the client's pain and bowel patterns, the nurse takes the client's vital signs and proceeds with the client's history. The nurse learns that the client has a first-degree relative who was diagnosed years ago with peptic ulcer disease.

The client is admitted for further testing. After testing is completed, the client receives a diagnosis of peptic ulcer disease (PUD) secondary to _H. pylori_ and family history. The physician prescribes a regimen of antiulcer and antibiotic combination medications. The client is then discharged home to follow up with the physician in 2 weeks. One week later, the client returns to the physician's office with complaints of an upper respiratory infection, loss of appetite, and constipation.

1. Given the client's diagnosis of PUD, what is the relationship between the client's current symptoms and his medication?

_____

_____

_____

2. What risk factors does the client have in relationship to developing PUD?

_____

_____

_____

3. What information would the nurse look for in her focused assessment of the client's pain and bowel patterns?

_____

_____

_____

4. How would aging and chronic stomach inflammation place this client at risk for pernicious anemia?

_____

_____

_____

SECTION 3:   GETTING READY FOR NCLEX

Activity I   _Answer the following questions._

1. The nurse assists the client experiencing nausea and vomiting to develop tolerance for fluids and foods. Which of the following nursing actions would help the client?
1. Advancing the diet slowly
2. Discouraging caffeinated or carbonated beverages
3. Recommending commercial over-the-counter beverages
4. Replacing dietary fat with medium-chain triglycerides (MCTs)

2. A nurse is preparing an intervention plan for a client who is receiving tube feedings after an oral surgery. Which of the following measures can prevent improper infusion and assist in preventing vomiting?
1. Consulting the physician and dietitian
2. Administering the feedings at room temperature
3. Changing the tube feeding container and tubing
4. Checking the tube placement and gastric residual prior to feedings

3. A client has diarrhea due to a high carbohydrate and electrolyte content of the fluid in the tube feeding. Which of the following nursing actions will be most appropriate?
1. Instructing the client to remain in a semi-Fowler's position
2. Consulting the physician about decreasing the infusion rate
3. Administering the tube feedings continuously
4. Maintaining the tube patency

4. The nurse needs to promote an easy passage of food to the stomach in an obese elderly client with hiatal hernia. Which of the following nursing actions in the care plan would help the client?
1. Encouraging frequent, small, well-balanced meals
2. Suggesting avoidance of foods that cause discomfort
3. Instructing to eat slowly and chew the food thoroughly
4. Instructing to avoid alcohol and tobacco products

5. A nurse is preparing an intervention plan for an older client who underwent esophageal surgery. The client frequently reports problems of gastric distention. Which of the following aspects will be the most essential in the client's intervention plan?
1. Supporting the surgical incision for coughing and deep breathing
2. Avoiding oral nourishment until bowel sounds resume and are active
3. Turning the client to perform deep breathing and coughing every 2 hours
4. Discouraging lying down immediately after eating

6. Which nursing actions will ensure tube placement and decrease the risk of bacterial infection as well as crusting or blockage of the tube?
1. Administering 10 to 40 mL of water before and after medications and feedings
2. Administering 15 to 30 mL of water before and after medications and feedings
3. Administering 30 to 40 mL of water before and after medications and feedings
4. Administering 5 to 10 mL of water before and after medications and feedings

7. The nurse needs to administer feedings to a client who has diarrhea due to gastroenteritis. Which of the following factors should the nurse consider?
1. Administer feedings at room temperature.
2. Administer cold feedings.
3. Administer bolus feedings.
4. Administer intermittent feedings.

8. The nurse is monitoring a client diagnosed with peptic ulcer disease for any signs of medical complications. Which of the following assessment measures is the most useful?
1. Assessing the client's bowel patterns and stool characteristics
2. Evaluating the client's skin for signs of infections
3. Evaluating the client's emotional status
4. Assessing the vital signs and fluid status

9. After esophageal surgery, a client exhibited the symptoms of dyspnea. What should a nurse do to minimize dyspnea?
1. Ensure the intake of soft foods or high-calorie, high-protein, semiliquid foods.
2. Advise avoidance of foods that contain significant air or gas.
3. Ensure frequent, small meals and discourage lying down immediately after eating.
4. Instruct client to take liquid supplements between meals.

10. A client has been experiencing difficulty swallowing and undergoes esophagoscopy, which reveals that the client has a stricture near the end of the client's esophagus. To help improve the client's ability to swallow, the best recommendation the nurse can make is to instruct the client to do which of the following?
1. Avoid drinking beverages while eating a meal.
2. Chew everything very thoroughly.
3. Eat a variety of foods containing a thickener.
4. Refrain from consuming milk and dairy products.

46 Caring for Clients With Disorders of the Lower Gastrointestinal Tract

LEARNING OBJECTIVES

1. List factors that contribute to constipation and diarrhea and describe nursing management for clients with these problems.
2. Explain the symptoms of irritable bowel syndrome.
3. Contrast Crohn's disease and ulcerative colitis.
4. Describe the features of appendicitis and peritonitis.
5. Describe nursing management for a client with acute abdominal inflammatory disorders.
6. Describe the nurse's role as related to care measures for the client with intestinal obstruction.
7. Differentiate diverticulosis and diverticulitis.
8. Identify factors that contribute to the formation of an abdominal hernia.
9. Discuss nursing management for a client requiring surgical repair of a hernia.
10. Describe warning signs of colorectal cancer.
11. List common problems that accompany anorectal disorders.

SECTION 1: ASSESSING YOUR UNDERSTANDING

Activity A *Fill in the blanks by choosing the correct word from the options given in parentheses.*

1. The _____ gastrointestinal tract includes the small and large intestines from the duodenum to anus. *(upper, lower, terminal)*

2. _____ results from increased peristalsis, which moves fecal matter through the GI tract much more rapidly than normal. *(Constipation, Diarrhea, An impaction)*

3. Medical treatment for _____ includes applying anesthetic creams, ointments, or suppositories; taking sitz baths and analgesics; and preventing constipation. *(anal fistula, anorectal abscess, anal fissure)*

4. _____ is a motility problem in which constipation and diarrhea are alternately present. *(Irritable bowel syndrome, Ulcerative colitis, Appendicitis)*

5. When _____ is present, the abdomen feels rigid and boardlike as it distends with gas and intestinal contents; bowel sounds typically are absent. *(ulcerative colitis, appendicitis, peritonitis)*

6. A _____ obstruction can occur when the intestine becomes adynamic from an absence of normal nerve stimulation to intestinal muscle fibers. *(mechanical, functional, dysfunctional)*

7. _____ are sacs or pouches caused by herniation of the mucosa through a weakened portion of the muscular coat of the intestine or other structure. *(Fissures, Strictures, Diverticula)*

8. When a _____ is performed, the protruding intestine is repositioned in the abdominal cavity and the defect in the abdominal wall is repaired. *(herniorrhaphy, hernioplasty, herniation)*

9. Symptoms of a _____ lesion include dull abdominal pain and melena. *(right-sided, left-sided, rectal)*

Activity B *Write the correct term for each description.*

1. This condition may result from insufficient dietary fiber and water, ignoring or resisting the urge to defecate, emotional stress, use of drugs that tend to slow intestinal motility, or inactivity. It may also stem from several disorders, either in the GI tract or systemically. _____

2. Refers to a cluster of symptoms that occur despite the absence of an identifiable disease process. Clients experience abdominal pain and cramping, bloating and flatus, as well as diarrhea and/or constipation, with or without the presence of mucus. _____

3. Antibiotics are prescribed to treat infection. A fistulotomy or fistulectomy are possible surgical options. _____

4. An obstruction that results from a narrowing of the bowel lumen with or without a space-occupying mass. _____

5. Medical management of this condition includes the client receiving nothing by mouth (NPO). Intravenous fluids with electrolytes are administered to correct fluid and electrolyte imbalances, and antibiotics are ordered to treat infection. _____

6. Asymptomatic diverticula are called diverticulosis. When the diverticula become inflamed, this term is used. _____

7. Signs and symptoms include constipation alternating with diarrhea, flatulence, pain and tenderness in the left lower quadrant (LLQ), fever, and rectal bleeding. A palpable mass may be felt in the lower abdomen. _____

8. Although this term refers to the protrusion of any organ from the cavity that normally confines it, it is most commonly used to describe the protrusion of the intestine through a defect in the abdominal wall. _____

Activity C *Match the anorectal disorders in Column A with the corresponding descriptions listed in Column B.*

Column A

_____ **1.** Anal fissure

_____ **2.** Anorectal abscess

_____ **3.** Anal fistula

_____ **4.** Hemorrhoids

_____ **5.** Pilonidal sinus

Column B

a. An inflamed tunnel that develops when the healing of an anorectal abscess is inadequate; the tunnel connects the area of the original abscess with perianal skin; purulent material drains from the opening.

b. An infection in the hair follicles in the sacrococcygeal area above the anus.

c. A linear tear in the anal canal tissue.

d. An infection with a collection of pus in an area between the internal and external sphincters.

e. Dilated veins outside or inside the anal sphincter.

Activity D *Briefly answer the following questions.*

1. Describe a normal bowel pattern.

_____

_____

_____

2. What are the major problems associated with diarrhea?

_____

_____

_____

3. How is a pilonidal sinus surgically managed?

_____

_____

_____

4. Describe the signs and symptoms of internal and external hemorrhoids.

_____

_____

_____

5. What is the pathophysiology of appendicitis?

_____

_____

_____

6. Identify common causes of peritonitis.

_____

_____

_____

7. What is the etiology of diverticula?

_____

_____

_____

8. How does a hernia develop?

_____

_____

_____

9. What are screening recommendations for colorectal cancer?

_____

_____

_____

SECTION 2: APPLYING YOUR KNOWLEDGE

Activity E   _Give rationale for each of the following questions._

1. Why is constipation a common problem for older adults?

_____

_____

_____

2. Why would constipation be misinterpreted as diarrhea?

_____

_____

_____

3. Why would pain medication be withheld when a client is suspected to have appendicitis?

_____

_____

_____

4. Why does dehydration occur more slowly with a large bowel obstruction?

_____

_____

_____

5. Why is intestinal decompression initiated with an intestinal obstruction?

_____

_____

_____

6. Why is it crucial to monitor urine output when caring for a client with an intestinal obstruction?

_____

_____

_____

7. Why would a hernioplasty be performed in addition to a herniorrhaphy?

_____

_____

_____

8. Why is a strangulated hernia an emergency?

_____

_____

_____

Activity F *Answer the following questions related to caring for clients with disorders of the lower gastrointestinal tract.*

1. What educational information will the nurse provide related to the medical management of constipation?

_____

_____

_____

2. What situations indicate that medical intervention is required for the treatment of diarrhea? What treatments are indicated in these situations?

_____

_____

_____

3. What are the assessment findings with acute appendicitis?

_____

_____

_____

4. Describe the pathophysiology of peritonitis.

_____

_____

_____

5. What signs and symptoms are associated with an intestinal obstruction?

_____

_____

_____

6. Describe the pathophysiology of diverticulitis.

_____

_____

_____

7. How are diverticulosis and diverticulitis medically and surgically managed?

_____

_____

_____

8. Identify the differences between reducible, irreducible, and strangulated hernias.

_____

_____

_____

Activity G *Think over the following questions. Discuss them with your instructor or peers.*

1. What high-priority nursing diagnoses and interventions would you identify for the client with altered bowel elimination?

_____

_____

_____

2. Irritable bowel disease results in periods of flare-ups and remissions. How would you assist the client in coping?

_____

_____

_____

3. Acute abdominal inflammatory disorders can be life threatening. What actions would you take to ensure early identification of the signs and symptoms associated with appendicitis and peritonitis?

_____

_____

_____

4. Describe the nursing management of an intestinal tube.

_____

_____

_____

Activity H *Read the following case study. Use critical thinking skills to discuss and answer the questions that follow.*

A 22-year-old client is seen in his physician's office by the nurse practitioner with complaints of abdominal pain, distention, and tenderness in the lower right abdomen. The client's vital signs indicate a low-grade fever. The nurse notes that the client's history indicates he is a smoker and has had past office visits for chronic diarrhea and fatigue. The client is sent for blood work and is scheduled for a sigmoidoscopy with biopsy. Upon completion of testing, a diagnosis of Crohn's disease is confirmed.

1. How do the signs and symptoms of this client differ from ulcerative colitis?

_____

_____

_____

2. Why would the nurse practitioner request a sigmoidoscopy instead of a barium enema?

_____

_____

_____

3. What precautions must the nurse be aware of for these procedures with this type of client?

_____

_____

_____

4. How could nutritional therapy induce remission of Crohn's disease for this client?

_____

_____

_____

SECTION 3:   GETTING READY FOR NCLEX

Activity I *Answer the following NCLEX-style questions.*

1. The nurse who is caring for a client with constipation is correct in recommending that the client slowly increase the intake of dietary fiber to which of the following amounts per day?
1. 25 g/day
2. 35 g/day
3. 45 g/day
4. 55 g/day

2. The nurse expects to find which of the following symptoms for a client with severe diarrhea?
1. The client's bowel sounds are hyperactive.
2. The client's stool has mucus and blood.
3. The client is experiencing tenesmus.
4. The client has a temperature of 38.5 C°.

3. When monitoring the food intake of a client with Crohn's disease, the nurse observes that the client does not eat most of the food served. The nurse learns that the client finds the food unappetizing. Which of the following steps should the nurse take to address this issue?
1. Explain to the client the benefits of eating the prescribed food.
2. Request the dietitian to suggest more acceptable food.
3. Provide the client total parenteral nutrition and lipid infusions.
4. Offer the client elemental diet formula and 5-ASA medications.

4. A client with ulcerative colitis who experiences severe diarrhea is prescribed a cleansing enema to relieve the symptoms. Which of the following interventions should the nurse consider at this stage?
   1. Question the physician about the use of the cleansing enema.
   2. Educate the client about the procedure of the cleansing enema.
   3. Position the client comfortably to receive the cleansing enema.
   4. Instruct the client to visit the toilet before receiving the enema.

5. A client is assessed for surgery for herniation. Why is it important that the nurse ask whether the client smokes?
   1. Smoking increases the risk for development of malnutrition and diabetes.
   2. Smoking interferes with lymphatic and venous blood flow.
   3. The required medications are contraindicated in the presence of nicotine.
   4. Sneezing and coughing due to smoking may increase intra-abdominal pressure.

6. Which of the following instructions should the nurse provide to a client who is asymptomatic of colonic cancer but whose stool test results are positive for blood?
   1. Add fiber to the diet.
   2. Undergo a colonoscopy.
   3. Use warm soaks.
   4. Use a stool softener.

7. A nurse enters the room of a client who is experiencing cramping, bloating, and flatus, as well as diarrhea and/or constipation, with or without the presence of mucus. What condition do the client's symptoms suggest?
   1. Peritonitis
   2. Irritable bowel syndrome
   3. Ulcerative colitis
   4. Appendicitis

8. An older client comes to the clinic for a physical examination. Which of the following screening tests would the nurse recommend the client have beginning at the age of 50 years, and every 10 years after?
   1. Colonoscopy
   2. Ultrasound of the kidney
   3. Mammogram
   4. Pap smear

9. A client is admitted to the hospital for a hemorrhoidectomy. Postoperatively, which of the following would a client's nurse be most concerned about?
   1. Pain at the incision site
   2. White blood count of 6500/mcL
   3. Client's refusal of a stool softener
   4. Excessive bloody drainage on the gauze dressing

10. Which of the following teaching strategies would the nurse plan for a client with an anal fissure?
    1. Teach the client strategies to relieve diarrhea.
    2. Instruct the client to not eat any fiber.
    3. Teach the client how to insert a suppository.
    4. Teach the client how to apply ice.

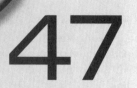

47 Caring for Clients With Disorders of the Liver, Gallbladder, or Pancreas

LEARNING OBJECTIVES

1. Explain possible causes of jaundice.
2. List common findings manifested by clients with cirrhosis.
3. Discuss common complications of cirrhosis.
4. Identify the modes of transmission of viral hepatitis.
5. Discuss nursing management for clients with a medically or surgically treated liver disorder.
6. Identify factors that contribute to, signs and symptoms of, and medical treatments for cholecystitis.
7. Name techniques for gallbladder removal.
8. Summarize the nursing management of clients undergoing medical or surgical treatment of a gallbladder disorder.
9. Describe the treatment and nursing management of pancreatitis.
10. Describe the treatment of pancreatic carcinoma.
11. Explain the nursing management of clients undergoing pancreatic surgery.

SECTION 1: ASSESSING YOUR UNDERSTANDING

Activity A   *Fill in the blanks by choosing the correct word from the options given in parentheses.*

1. _____ accompanies many diseases that directly or indirectly affect the liver and is probably the most common sign of a liver disorder. *(Jaundice, Pallor, Cyanosis)*

2. Serum bilirubin levels increase when the liver cannot excrete bilirubin normally or there is excessive destruction of _____. *(RBCs, WBCs, platelets)*

3. _____ may be performed to remove ascitic fluid. *(balloon tamponade, Sclerotherapy, abdominal paracentesis)*

4. Disorders of the _____ can affect both exocrine and endocrine functions. *(liver, gallbladder, pancreas)*

5. Pancreatitis results in the accumulations of the enzymes _____ and _____. As the enzymes accumulate in the gland, they begin to digest the pancreatic tissue itself. *(bilirubin and bile salts, amylase and lipase, albumin and ammonia)*

6. _____ is usually the cause of chronic pancreatitis. *(Trauma, Infection, Alcohol)*

Activity B   *Write the correct term for each description.*

1. The hepatic duct joins with the cystic duct from the gallbladder to form this duct, which empties into the small intestine. _____

2. If a tumor is confined to a single lobe of the liver, this procedure may be attempted to remove primary malignant or benign tumors. _____

3. Occur more frequently in women than in men, particularly women who are middle-aged or have a history of multiple pregnancies, diabetes, and obesity or frequent weight changes. _____

4. Develops when there is reflux of bile and duodenal contents into the pancreatic duct, which activates the exocrine enzymes that the pancreas produces.

_____

5. The most common complaint of clients with this disorder is severe midabdominal to upper abdominal pain, radiating to both sides and straight to the back. Nausea, vomiting, and flatulence usually are present. The client may describe the stools as being frothy and foul-smelling, a sign of steatorrhea.

The symptoms worsen after the client eats fatty foods or drinks alcohol and are relieved when the client sits up and leans forward or curls into a fetal position. _____

6. A surgical procedure that involves removing the head of the pancreas, resecting the duodenum and stomach, and redirecting the flow of secretions from the stomach, gallbladder, and pancreas into the jejunum. _____

Activity C *Match the phases of hepatitis in Column A with their corresponding signs and symptoms in Column B.*

Column A

_____ **1.** Incubation phase

_____ **2.** Preicteric or prodromal phase

_____ **3.** Icteric phase

_____ **4.** Posticteric phase

Column B

a. Jaundice, pruritus, clay-colored or light stools, dark urine, fatigue, anorexia, and RUQ discomfort; symptoms of the preicteric phase may continue.

b. The virus replicates within the liver; the client is asymptomatic. Late in this phase, the virus can be found in blood, bile, and stools (for hepatitis A). At this point, the client is considered infectious.

c. Liver enlargement, malaise, and fatigue; other symptoms subside; liver function tests begin to return to normal.

d. Nausea; vomiting; anorexia; fever; malaise; arthralgia; headache; right upper quadrant (RUQ) discomfort; enlargement of the spleen, liver, and lymph nodes; weight loss; rash; and urticaria.

Activity D *The following table lists the complications associated with cirrhosis. Provide the description for each and its related treatments.*

Complication	Description	Treatments
Portal hypertension		
Esophageal varices		
Ascites		
Hepatic encephalopathy		

Activity E *Briefly answer the following questions.*

1. What are the causes of hemolytic jaundice, hepatocellular jaundice, and obstructive jaundice?

2. What are the causes of alcoholic cirrhosis, postnecrotic cirrhosis, and biliary cirrhosis?

3. Acute hemorrhage from esophageal varices is life threatening. Describe the care for an acute hemorrhage.

4. How does ascites develop?

5. Describe the treatment for hepatitis.

_____

_____

_____

6. Differentiate between the following terms: cholelithiasis, choledocholithiasis, and cholecystitis.

_____

_____

_____

7. Describe the signs and symptoms of cholecystitis.

_____

_____

_____

SECTION 2: APPLYING YOUR KNOWLEDGE

Activity F   _Give rationale for the following questions._

1. Why do older adults need to be carefully screened for alcohol use?

_____

_____

_____

2. Why can disorders of the liver lead to coagulopathies?

_____

_____

_____

3. Why are metastatic liver tumors usually considered inoperable?

_____

_____

_____

_____

4. Why is a client with pancreatitis usually NPO with a nasogastric tube connected to suction?

_____

_____

_____

5. Why would a client with pancreatitis become hypotensive?

_____

_____

_____

6. Why is it important for the client with pancreatitis to remain on bed rest and receive adequate pain relief?

_____

_____

_____

Activity G   _Answer the following questions related to caring for clients with disorders of the liver, gallbladder, and pancreas._

1. How does jaundice develop?

_____

_____

_____

2. Describe the pathophysiology of cirrhosis.

_____

_____

_____

3. What are the signs and symptoms of cirrhosis?

_____

_____

_____

4. Describe the medical and surgical management of cholecystitis.

_____

_____

_____

5. Describe the medical management of pancreatitis.

_____

_____

_____

Activity H   _Think over the following questions. Discuss them with your instructor or peers._

1. What high-priority nursing diagnoses and interventions would you identify for a client with hepatitis?

_____

_____

_____

2. How would you provide support to a client diagnosed with pancreatic cancer?

_____

_____

_____

3. How would you prepare a client who will be having a same-day surgery laparoscopic cholecystectomy?

_____

_____

_____

4. A client taking multiple medications associated with liver disease does not understand their significance to the disorder. What educational information would you provide?

_____

_____

_____

SECTION 3:   GETTING READY FOR NCLEX

Activity I   _Answer the following NCLEX-style questions._

1. When a client undergoes a cholecystectomy, if the client drains more than _____, the nurse notifies the physician.
1. 250 mL
2. 500 mL
3. 750 mL
4. 1000 mL

2. When assessing clients for chronic hepatitis, in which group of clients will the nurse observe the pain to be mild or absent?
1. Women nearing menopause
2. Children
3. Young adults
4. Older adults

3. For a client with symptomatic gallstones, which of the following should a nurse instruct the client to avoid?
1. Fatty foods
2. Fruits and fruit juices
3. Milk and milk products
4. Potassium-rich foods

4. A client with pancreatitis experiences a seizure due to alcohol withdrawal. Which of the following interventions should a nurse consider to minimize the risk for injury in such a client?
1. Initiate precautions by restraining the client.
2. Observe the client throughout the seizure.
3. Administer oxygen throughout the seizure.
4. Administer an analgesic during the seizure.

5. When assessing a client for acute pancreatitis, which of the following symptoms will the nurse observe?
   1. Increased thirst and urination
   2. Hypertension and nausea
   3. Rapid breathing and pulse rate
   4. Frothy, foul-smelling stools

6. Which of the following dietary interventions should a nurse consider immediately after the removal of the nasogastric tube in a client who has undergone surgery for a liver disorder?
   1. Provide small sips of clear liquids.
   2. Provide small sips of fruit juice or soup.
   3. Provide small meal of soft foods.
   4. Provide meal of protein-rich foods.

7. A nurse identifies that the skin of an elderly client with liver cancer is yellow. Which of the following is the cause of jaundice?
   1. Abnormally high concentration of bilirubin in the blood
   2. Abnormally low concentration of bilirubin in the blood
   3. Excessive production of RBCs
   4. Excessive production of platelets

8. A client who is experiencing alcohol withdrawal is diagnosed with cirrhosis of the liver. The nurse recognizes that which of the following physiologic changes occurs in cirrhosis of the liver?
   1. Adequate ability to metabolize hormones
   2. Absorption of fat-soluble vitamins
   3. Impaired ability to detoxify chemicals
   4. Malabsorption of water-soluble vitamins

9. A nurse is giving discharge instructions to a client with pancreatitis. Which of the following instructions is correct?
   1. Eat two meals a day.
   2. If alcohol abuse is known, limit alcohol to one drink per day.
   3. Follow written instructions for a high-carbohydrate, high-fat diet.
   4. Follow the written instructions for a bland, low-fat, calorie-controlled diet.

10. A nurse is giving a presentation to a group of colleagues about the prevention of hepatitis transmission. Which of the following recommendations would the nurse suggest a healthcare worker follow when working in the hospital?
    1. Perform handwashing even after removing gloves.
    2. Drink tap water in developing countries.
    3. Use bar soap and cloth towels in public restrooms.
    4. Perform CPR without a pocket mask.

48 Caring for Clients With Ostomies

LEARNING OBJECTIVES

1. Differentiate between ileostomy and colostomy.
2. Discuss preoperative nursing care of a client undergoing ostomy surgery.
3. List complications associated with ostomy surgery.
4. Discuss postoperative nursing management of a client with an ileostomy.
5. Describe the components used to apply and collect stool from an intestinal ostomy.
6. Cite reasons for changing an ostomy appliance.
7. Summarize how to change an ostomy appliance.
8. Explain how stool is released from a continent ileostomy.
9. Describe the two-part procedure needed to create an ileoanal reservoir.
10. Discuss various types of colostomies.
11. Explain ways that clients with descending or sigmoid colostomies may regulate bowel elimination.

SECTION 1: ASSESSING YOUR UNDERSTANDING

Activity A Fill in the blanks by choosing the correct word from the options given in parentheses.

1. A(n) _____ refers to an opening between an internal body structure and the skin. *(ostomy, ileostomy, colostomy)*

2. Irrigation for a single-barrel colostomy begins on the _____ postoperative day. *(1st or 2nd, 4th or 5th, 7th or 8th)*

3. In the usual surgical procedure for a conventional _____, the entire colon and rectum are removed. *(ileostomy, single-barrel colostomy, double-barrel colostomy)*

4. Clients with _____ always wear an appliance, which requires frequent emptying. *(a continent ileostomy, an ileoanal reservoir, an ileostomy)*

5. Following an ileostomy, the rectal pack is removed after _____. *(1 to 2 days, 5 to 7 days, 10 to 14 days)*

6. After ileostomy surgery, the client is shown how to prepare the drainage pouch for a secure fit around the stoma, leaving an extra _____ inch in the appliance opening, which provides room for stoma clearance and potential swelling. *(1/8, 1/2, 1)*

Activity B Write the correct term for each description.

1. An opening on the exterior abdominal surface. _____

2. The collection device worn over a stoma. _____

3. When this procedure is performed, the stoma continually releases stool and gas. _____

4. A certified nurse who assists with marking placement of the stoma and collaborates with the surgeon regarding placement and the client's educational needs. _____

5. How types of colostomies are described. _____

6. This type of ileostomy is performed in two stages. _____

Activity C *Match the types of colostomy in Column A with the appearances of feces in Column B.*

Column A

_____ 1. Conventional and continent ileostomy

_____ 2. Ascending and transverse colostomy

_____ 3. Descending colostomy

_____ 4. Sigmoid colostomy

Column B

a. Semiliquid

b. Formed

c. Liquid

d. Soft

Activity D *Listed are the various ileostomy and colostomy procedures. Differentiate the procedures by identifying characteristics of each type.*

Procedure	Description
Ileostomy	
Continent ileostomy (Kock pouch)	
Ileoanal reservoir (ileoanal anastomosis)	
Colostomy	
Single-barrel colostomy	
Double-barrel colostomy	
Loop colostomy	

Activity E *Briefly answer the following questions.*

1. Describe an appliance worn by an ostomate.

_____

_____

_____

2. What issues with sexuality and reproduction may result from a colectomy?

_____

_____

_____

3. What are the possible postoperative complications associated with ileostomy surgery?

_____

_____

_____

4. Following a double-barrel colostomy, what essential information is recorded by the physician?

_____

_____

_____

5. What is the benefit of a loop colostomy?

_____

_____

_____

6. What interventions can the nurse use to promote adequate learning of the required information for ostomy care?

_____

_____

_____

SECTION 2: APPLYING YOUR KNOWLEDGE

Activity F   *Give rationale for the following questions.*

1. Why is a disposable, or temporary, appliance preferred in the immediate postoperative phase?

_____

_____

_____

2. Why would karaya gum be preferred over an adhesive in the immediate postoperative period?

_____

_____

_____

3. Why should clients with an ileostomy avoid enteric-coated products and some modified-release drugs?

_____

_____

_____

4. Why would clients with an ileostomy need vitamin B_{12} injections or intranasal vitamin B_{12}?

_____

_____

_____

5. Why is a double-barrel colostomy usually performed?

_____

_____

_____

Activity G   *Answer the following questions related to caring for clients with ostomies.*

1. Describe a typical reusable appliance.

_____

_____

_____

2. What is the preoperative care for ileostomy surgery?

_____

_____

_____

3. What is the postoperative care for ileostomy surgery?

_____

_____

_____

4. Identify the steps for changing an appliance.

_____

_____

_____

5. Describe the irrigation process of a single-barrel colostomy.

_____

_____

_____

6. Describe the two-stage procedure for an ileoanal reservoir.

_____

_____

_____

Activity H *Think over the following questions. Discuss them with your instructor or peers.*

1. When caring for an ostomy, what interventions will you take to prevent bowel leaking from around the appliance?

_____

_____

_____

2. When caring for an ostomy, what interventions will you take to promote skin integrity around the ostomy site?

_____

_____

_____

3. When caring for the client with an ostomy, what interventions will you take to promote coping and a positive body image?

_____

_____

_____

SECTION 3: GETTING READY FOR NCLEX

Activity I *Answer the following NCLEX-style questions.*

1. Which of the following instructions should a nurse provide to a client with a continent ileostomy when using the catheter?
   1. Avoid warming the catheter before inserting it into the ileal pouch.
   2. Report if there is resistance when the catheter reaches the nipple valve.
   3. Avoid coughing when the catheter is being inserted into the ileal pouch.
   4. Clean catheter with soapy water and store it in a plastic bag after use.

2. The nurse should urge a client with an ileoanal anastomosis to do perineal exercises four to six times a day for _____ repetitions.
   1. 5
   2. 10
   3. 15
   4. 20

3. Compounds containing aspirin are discontinued at least _____ week(s) before ileostomy surgery.
   1. 1
   2. 2
   3. 3
   4. 4

4. The nurse has performed nasogastric decompression for a client who has undergone colostomy surgery. Which of the following related interventions should a nurse consider for this client?
   1. Inspect the swelling of joints.
   2. Inspect the bleeding wound.
   3. Monitor pulse pressure and rate.
   4. Measure the amount of fluids lost.

5. A client with an ileostomy wants to know why to avoid nuts. What should be the nurse's response?
   1. They cause gas formation.
   2. They cause stomal obstruction.
   3. They are difficult to digest.
   4. They increase the risk of diarrhea.

6. Why should a nurse instruct a client with an ileostomy to avoid enteric-coated products?
   1. The coating prevents the absorption of the product.
   2. The coating adversely affects an ileostomy.
   3. The coating affects the absorption of vitamins.
   4. The coating causes particularly strong odors.

7. The nurse tells the client that the surgery involves an opening in the large bowel created by bringing a section of large intestine out to the abdomen and creating a stoma. Which procedure is the nurse describing?
   1. Continent ileostomy
   2. Colostomy
   3. Ileostomy
   4. Ileoanal reservoir

8. A client is visited by the dietitian following a colostomy procedure. Which of the following is the primary nutrition concern for this type of client?
   1. Fiber
   2. Small, frequent meals
   3. Chewing food thoroughly
   4. Fluids and electrolytes

9. A nurse is doing discharge teaching with a client who has undergone a colostomy. What would the nurse convey to the client regarding the best time to perform irrigation?
   1. After a meal
   2. After a bowel movement
   3. During a meal
   4. Two hours before a meal

10. The nurse is teaching a client about sexual modifications for clients with an ostomy. Which of the following strategies would the nurse suggest for times when the client is anticipating sexual activity?
    1. Leave the stoma open to air and cover with a towel.
    2. Instruct the client to limit foods that activate the bowel.
    3. Bathe and apply a fresh pouch after having sex.
    4. Consult with members of a local ostomy group.

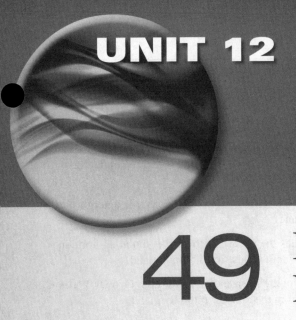

49 Introduction to the Endocrine System

LEARNING OBJECTIVES

1. Identify the chief function of the endocrine glands.
2. Describe the general function of hormones.
3. Explain the relationship between the hypothalamus and the pituitary gland.
4. Discuss the regulation of levels of hormones.
5. List endocrine glands and the hormones they secrete.
6. Name other organs that are not classified as endocrine glands but secrete hormones.
7. Outline information to include when taking the health history of a client with an endocrine disorder.
8. Describe physical assessment findings that suggest an endocrine disorder.
9. List examples of laboratory and diagnostic tests that identify endocrine disorders.
10. Discuss the nursing management of clients undergoing diagnostic tests to detect endocrine dysfunction.

SECTION 1: ASSESSING YOUR UNDERSTANDING

Activity A   *Fill in the blanks by choosing the correct word from the options given in parentheses.*

1. Hormones circulate in the blood until they reach _____ in target cells or other endocrine glands. *(receptors, exocrine glands, the nuclei)*

2. The _____ gland is attached to the thalamus in the brain. It secretes melatonin, which aids in regulating sleep cycles and mood. *(thymus, pineal, thyroid)*

3. Insulin is a hormone released by _____. It lowers the level of blood glucose when it rises beyond normal limits. *(alpha islet cells, delta islet cells, beta islet cells)*

Activity B   *Write the correct term for each description.*

1. Chemicals that accelerate or slow physiologic processes, secreted directly into the bloodstream by the endocrine glands. _____

2. The hormone-secreting cells of the pancreas, which release insulin, glucagon, somatostatin, and pancreatic polypeptide. _____

3. A hormone released by alpha islet cells that raises blood sugar levels by stimulating glycogenolysis, the breakdown of glycogen into glucose, in the liver. _____

Activity C
Match the hypothalamic hormones given in Column A to their associated functions given in Column B.

Column A

_____ **1.** Thyrotropin-releasing hormone (TRH)

_____ **2.** Corticotropin-releasing hormone (CRH)

_____ **3.** Gonadotropin-releasing hormone (GnRH)

_____ **4.** Growth hormone–releasing hormone (GHRH)

_____ **5.** Somatostatin

_____ **6.** Hypothalamic dopamine

Column B

a. Triggers sexual development at the onset of puberty and continues to cause the anterior pituitary gland to secrete luteinizing hormone (LH) and follicle-stimulating hormone (FSH).

b. Inhibits the release of prolactin from the anterior pituitary gland.

c. Stimulates the release of thyroid-stimulating hormone (TSH) from the anterior pituitary gland.

d. Results in the release of somatotropin (growth hormone [GH]) from the anterior pituitary gland.

e. Causes the anterior pituitary gland to secrete adrenocorticotropic hormone (ACTH).

f. Inhibits GHRH and TSH and blocks the secretion of several gastrointestinal hormones, lowers the blood flow within the intestine, suppresses the release of insulin and glucagon from the pancreas, and suppresses the release of exocrine enzymes from the pancreas.

Activity D
Compare the following diagnostic tests used to evaluate endocrine function based on the given criteria.

Diagnostic Test	Description/Purpose of Test
Hormone levels	
Radiography, computed tomography, and magnetic resonance imaging	
Radionuclide studies	
Radioimmunoassay	
Nuclear scan	

Activity E
Briefly answer the following questions.

1. Describe the function of the hypothalamus.

_____

_____

_____

2. Describe a feedback loop.

_____

_____

_____

3. Identify fight-or-flight responses.

_____

_____

_____

SECTION 2: APPLYING YOUR KNOWLEDGE

Activity F *Give rationale for the following questions.*

1. Why is a complete family history essential when obtaining a health history from a client in relation to endocrine disorders?

_____

_____

_____

2. Why is it essential to obtain a medication history before a diagnostic examination from an older adult in relation to endocrine disorders?

_____

_____

_____

3. Why is the pancreas considered to be both an exocrine *and* endocrine gland?

_____

_____

_____

4. Why does the nurse not palpate the thyroid repeatedly or forcefully if a hyperactive thyroid is suspected?

_____

_____

Activity G *Answer the following questions related to the endocrine system.*

1. Describe the thyroid gland and the hormones it secretes.

_____

_____

2. Describe the adrenal glands and the hormones they secrete.

_____

_____

_____

3. Describe the organs that are not typically considered endocrine glands but secrete hormones, and the functions of the hormones that these organs secrete.

_____

_____

_____

4. What assessments and findings may the nurse identify when performing a physical examination on the client with an endocrine disorder?

_____

_____

_____

Activity H *Think over the following questions. Discuss them with your instructor or peers.*

1. How will you prepare clients for diagnostic testing related to the endocrine system?

_____

_____

2. What information will you include in the health history for a client with an endocrine disorder?

_____

_____

SECTION 3: GETTING READY FOR NCLEX

Activity I   *Answer the following questions.*

1. Arrange the following in the correct sequence of hormone secretion:
   1. Anterior pituitary gland
   2. Corticosteroids
   3. Hypothalamus
   4. Adrenal cortex

2. Before the nurse schedules a client for a diagnostic test involving contrast medium, an allergy to which substance should be identified?
   1. Eggs
   2. Seafood
   3. Peanuts
   4. Wheat

3. Which nursing strategies are appropriate when caring for an older client who is scheduled for a diagnostic test? Select all that apply.
   1. Verbally explain the test.
   2. Provide a printed pamphlet.
   3. Include a family member.
   4. Escort the client to the test.

4. Which of the following drugs will the physician most likely order the nurse to administer in the case of an allergic reaction to contrast medium?
   1. morphine sulfate
   2. aminophylline (Truphylline)
   3. epinephrine (Adrenalin)
   4. atropine sulfate

5. After the nurse obtains a drug history from a client, which drug category has the potential to affect the accuracy of a thyroid test?
   1. Cough syrup
   2. Calcium supplement
   3. Bulk forming laxative
   4. Antidiarrheal

6. Which one of the following is an appropriate nursing intervention when preparing a client for a CT scan?
   1. Consult the physician for the special preparation.
   2. Provide a general explanation to the client.
   3. Inform client to temporarily eliminate salt.
   4. Instruct the client to fast for 8 hours beforehand.

7. How can the nurse allay a client's fear about a test that involves a radioactive substance?
   1. Have the client wear a lead apron during the diagnostic test.
   2. Tell the client that a geiger counter will measure his radiation level.
   3. Reassure the client that the substance poses no danger.
   4. Ask the physician to premedicate the client with a sedative.

8. A client who is scheduled for a thyroid panel consisting of measurements of TSH, T3, and T4 asks the nurse what type of specimen is required. What is the most accurate answer?
   1. Urine
   2. Saliva
   3. Blood
   4. Serum

9. A client who has amenorrhea asks the nurse what hormone deficiency would be tested. The nurse is correct in identifying which one of the following?
   1. Melatonin
   2. Oxytocin
   3. Follicle stimulating hormone (FSH)
   4. Adrenocorticotropic hormone (ACTH)

10. A client with a disorder affecting the adrenal medulla must collect a 24 hour urine specimen. What nursing instruction is accurate when the client voids for the first time?
    1. Discard the urine and note the time.
    2. Save the urine in a large container.
    3. Mix the urine with a preservative.
    4. Refrigerate the urine and all others.

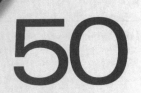

50 Caring for Clients With Disorders of the Endocrine System

LEARNING OBJECTIVES

1. Describe the physiologic effects of hyposecretion and hypersecretion of the pituitary, thyroid, parathyroid, and adrenal glands.
2. Describe the nursing management of clients with pituitary disorders.
3. Describe thyroid disorders and nursing management of clients with these disorders.
4. Compare the differences in physiologic effects, assessment findings, and management of disorders affecting the parathyroid glands.
5. Identify disorders of the adrenal glands and describe nursing management of clients with these disorders.
6. Identify symptoms of emergency conditions resulting from endocrine disorders.

SECTION 1: ASSESSING YOUR UNDERSTANDING

Activity A *Fill in the blanks by choosing the correct word from the options given in parentheses.*

1. Growth hormone (GH) is overproduced when the pituitary gland is insensitive to feedback of _____ hormones. Overproduction may result from hypersecretion caused by hyperplasia. *(stimulating, sensitizing, inhibiting)*

2. Tetany and severe hypoparathyroidism are treated immediately by the administration of IV _____. *(calcium, potassium, phosphorus)*

3. Untreated hypothyroidism becomes a risk factor for _____. *(diabetes, coronary artery disease, insomnia)*

4. _____ is an enlarged thyroid, usually with no symptoms of thyroid dysfunction. *(A nontoxic goiter, An endemic goiter, A nodular goiter)*

5. Clients with primary adrenal insufficiency require daily _____ replacement therapy for the rest of their lives. *(growth hormone, corticosteroid, calcium)*

6. The cause of primary hyperaldosteronism may be a benign aldosterone-secreting adenoma of the _____. *(adrenal glands, thyroid gland, parathyroid glands)*

7. Excessive secretion of _____ results in increased reabsorption of sodium and water, and excretion of potassium by the kidneys. *(mineralocorticoids, aldosterone, glucocorticoids)*

Activity B *Write the correct term for each description.*

1. The treatment of choice for acromegaly (hyperpituitarism). _____

2. An enlarged thyroid gland. _____

3. Medications such as propylthiouracil (PTU, Propyl-Thyracil) and methimazole (Tapazole). _____

4. A surgery that involves partial removal of the thyroid gland. _____

5. A chronic form of thyroiditis believed to be an autoimmune disorder. _____

6. The main symptom of acute and sudden hypoparathyroidism. _____

7. Secondary adrenal insufficiency can result from discontinuation of this type of therapy. _____

8. This is usually a benign tumor. Hyperfunction causes the adrenal medulla to secrete the catecholamines epinephrine and norepinephrine excessively. _____

Activity C

Match these life-threatening endocrine conditions listed in Column A with their signs and symptoms in Column B.

Column A

____ **1.** Simmonds' disease (panhypopituitarism)

____ **2.** Thyrotoxic crisis (thyroid storm)

____ **3.** Myxedemic crisis

____ **4.** Acute adrenal crisis (Addisonian crisis)

Column B

a. Onset may be sudden or gradual. It may begin with anorexia, nausea, vomiting, diarrhea, abdominal pain, profound weakness, headache, intensification of hypotension, restlessness, or fever. The BP markedly decreases and shock develops. Without treatment, the client's condition will deteriorate and death may occur from hypotension and vasomotor collapse.

b. The temperature may be as high as 106° F (41° C). The pulse rate is rapid, and cardiac dysrhythmias are common. The client may experience persistent vomiting, extreme restlessness with delirium, chest pain, and dyspnea.

c. The gonads and genitalia atrophy. Because of the impaired pituitary stimulus, the thyroid and adrenals fail to secrete adequate hormones. Signs and symptoms of hypothyroidism, hypoglycemia, and adrenal insufficiency are apparent. The client ages prematurely and becomes extremely cachectic.

d. A client with hypothyroidism experiencing infection, trauma, or excessive chills, or taking narcotics, sedatives, or tranquilizers, may develop this condition. Signs of this life-threatening event are hypothermia, hypotension, and hypoventilation.

Activity D

Briefly answer the following questions.

1. Describe Simmonds' disease (panhypopituitarism).

_____

_____

_____

2. What are the nursing priorities when caring for the client with acromegaly?

_____

_____

_____

3. Describe the nursing management of Simmonds' disease.

_____

_____

_____

4. Describe the function of antidiuretic hormone (ADH), also called vasopressin.

_____

_____

_____

5. Describe the medical management of the syndrome of inappropriate antidiuretic hormone.

_____

_____

_____

6. Describe the signs and symptoms of a goiter.

_____

_____

_____

7. What conditions may cause acute adrenal crisis?

_____

_____

_____

8. What is the nursing management of a client with pheochromocytoma?

_____

_____

_____

SECTION 2: APPLYING YOUR KNOWLEDGE

Activity E _Give rationale for the following questions._

1. Why are thyroid disorders difficult to diagnose?

_____

_____

_____

2. Why might hyperthyroidism be overlooked in an older adult?

_____

_____

_____

3. Why are antithyroid medications avoided during pregnancy?

_____

_____

_____

4. Why is a client receiving antithyroid medication instructed to report sore throat, fever, chills, headache, malaise, or weakness?

_____

_____

_____

5. Why is hypothyroidism difficult to identify in the older client?

_____

_____

_____

Activity F _Answer the following questions related to caring for clients with disorders of the endocrine system._

1. How is the treatment for neurogenic diabetes insipidus different from that for nephrogenic diabetes insipidus?

_____

_____

_____

2. Describe the nursing management for the client with SIADH.

_____

_____

_____

3. What are potential complications of thyroid surgery?

_____

_____

_____

4. Describe the pathophysiology of thyroiditis.

_____

_____

_____

5. Describe the nursing management for a client with hyperparathyroidism.

_____

_____

_____

6. How is hypoparathyroidism medically managed?

_____

_____

_____

7. Describe the medical and surgical management of Cushing's syndrome/cushingoid syndrome.

_____

_____

_____

8. What are the signs and symptoms of hyperaldosteronism?

_____

_____

_____

Activity G *Think over the following questions. Discuss them with your instructor or peers.*

1. You are caring for a client diagnosed with SIADH. What signs and symptoms will you closely monitor?

_____

_____

_____

2. What high-priority nursing diagnoses and interventions will you identify for the client with hypothyroidism?

_____

_____

_____

3. You are providing postoperative care to a client who has undergone a total thyroidectomy. What high-priority assessment and interventions will you identify?

_____

_____

_____

4. Your client is diagnosed with pheochromocytoma. What priority interventions will you implement to care for this client?

_____

_____

_____

5. Your client is diagnosed with cushingoid syndrome secondary to corticosteroid therapy. The client is receiving corticosteroids to prevent organ transplant rejection and these will not be discontinued. What interventions will you implement to assist the client in dealing with the issues associated with cushingoid syndrome?

_____

_____

_____

Activity H *Read the following case study. Use critical thinking skills to discuss and answer the questions that follow.*

A 42-year-old male client is seen by his primary care physician. The client has multiple symptoms such as painful joints, muscle weakness, and headaches with partial blindness. The client was tested for various joint disorders and arthritis, all of which came back negative. The client is referred to an endocrinologist where he is seen initially by a nurse practitioner. The nurse begins with a focused assessment about the client's pain and gathers historical data about the client's past medical issues. The nurse then begins a physical assessment and notes that the client has a large lower jaw, thick lips, a thickened tongue, a bulbous nose, and large hands and feet. The nurse asks the client if he has a photograph of how he looked several years prior. The client retrieves a 5-year-old picture from his wallet. The nurse practitioner reported the assessment findings to the physician. After the physician examined the client, several diagnostic tests were ordered.

1. Given the client's symptoms and history, what is the likely cause of the client's illness?

_____

_____

_____

2. Why did the nurse practitioner ask to see a photograph of the client from several years prior?

_____

_____

_____

3. What is the relationship between a blood sugar test (glucose tolerance) and acromegaly?

_____

_____

_____

4. This client chose to have a series of radiation treatments over 4 to 6 weeks to remove the tumor. What other treatment is available to him?

_____

_____

_____

SECTION 3:   GETTING READY FOR NCLEX

Activity I   *Answer the following questions.*

1. Which of the following postoperative nursing actions should the nurse perform when a client with acromegaly has nasal packing?
   1. Monitor for signs of increased intracranial pressure.
   2. Observe for the presence of cerebrospinal fluid.
   3. Assess for signs of hypoglycemia.
   4. Examine the face for swelling.

2. Which of the following is best for the nurse to suggest to a client with diabetes insipidus to reduce fluid loss during hot and humid weather?
   1. Remain in air-conditioned areas.
   2. Increase your use of table salt.
   3. Walk outside in shaded locations.
   4. Avoid drinking caffeinated beverages.

3. When the nurse assesses a client with a thyroid disorder, which of the following findings are associated with hyperthyroidism? Select all that apply.
   1. Tremors of the hands
   2. Heat intolerance
   3. Physical sluggishness
   4. Weight gain
   5. Decreased vital signs
   6. Insomnia

4. While awaiting surgery to remove an enlarged thyroid gland, the physican orders potassium iodide. What is the best nursing rationale for this drug order?
   1. Potassium iodide thins respiratory secretions.
   2. Potassium iodide replaces serum potassium.
   3. Potassium iodide suppresses thyroid releasing hormone.
   4. Potassium iodide prevents possible hypokalemia.

5. Following a thyroidectomy, which of the following should the nurse suspect as being the result of laryngeal nerve damage?
   1. Numbness over the neck
   2. Inability to flex the neck
   3. Tingling in the throat
   4. Hoarse vocalization

6. When the nurse taps over a client's facial nerve, what response is indicative of hypocalcemia due to accidental removal of the parathyroid glands during a thyroidectomy?
   1. The client's eyes flutter and tear.
   2. The client's facial muscles spasm.
   3. The client stutters when speaking.
   4. The client's tongue protrudes.

7. Which of the following nursing actions are essential for identifying hemorrhage following a thyroidectomy. Select all that apply.
   1. Observe the ability to swallow.
   2. Check vital signs frequently.
   3. Attend to complaints of neck fullness.
   4. Feel the posterior neck area.
   5. Inspect the neck dressing.
   6. Note straining of neck muscles.

8. Which of the following nursing assessment data is the nurse likely to detect when caring for a client with Cushing's syndrome? Select all that apply.
   1. Moon face
   2. Emaciation
   3. Buffalo hump
   4. Bronzed skin
   5. Abdominal striae
   6. Hirsuitism in females

9. A physician orders levothyroxine (Synthroid) 125 mcg p.o. daily 1 hr. a.c. in AM. If the medication is supplied in 50 mcg scored tablets, calculate the number of tablets the nurse should administer.

_____

10. A client is receiving an IV containing 250 mL of solution to which calcium gluconate has been added to treat tetany. The IV is to infuse in 2 hours. Calculate the rate of infusion (drops per minute/gtt/min) if the drop factor for the IV tubing is 10 gtt/mL. Round your answer to the nearest whole number.

_____

_____

51 Caring for Clients With Diabetes Mellitus

LEARNING OBJECTIVES

1. Define and distinguish the two types of diabetes mellitus.
2. Identify the three classic symptoms of diabetes mellitus.
3. Name three laboratory methods used to diagnose diabetes mellitus.
4. Describe the methods used to treat diabetes mellitus.
5. Discuss the nursing management of the client with diabetes mellitus.
6. Explain the source of ketones and cause of diabetic ketoacidosis.
7. List three main goals in the treatment of diabetic ketoacidosis.
8. Identify two physiologic signs of hyperosmolar hyperglycemic nonketotic syndrome.
9. Describe the treatment of hyperosmolar hyperglycemic nonketotic syndrome.
10. Explain the cause and treatment of hypoglycemia.
11. Differentiate between the symptoms of hypoglycemia and hyperglycemia.
12. Describe common chronic complications of diabetes mellitus.

SECTION 1: ASSESSING YOUR UNDERSTANDING

Activity A *Fill in the blanks by choosing the correct word from the options given in parentheses.*

1. Although no age group is exempt from diabetes, the National Diabetes Information Clearinghouse [NDIC] (2011) indicates that _____ of affected people acquire the disease as adults. *(70% to 80%, 75% to 80%, 90% to 95%)*

2. The onset for rapid-acting insulin is _____ minutes. *(1 to 2, 5 to 15, 20 to 30)*

3. All clients with _____ diabetes must rely on insulin therapy. *(type 1, type 2, type 1 and type 2)*

4. The buildup of subcutaneous fat at the site of repeated injections that eventually interferes with insulin absorption in the tissue is called _____. *(lipoatrophy, lipohypertrophy, liposuction)*

5. _____ and _____ are described as "insulin releasers" because they stimulate the pancreas to secrete more insulin. *(Thiazolidinediones and biguanides, Alpha-glucosidase inhibitors and thiazolidinediones, Sulfonylureas and meglitinides)*

6. _____ refers to the progressive decrease in renal function that occurs with diabetes mellitus. *(Sensory neuropathy, Diabetic nephropathy, Motor neuropathy)*

Activity B *Write the correct term for each description.*

1. A syndrome that includes obesity, especially in the abdominal area; high blood pressure (BP); elevated triglyceride, low-density lipoprotein, and blood glucose levels; and a low high-density lipoprotein level. _____

2. An elevated blood glucose level. _____

3. This system attempts to neutralize ketones. _____

4. The peak for Lantus insulin. _____

5. The breakdown of subcutaneous fat at the site of repeated injections. _____

6. Always a potential adverse reaction when administering medications for diabetes. _____

7. Clients may not experience any visual changes for some time. When symptoms do occur, clients report blurred vision, no vision in spotty areas, or seeing debris floating about the visual field. _____

Activity C *Match the diagnostic tests in Column A with their descriptions given in Column B.*

Column A

_____ **1.** Glucometer testing

_____ **2.** Glycosylated hemoglobin (hemoglobin A1c)

_____ **3.** Urine screening

_____ **4.** Oral glucose tolerance test

_____ **5.** Postprandial glucose

_____ **6.** Fasting blood glucose

Column B

a. Blood specimen is obtained after abstaining from eating for 8 hours. In the nondiabetic client, the glucose level will be between 70 and 110 mg/dL.

b. Normally contains no detectable glucose or ketones; in diabetes, one or both may be present.

c. The results of this test reflect the amount of glucose that is stored in the hemoglobin molecule during its life span of 120 days.

d. Measures capillary blood glucose from blood sampled from a finger stick.

e. Blood is drawn at 30 minutes and at 1-, 2-, and 3-hour intervals after the ingestion of glucose solution.

f. Blood sample is taken 2 hours after a high-carbohydrate meal.

Activity D *Compare and contrast the signs, symptoms, and treatments for acute complications of diabetes.*

Acute Complication	Signs and Symptoms	Treatment
Diabetic ketoacidosis (DKA)		
Hyperosmolar hyperglycemic nonketotic syndrome (HHNKS)		
Hypoglycemia		

Activity E *Briefly answer the following questions.*

1. Incidence of diabetes is increased among which ethnic groups?

2. What is the criterion to identify people with pre-diabetes?

3. How can individuals with pre-diabetes avoid or delay the onset of type 2 diabetes?

4. Identify the three functions of insulin.

5. Name three methods used for diet control and weight management with the diabetic client.

_____

_____

_____

6. Identify and describe the three important properties of insulin.

_____

_____

_____

7. Describe the procedure for mixing two types of insulin in a syringe.

_____

_____

_____

8. How does diabetic nephropathy result in swelling of the hands and feet?

_____

_____

_____

SECTION 2: APPLYING YOUR KNOWLEDGE

Activity F _Give rationale for the following questions._

1. Why does exercise reduce blood sugar levels in those with type 2 diabetes?

_____

_____

2. Why is a client with type 1 diabetes more likely to develop ketoacidosis and a client with type 2 diabetes more likely to develop hyperosmolar hyperglycemic nonketotic syndrome?

_____

_____

_____

3. Why do infection, failure to eat, vomiting, and stress increase the risk of ketosis?

_____

_____

_____

4. Why do clients with diabetes often develop skin, urinary tract, and vaginal infections?

_____

_____

5. Why might human insulin be preferred to pork or beef insulin?

_____

_____

6. Why are clients with type 2 diabetes not offered the option of a pancreas transplant?

_____

_____

_____

7. Why are steroids not used to prevent rejection of islet cell transplantation?

_____

_____

_____

Activity G *Answer the following questions related to caring for clients with diabetes mellitus.*

1. Differentiate between type 1 and type 2 diabetes.

_____

_____

_____

2. How does ketoacidosis develop in type 1 diabetes?

_____

_____

_____

3. Describe the pathophysiology of type 2 diabetes.

_____

_____

_____

4. The three classic signs of diabetes are polyuria, polydipsia, and polyphagia. What causes these three signs to develop in the diabetic client?

_____

_____

_____

5. Differentiate between an insulin pen, jet injector, and insulin pump. Describe how each distributes insulin.

_____

_____

_____

6. Compare and contrast motor, sensory, and autonomic neuropathy.

_____

_____

7. In addition to neuropathy, nephropathy, and retinopathy, what other vascular changes occur with diabetes?

_____

_____

_____

Activity H *Think over the following questions. Discuss them with your instructor or peers.*

1. Your client is a brittle (difficult to control) diabetic; what signs and symptoms would you expect to see if the client is experiencing a hypoglycemic reaction? What treatment would you provide?

_____

_____

2. Your neighbor asks you to provide assistance to her spouse, who is diabetic. You take a glucometer reading, and the result is a measurement of 360 mg/dL. What symptoms would you expect this person to be exhibiting? What treatment would you provide? What signs and symptoms would indicate further medical intervention is required?

_____

_____

_____

3. What educational information would you provide about foot care to a diabetic client?

_____

_____

_____

4. A diabetic client describes visual changes she is experiencing. How would you advise her?

_____

_____

_____

5. A client asks you how he can reduce his risk of long-term complications associated with diabetes. What educational information would you provide?

_____

_____

SECTION 3: GETTING READY FOR NCLEX

Activity I _Answer the following questions._

1. A client with type 1 diabetes mellitus asks a nurse to identify the goal of a pancreas and islet cell transplant. What is the nurse's most accurate answer?
1. The transplant reduces the amount of insulin you require.
2. The transplant reduces the number of daily injections.
3. The transplant prevents fewer episodes of ketoacidosis.
4. The transplant eliminates the need for insulin injections.

2. Which of the following actions is most appropriate when a nurse cares for a client with diabetes mellitus is on the hospital unit?
1. Insert an indwelling urinary catheter.
2. Stock quick-acting carbohydrates.
3. Arrange for an insulin pump.
4. Administer insulin by the IV route.

3. Which of the following nursing actions helps the nurse to detect evidence of albuminuria when caring for a client with diabetic neuropathy?
1. Check the urine with a test strip.
2. Check the hemoglobin A1c results.
3. Check the postprandial glucose test results.
4. Check the fasting blood glucose test results.

4. A client is brought to the emergency department with suspected diabetic ketoacidosis. What assessment findings will the nurse identify with this condition?
1. Diaphoresis
2. Drowsiness
3. Fruity breath
4. Shakiness
5. Flushed skin
6. Deep breathing

5. How can the nurse anticipate thtat the client with diabetic ketoacidosis will be treated?
1. Administration of glucose tablets
2. Administration of regular insulin
3. Give 50% glucose intravenously
4. Provide a high carbohydrate diet

6. A nurse administers NPH insulin, which is classified as intermediate acting. At what time should the nurse expect the client to most likely to experience hypoglycemia?
1. Before breakfast
2. During mid-day
3. During the night
4. Before bedtime

7. A nurse should have a client's dietary tray immediately available when administering which of the following types of insulin?
1. glargine (Lantus)
2. lispro (Humalog)
3. detemir (Levemir)
4. zinc suspension (Lente)

8. When the nurse administers an alpha-glucosidase inhibitor like miglitol (Glyset), how should the nurse manage hypoglycemia if it occurs?
1. Give the client 1/2 cup of grape juice.
2. Give a rapid acting type of insulin like glulisine (Apidra).
3. Have the client consume graham crackers and milk.
4. Administer oral glucose tablets.

9. There is a standing order to give 15 g of glucose to a client experiencing hypoglycemia. Calculate the number of tablets to administer if the label indicates each tablet contains 5 g.

_____

10. What is the best method the nurse can use to avoid a medication error when administering insulin?
   1. Consult the pharmacist about the usual type and dose of insulin.
   2. Ask the client his usual insulin dose.
   3. Look up the amount of the previous insulin injection.
   4. Have another nurse check the amount and type of insulin against the order.

CARING FOR CLIENTS WITH BREAST AND REPRODUCTIVE DISORDERS

52 Introduction to the Reproductive System

LEARNING OBJECTIVES

1. Name the major external structures of the female reproductive system.
2. Name and give the function of four internal female reproductive structures.
3. Discuss the process of ovulation.
4. Explain the physiologic changes that lead to menstruation.
5. List at least five types of reproductive data that are obtained when taking a female's health history.
6. Discuss the purpose for the cytologic test known as a Papanicolaou test.
7. Review the instructions the nurse provides for a client who is scheduling a gynecologic examination and Papanicolaou test.
8. Name diagnostic tests used for diagnosing disorders of the female reproductive system.
9. Describe the anatomy and physiology of the breast.
10. Explain the differences between a clinical breast examination and breast self-examination.
11. Discuss the advantage of a mammographic examination.
12. Name three techniques for performing a breast biopsy.
13. Identify the major external structures of the male reproductive system.
14. Name and give the function of the chief internal male reproductive structures.
15. List three accessory structures of the male reproductive system.
16. Explain the terms: erection, emission, and ejaculation.
17. List at least five types of reproductive data that are obtained when taking a male's health history.
18. Name techniques for physically assessing male reproductive structures.
19. List methods that are used to diagnose prostate cancer.
20. Name two tests for determining infertility problems in males.

SECTION 1: ASSESSING YOUR UNDERSTANDING

Activity A
Fill in the blanks by choosing the correct word from the options given in parentheses.

1. _____ causes the mature follicle to rupture, thereby releasing an ovum from the ovary. (*Luteinizing hormone, Follicle-stimulating hormone, Growth hormone*)

2. _____ is a test that is used primarily to detect early cancer of the cervix and secondarily to determine estrogen activity as it relates to menopause or endocrine abnormalities. (*Endometrial smear, Papanicolaou test, Culdoscopy*)

3. _____ is performed when results from a Pap test are positive or questionable. (*Cervical biopsy, Endometrial smear, Culdoscopy*)

4. _____ refers to the manual palpation of the breast performed by a physician, nurse, or physician's assistant. It is performed during a client's gynecologic examination, before a mammogram, or during an annual physical examination. (*Mammography, Breast self-examination, Clinical breast examination*)

5. The _____ lie within the scrotum and are responsible for spermatogenesis, or sperm production, and secretion of testosterone. *(ductus deferens, epididymis, testes)*

6. The _____ loops through the inguinal canal and into the pelvic cavity before it descends to the prostate gland. The wall of the ductus deferens contains smooth muscle that moves sperm along the ductal pathway. *(spermatic cord, testes, epididymis)*

Activity B   *Write the correct term for each description.*

1. Time when the reproductive system becomes active and functional. _____

2. The anterior pituitary hormone known as follicle-stimulating hormone (FSH) initiates this process monthly. _____

3. Begins about 2 weeks after ovulation; usually lasts 4 to 5 days, with a normal loss of 30 to 60 mL of blood. _____

4. Age of the first menstruation. _____

5. A procedure used to visualize the cervix and vagina. A speculum is inserted into the vagina, and the surface areas are examined with a light and magnifying lens. _____

6. The testes are subdivided into lobules containing coiled _____ tubules within which spermatocytes (immature spermatozoa) form.

Activity C   *Match the examination procedures and diagnostic tests performed to evaluate the male genitourinary tract given in Column A with their descriptions given in Column B.*

Column A

_____ **1.** Transrectal ultrasonography (TRUS)

_____ **2.** Cystoscopy

_____ **3.** Needle biopsy of prostatic tissue

_____ **4.** Testicular biopsy

_____ **5.** Digital rectal examination (DRE)

_____ **6.** Fertility studies

_____ **7.** Transillumination

_____ **8.** Prostate-specific antigen (PSA)

_____ **9.** Cultures

Column B

a. Obtained to definitively diagnose cancer of the prostate when other assessment findings appear suspiciously abnormal.

b. Evaluates spermatozoa production for diagnosing infertility problems or testicular malignancy.

c. A test in which a lubricated probe is inserted into the rectum to obtain a view of the prostate gland from various angles.

d. An illuminated optical instrument is inserted into the urinary meatus to inspect the bladder, prostate, and urethra.

e. Performed to assess the prostate for size as well as evidence of tumor.

f. A blood test that, when elevated over 4 ng/mL, may correspond with prostate cancer.

g. Performed on urethral secretions, skin lesions, or urine.

h. Includes a semen analysis to determine sperm count, sperm motility, and abnormal sperm.

i. Shining a light through the scrotum to assess the density of scrotal tissue.

Activity D *Provide the description and purpose of the following diagnostic tests used to evaluate the female breasts.*

Diagnostic Test	Description	Purpose
Mammography		
Ultrasonography		
Breast biopsy		
Incisional biopsy (*description only*)		
Excisional biopsy (*description only*)		
Aspiration biopsy (*description only*)		

Activity E *Briefly answer the following questions.*

1. Provide a description for each of the major female external structures: mons pubis, vaginal orifice, Bartholin's glands, labia majora, labia minora, clitoris, fourchette, and hymen.

2. Describe the procedure for a gynecologic examination.

3. What instructions will the nurse provide to a client scheduling a Papanicolaou test?

4. What is a hysterosalpingogram? What is it used for?

5. What are the recommendations for clinical and self-breast examinations by the American Cancer Society (ACS)?

6. How does the scrotum maintain the temperature of the testes at 3° cooler than body temperature?

SECTION 2: APPLYING YOUR KNOWLEDGE

Activity F *Provide rationale for the following questions.*

1. Why is routine douching of the vagina discouraged?

2. Why does the endometrium become thick and vascular during ovulation?

3. Why is it important that each gynecologic specimen sent to the laboratory be marked with the date of the beginning of the client's last menstrual period (LMP)?

_____

_____

_____

4. Why are breast self-examinations (BSEs) encouraged even though they play a small role in the detection of breast cancer?

_____

_____

_____

5. Why may the older male experience difficulty with urination?

_____

_____

_____

_____

Activity G *Answer the following questions related to the reproductive system.*

1. Identify the internal female structures and describe their function.

_____

_____

_____

2. Describe the process of fertilization and implantation.

_____

_____

_____

3. What are the recommendations by the American Cancer Society for the Papanicolaou test? What are additional recommendations for testing?

_____

_____

_____

4. Provide a description and identify the major function of the female breasts.

_____

_____

_____

5. Describe the external structures of the male reproductive system.

_____

_____

_____

6. Describe the accessory structures of the male reproductive system.

_____

_____

_____

Activity H *Think over the following questions. Discuss them with your instructor or peers.*

1. A married couple is trying to conceive and asks your advice about how to increase their chances of conception. Based on your knowledge of the female and male reproductive systems, how would you advise them?

_____

_____

_____

2. A male client is being seen by the physician about erectile dysfunction. What information is significant for you to obtain about the client's history and reproductive health?

_____

_____

_____

3. A female client is being seen by the physician about irregular menstruation. What essential information will you obtain about the client's history and reproductive health?

_____

_____

_____

_____

_____

_____

_____

_____

SECTION 3: GETTING READY FOR NCLEX

Activity I *Answer the following questions.*

1. What information is most accurate for the nurse to provide to a client who is concerned about the hymen and its relation to virginity?
1. The hymen is not affected by any sexual activity
2. The hymen's absence does not confirm the loss of virginity
3. The hymen is ruptured the first time a person menstruates
4. The hymen may be ruptured even when doing strenuous exercises

2. Which of the following assessments does a nurse obtain to ensure a thorough baseline reproductive history of a female client? Select all that apply.
1. Age of menarche
2. Pregnancy history
3. Mother's menstrual disorders
4. Frequency of sexual activities
5. Contraceptive practices
6. Menstrual pattern

3. Which of the following reasons should a nurse provide a client when asked about the primary purpose of a Papanicolaou test?
1. It is used to detect early ovarian cancer.
2. It is used to detect cancer of the cervix.
3. It is used to detect fertility status.
4. It is used to detect sexually transmitted infections.

4. How can the nurse best relieve the anxiety of a client scheduled for an endometrial biopsy who is fearful of undergoing surgery?
1. Explain that the test will not require prolonged anesthesia.
2. Explain that anesthesia will result in being pain free.
3. Explain that the procedure will be done by experts.
4. Explain that a specimen can be obtained nonsurgically.

5. What complications should be the focus of the nurse's immediate assessments when caring for a client who has undergone a culdoscopy?
1. Chest pain that radiates to the shoulder.
2. Shock secondary to internal bleeding.
3. Infection manifested by a fever over 101° F.
4. Bladder perforation evidenced anuria.

6. When assisting with a pelvic examination, what nursing actions are appropriate? Select all that apply.
1. Have the client void beforehand.
2. Place the client in Sims' position.
3. Cover the client with a drape.
4. Obtain a bivalved speculum.

7. Which of the following instructions are essential to give a client who will be having a mammography
1. Wear a comfortable bra.
2. Avoid using a deodorant.
3. Wash the breasts with soap.
4. Powder the breasts with talc.

8. A male client reports that he and his wife have not been able to become pregnant. The nurse is correct in identifying which of the following tests to help identify male infertility?
1. Prostatic-specific antigen test
2. Transrectal ultrasonography
3. Transillumination of scrotum
4. Semen collection for analysis

9. What reproductive examination is most appropriate for the nurse to tell a male client he will have during a routine physical?

1. Testicular biopsy
2. Digital rectal exam
3. Prostatic ultrasound
4. Erection analysis

10. Before discharging a client who has had a biopsy of the prostate gland, what can the nurse suggest for relieving discomfort? Select all that apply.

1. Take acetaminophen (Tylenol) as directed.
2. Take a sitz bath whenever desired.
3. Insert an aspirin suppository for relief.
4. Sit on a synthetic sheepskin pad.

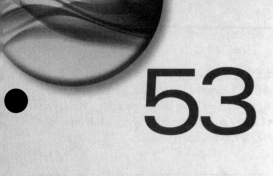

53 Caring for Clients With Disorders of the Female Reproductive System

LEARNING OBJECTIVES

1. Describe at least four conditions that deviate from normal menstrual patterns.
2. Describe the purpose of and how to keep a menstrual diary.
3. Give two examples of disorders characterized by amenorrhea and oligomenorrhea.
4. Discuss therapeutic techniques and nursing management for menstrual disorders.
5. List several physiologic consequences of menopause.
6. Give reasons for and against hormone replacement therapy.
7. Name four infectious and inflammatory conditions common in women and one cause for each.
8. Describe the signs and symptoms that differentiate three types of vaginal infections.
9. Discuss methods that may help prevent vaginal infections or their recurrence.
10. Describe the technique for inserting vaginal medications.
11. Name at least four aspects of nursing care for clients with pelvic inflammatory disease.
12. Give at least two suggestions that can help women avoid toxic shock syndrome.
13. List four structural abnormalities of the female reproductive system and their effects on fertility or sexuality.
14. Discuss methods the nurse can use to help a client select an appropriate treatment for endometriosis.
15. List three problems experienced by women who develop vaginal fistulas, and related nursing management.
16. Give examples of appropriate information when teaching a client to use a pessary.
17. Explain the term *carcinoma in situ* and how it applies to the prognosis of women with gynecologic malignancies.
18. Identify the most common reproductive cancers and methods for early diagnosis.
19. Discuss nursing diagnoses and potential complications among clients who undergo a hysterectomy and nursing interventions important to include in their care.
20. Give two reasons that explain the high lethality associated with ovarian cancer.
21. Name three possible causes of vaginal cancer.
22. Discuss the nursing management of and appropriate discharge instructions for a client who has a radical vulvectomy for vulvar cancer.

SECTION 1: ASSESSING YOUR UNDERSTANDING

Activity A *Fill in the blanks by choosing the correct word from the options given in parentheses.*

1. Treatment of _____ includes IV fluids to support circulation while combating the infection with IV antibiotic therapy. Potent adrenergic drugs are given to counteract peripheral vasodilation and maintain renal perfusion. Oxygen is given to promote aerobic metabolism at the cellular level. *(vaginitis, pelvic inflammatory disease, toxic shock syndrome)*

2. _____ is a condition in which tissue with a cellular structure and function resembling that of the endometrium is found outside the uterus. *(Endometriosis, Vaginal fistula, Pelvic organ prolapse)*

3. A(n) _____ is an unnatural opening between two structures. *(prolapse, fistula, abscess)*

4. A _____ is a firm, doughnut-shaped or ring device, which may be inserted in the upper vagina to reposition and give support to the uterus when surgery cannot be done or the client declines surgery. *(Kegel, pessary, colporrhaphy)*

5. A(n) _____ (also called myoma) is a benign uterine growth principally consisting of smooth muscle and fibrous connective tissue. Myomas, which are the most common tumor in the female pelvis, often are referred to as fibroid tumors. *(leiomyoma, endometriosis, vaginal fistula)*

6. A localized malignancy is referred to as _____. (*premalignant, nonmalignant, carcinoma in situ*)

7. Cancer of the _____ is relatively rare. It usually occurs in women older than 60 years of age, but cases among younger women have arisen recently. This type of cancer is highly curable when diagnosed in an early stage. (*ovaries, cervix, vulva*)

Activity B *Write the correct term for each description.*

1. Deficiency of this hormone causes thinning of the vaginal walls, breast and uterine atrophy, and loss of bone density. The risks of heart disease and stroke increase with reduction in this hormone. _____

2. Hospitalization with complete bed rest often is necessary. Parenteral or oral antibiotics are administered as soon as culture and sensitivity tests are obtained. Intravenous (IV) fluids are ordered if the client is dehydrated, and antipyretics are used if the temperature is elevated. A ruptured pelvic abscess requires emergency surgery. _____

3. Severe dysmenorrhea and copious menstrual bleeding are typical symptoms. The client may experience dyspareunia and pain on defecation. Rupture of a chocolate cyst results in severe abdominal pain that can mimic other abdominal pathologies such as appendicitis or bowel obstruction. _____

4. They result in the continuous drainage of urine or feces from the vagina. The vaginal wall and the external genitalia become excoriated and often infected. The client may not void through the urethra because urine does not accumulate in the bladder. _____

5. These exercises are also known as pelvic floor strengthening exercises. They are recommended when there is stress incontinence. _____

6. When symptoms exist, menorrhagia is most common. There can be a feeling of pressure in the pelvic region, dysmenorrhea, anemia (from loss of blood), and malaise. _____

7. The incidence of this type of cancer is higher among women infected with human papilloma virus (HPV), a sexually transmitted microorganism, and among those who use a pessary but neglect to remove and clean it. _____

Activity C *Briefly answer the following questions.*

1. What is a menstrual diary? What is it used for?

_____

_____

_____

2. What is the nurse's role when caring for the client with a menstrual disorder?

_____

_____

_____

3. Describe the treatment for infectious vaginitis.

_____

_____

_____

4. Describe the types of uterine displacements. What are the typical causes?

_____

_____

_____

5. What are the signs and symptoms of cervical and endometrial cancer?

_____

_____

_____

6. What is an important role of the nurse in the prevention and early diagnosis of cervical and endometrial cancer?

_____

_____

_____

7. Describe the medical and surgical management of an ovarian cyst.

_____

_____

_____

SECTION 2: APPLYING YOUR KNOWLEDGE

Activity D *Give rationale for the following questions.*

1. If hormone replacement therapy (HRT) or estrogen replacement therapy (ERT) is indicated for the treatment of menopause, why is it prescribed in the lowest appropriate dose for the shortest time necessary?

_____

_____

_____

2. Why are low-dose androgens given to women who are menopausal?

_____

_____

_____

3. Why are women taking HRT instructed to contact the physician if tenderness, pain, swelling, or redness occurs in the legs?

_____

_____

_____

4. Why are older women predisposed for development of vaginitis?

_____

_____

_____

5. Historically, why has ovarian cancer been so lethal?

_____

_____

_____

6. Why are clients with HPV and herpes simplex virus type 2 at lifelong risk for genital cancer?

_____

_____

_____

Activity E *Answer the following questions related to caring for the client with disorders of the female reproductive system.*

1. Describe the process of menopause.

_____

_____

2. Describe the pathophysiology of endometriosis.

_____

_____

_____

3. What are the treatment options for endometriosis?

_____

_____

4. Describe the pathophysiology of pelvic organ prolapse.

_____

_____

_____

5. What are the instructions for use of a pessary?

_____

_____

_____

6. What are the risk factors associated with cervical and endometrial cancer?

_____

_____

_____

7. What preventive measures are recommended for women at high risk for ovarian cancer?

_____

_____

_____

Activity F   *Think over the following questions. Discuss them with your instructor or peers.*

1. A client asks you how to prevent vaginal infections. What educational information will you provide?

_____

_____

_____

2. What high-priority nursing diagnoses and interventions will you identify for the client undergoing a hysterectomy?

_____

_____

_____

3. What educational information will you provide to the client undergoing a hysterectomy?

_____

_____

_____

4. What nutritional information will you provide to the client with premenstrual syndrome?

_____

_____

_____

Activity G   *Read the following case study. Use critical thinking skills to discuss and answer the questions that follow.*

A 53-year-old female client is seen in her physician's office. The client is experiencing menopause but is currently seeking treatment for symptoms of vaginal discharge with itching and burning. The nurse takes the client's vital signs and begins a more focused assessment of the client's discharge. The nurse asks the client about the color, consistency, and odor of the discharge. The client states that the discharge is yellow white, foamy, and has a foul odor. The nurse prepares the client for a physical examination by the physician. After examination, the physician diagnoses the client with a vaginal infection.

1. Due to the symptoms the client is experiencing, what type of microorganism is likely responsible for the client's vaginal infection?

_____

_____

_____

2. What role does this client's menopausal status play in the development of this disorder?

_____

_____

_____

3. How do excess glycogen levels contribute to the occurrence of vaginitis?

_____

_____

_____

4. The client is prescribed metronidazole (Flagyl). What education should the nurse provide to this client in reference to the side effects and implications of this medication?

_____

_____

_____

SECTION 3: GETTING READY FOR NCLEX

Activity H *Answer the following questions.*

1. Which of the following is the best suggestion the nurse can recommend to a client diagnosed with vaginitis to relieve itching, burning, and swelling of the vulva and perineum?
   1. Douche with vinegar.
   2. Eat unpasteurized yogurt.
   3. Take frequent sitz baths.
   4. Wear an absorbent pad.

2. The nurse advocates that pre-teens and teenagers receive human papilloma virus vaccination to reduce the risk for which reproductive disorder?
   1. Uterine fibroids
   2. Cervical cancer
   3. Ovarian cysts
   4. Endometriosis

3. What information is appropriate when a nurse explains the use of a pessary to a client? Select all that apply.
   1. Wash, rinse, and dry the pessary before reinsertion.
   2. Apply antibacterial ointment to the pessary surface.
   3. Insert the pessary as far back in the vagina as possible.
   4. Remove the pessary if discomfort develops.

4. Which type of infection transmission precautions is best for the nurse to follow when caring for a client with pelvic inflammatory disease?
   1. Contact precautions
   2. Airborne precautions
   3. Droplet precautions
   4. Standard precautions

5. Which of the following should be the most important nursing assessment when caring for a client with uterine fibroids?
   1. Monitoring for anemia
   2. Monitoring for infection
   3. Monitoring for pain
   4. Monitoring for thrombi

6. The nurse advises clients regarding the increased the potential for developing toxic shock by avoiding which of the following? Select all that apply.
   1. Exercising during menstruation.
   2. Taking analgesics for menstrual discomfort.
   3. Using superabsorbent tampons.
   4. Leaving internal contraceptive devices in place.

7. Which of the following interventions should the nurse take to promote healing and to lessen discomfort of a client who has just undergone surgical repair of a rectovaginal fistula?
   1. Provide warm perineal irrigations.
   2. Administer kanamycin (Kantrex).
   3. Insert an indwelling catheter.
   4. Change bed linens promptly.

8. The physician prescribes ampicillin (Polycillin) 1 g IM q 6h for a client with toxic shock syndrome. The accompanying literature says an adult client may have 25 mg to 100 mg per kg in 4 equally divided doses. Calculate the safe range of doses for the client who weighs 164 lbs. Round your answer to the nearest tenth.

   _____

   _____

9. A client asks a nurse to identify what sign or symptom suggests cervical cancer. The nurse is most correct in identifying which of the following?
   1. Unexplained vaginal bleeding.
   2. Vaginal drainage that has an odor.
   3. Pain experienced during intercourse.
   4. Intense cramping during menses.

10. Following an abdominal hysterectomy, what nursing measures help to prevent the development of thrombo-phlebitis? Select all that apply.
    1. Report scant incisional drainage.
    2. Ambulate the client frequently.
    3. Keep the knees flexed.
    4. Apply antiembolic stockings.
    5. Supervise active leg exercises.

54 Caring for Clients With Breast Disorders

LEARNING OBJECTIVES

1. List four signs and symptoms common in breast disorders.
2. Name two infectious and inflammatory breast disorders and explain how they are acquired.
3. Discuss health teaching that may help prevent or eliminate infectious and inflammatory breast disorders.
4. Compare and contrast two benign breast disorders.
5. Name groups at high risk for developing breast cancer.
6. List common signs and symptoms of breast cancer.
7. Describe four methods for treating cancer, including six surgical techniques used to remove a malignant breast tumor.
8. Give two criteria that are used when selecting a mastectomy procedure.
9. Name a serious complication of breast cancer treatment.
10. Discuss the nursing management of clients who undergo surgical treatment for breast cancer.
11. List four sites to which breast cancer commonly metastasizes.
12. Describe three elective cosmetic breast procedures for clients with a mastectomy.
13. Describe three cosmetic breast procedures that women with nondiseased breasts may elect.

SECTION 1: ASSESSING YOUR UNDERSTANDING

Activity A   Fill in the blanks by choosing the correct word from the options given in parentheses.

1. The breasts' primary function is the production of milk, a process referred to as _____. (gestation, lactation, ovulation)

2. Signs and symptoms of _____ include fever and malaise, along with breast tenderness, pain, and redness. The breast later becomes swollen, firm, and hard. A crack in the nipple or areola develops, and the axillary lymph nodes enlarge. (mastitis, breast abscess, fibroadenoma)

3. _____ is a benign breast condition that affects women primarily between the ages of 30 and 50 years. (Mastitis, Fibroadenoma, Fibrocystic breast disease)

4. One in _____ women develops breast cancer. (five, eight, ten)

5. Side effects of _____ include nausea, vomiting, changes in taste, alopecia (hair loss), mucositis, dermatitis, fatigue, weight gain, and bone marrow suppression. (radiation, chemotherapy, radial breast mastectomy)

6. _____ are most commonly involved in metastasis. Skeletal and pulmonary systems may also be involved (in that order). In addition, metastases may be found in the brain, adrenals, and liver. (Lymph nodes, Cardiac tissues, Skin tissues)

Activity B   Write the correct term for each description.

1. It is most common in women who are breastfeeding. Although inflammation can occur at any time, it is most common during the 2nd or 3rd week postpartum. _____

2. Most frequently occurs as a complication of postpartum mastitis. Purulent exudate accumulates in a confined, local area of breast tissue. The client is usually started on intravenous (IV) antibiotic therapy and may require incision, drainage, and packing. _____

3. This condition may produce no symptoms. However, many women report having tender or painful breasts and feeling one or, more often, multiple lumps within breast tissue. The symptoms are most noticeable just before menstruation and usually abate during menstruation. _____

4. A solid, benign breast mass composed of connective and glandular tissue. This type of breast lesion usually occurs in women during late adolescence and early adulthood, but occasionally, it is found in older women. _____

5. Soft-tissue swelling from accumulated lymphatic fluid that occurs in some women after they have undergone breast cancer surgery. The condition, a consequence of removing or irradiating the axillary lymph nodes, is evidenced by temporary or permanent enlargement of the arm and hand on the side of the amputated breast. _____

6. The migration of cancer cells from one part of the body to another. Malignant cells are spread by direct extension, through the lymphatic system, bloodstream, and cerebrospinal fluid. _____

Activity C *Match the surgical procedures for breast cancer given in Column A with their descriptions in Column B.*

Column A

_____ 1. Lumpectomy

_____ 2. Partial or segmental mastectomy

_____ 3. Simple or total mastectomy

_____ 4. Subcutaneous mastectomy

_____ 5. Modified radical mastectomy

_____ 6. Radical mastectomy

Column B

a. The breast, the axillary lymph nodes, and pectoralis major and minor muscles are removed. In some instances, sternal lymph nodes are also removed.

b. The tumor and some breast tissue and some lymph nodes are removed.

c. The breast, some lymph nodes, the lining over the chest muscle, and the pectoralis minor muscle are removed.

d. All breast tissue is removed, but the skin and nipple are left intact.

e. Only the tumor is removed; some axillary lymph nodes may be excised at the same time for microscopic examination.

f. All breast tissue is removed. No lymph node dissection is performed.

Activity D *Briefly answer the following questions.*

1. Describe the pathophysiology of mastitis.

_____

_____

_____

2. What is the cause of fibrocystic disease?

_____

_____

_____

3. How does breast cancer spread to distant areas?

_____

_____

_____

4. What are the signs and symptoms of breast cancer?

_____

_____

_____

5. What is the treatment for breast cancer?

_____

_____

_____

6. What options are available for women at increased risk of developing breast cancer?

_____

_____

_____

SECTION 2: APPLYING YOUR KNOWLEDGE

Activity E *Give rationale for the following questions.*

1. Why are clients who are diagnosed with a breast abscess placed in contact isolation precautions?

_____

_____

_____

2. Why are the arms and shoulders of the client with a breast abscess supported on pillows?

_____

_____

_____

3. Why might older women mistake changes in their breasts due to aging for signs of breast cancer?

_____

_____

_____

4. Why can lymphedema be a serious complication following breast cancer surgery?

_____

_____

_____

5. Why are antiemetics and anxiolytic medications administered before chemotherapy?

_____

_____

_____

6. Why would taking nonsteroidal anti-inflammatory drugs (NSAIDs) be beneficial to the client at risk for the development of breast cancer?

_____

_____

_____

Activity F *Answer the following questions related to caring for clients with breast disorders.*

1. What educational information will the nurse provide to the client with mastitis?

_____

_____

_____

2. What educational information will the nurse provide to the client with fibrocystic breast disease?

_____

_____

_____

3. What are the risk factors associated with breast cancer?

_____

_____

_____

4. What instructions will the nurse provide to the client with fibroadenoma?

_____

_____

_____

5. What information must the nurse commonly address with clients following breast cancer surgery?

_____

_____

_____

6. Identify the action/purpose of each of the following medications used in the treatment of breast cancer: antiestrogen drugs, aromatase inhibitors (AIs), antiprogestin drugs, androgen therapy, and single or combined antineoplastic agents.

_____

_____

_____

Activity G   *Think over the following questions. Discuss them with your instructor or peers.*

1. You are providing postoperative instruction to a client following breast cancer surgery. What information will you provide about postoperative arm exercises?

_____

_____

_____

2. What high-priority nursing diagnoses and intervention will you identify for the client with infectious and inflammatory breast disorders?

_____

_____

_____

3. What educational information will you provide to the client following breast cancer surgery?

_____

_____

_____

4. What high-priority nursing diagnoses and interventions will you identify for the client following breast cancer surgery?

_____

_____

_____

Activity H   *Read the following case study. Use critical thinking skills to discuss and answer the questions that follow it.*

A new mother goes to the local clinic with complaints that she is no longer able to breastfeed her infant due to a cracked nipple. The client explains to the nurse that she has been breastfeeding her new baby for approximately 3 weeks. The client states that, over a period of days, her left breast has gone from being tender and painful to now being swollen and firm. The nurse determines the client's allergies, completes the health history, and prepares the client for a physical exam and possible specimen collection of expressed milk. When preparing the client for the physical exam, the nurse notes that the client has not bathed recently and is unkempt in appearance. The physician examines the client and finds the left breast swollen, firm to the touch, and with a cracked nipple. The diagnosis is mastitis. A collected specimen shows a penicillin-resistant microorganism responsible for the infection.

1. Because the typical drug therapy treatment for mastitis involves 10 days of an antibiotic from the penicillin group, what options does this client have for treatment with a microorganism that is penicillin resistant?

_____

_____

_____

2. How can the nurse differentiate the symptoms of mastitis from those of an abscess?

_____

_____

3. What information in the case study indicates a possible cause for the infectious process?

_____

_____

_____

SECTION 3: GETTING READY FOR NCLEX

Activity I   *Answer the following questions.*

1. Which one of the following adverse reactions is the nurse most likely to detect when administering danazol (Danocrine) for fibrocystic breast disease?
   1. Nausea
   2. Confusion
   3. Amenorrhea
   4. Hypotension

2. When the nurse assesses the breasts of a postpartum client, which finding suggests that the client has mastitis?
   1. A crack in the nipple or the areola
   2. Multiple lumps within the breast
   3. Breasts engorged with milk
   4. Breast tenderness, without any pain

3. Which of the following is the best reason for the nurse to provide early discharge instructions and home care arrangements for clients undergoing mastectomy?
   1. The adverse effects of mastectomy are immediate.
   2. Wound care requires skill and practice.
   3. Most clients are not hospitalized long after a mastectomy.
   4. Depression and suicide are high postoperatively.

4. Which of the following suggestions should a nurse give breastfeeding mothers to prevent or eliminate mastitis and breast abscess?
   1. Offer the opposite breast at each feeding of the infant.
   2. Minimize the frequency of feedings to the infants.
   3. Use a breast shield when not breastfeeding.
   4. Avoid using a breast pump to save milk.

5. Which of the following nursing interventions is appropriate to avoid maceration from irritating drainage in a client with a breast abscess?
   1. Apply zinc oxide to the surrounding skin.
   2. Use a binder to hold the dressing in place.
   3. Cover the dressing with clear plastic.
   4. Shave the axillary hair on the side with the abscess.

6. When teaching a group about detecting breast cancer, which one of the following is the nurse correct in identifying as the primary sign of this malignancy?
   1. A bloody discharge from the nipple
   2. A dimpling of the skin over the lesion
   3. A retraction of the nipple
   4. A painless mass in the breast

7. When a nurse is educating a group of women about the risks of breast cancer, she includes which of the following as one of the most common risk factors?
   1. Older than 30 years of age
   2. Family history of breast cancer
   3. African American heritage
   4. Early menarche or menopause

8. Besides mammography, which additional test should the nurse advocate be done for women at high risk for breast cancer?
   1. Excisional breast biopsy
   2. Magnetic resonance imaging (MRI)
   3. Chest radiography
   4. Computed tomography (CT) scan

9. A client is undergoing sentinel lymph node mapping. A nurse explains that this technique offers which of the following advantages? Select all that apply.
   1. Avoids unnecessary removal of axillary lymph nodes
   2. Detects severity of axillary lymph node metastasis
   3. Prevents postoperative wound dehiscence
   4. Preserves more breast, axillary tissue, and chest muscle
   5. Reduces the potential for lymphedema of the arm

10. A nurse is working with a client who has undergone chemotherapy for breast cancer. The client is experiencing body image disturbances. Which of the following would contribute to this psychosocial issue?
   1. Fatigue
   2. Vomiting
   3. Alopecia
   4. Nausea

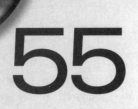

55 Caring for Clients With Disorders of the Male Reproductive System

LEARNING OBJECTIVES

1. Give four examples of structural disorders that affect the male reproductive system.
2. Explain the technique and purpose for performing testicular self-examination.
3. List three infectious or inflammatory conditions and how they are acquired.
4. Discuss two erectile disorders and explain their effects on fertility and sexuality.
5. Identify two methods for treating erectile dysfunction.
6. Describe nursing care for a client being treated for erectile dysfunction.
7. Explain how prostatic hyperplasia compromises urinary elimination, and the symptoms it produces.
8. Discuss the nursing management of a client undergoing a prostatectomy.
9. Compare and contrast three male reproductive cancers in terms of age of onset, incidence, and treatment outcomes.
10. List home care instructions after a vasectomy.

SECTION 1:   ASSESSING YOUR UNDERSTANDING

Activity A   *Fill in the blanks by choosing the correct word from the options given in parentheses.*

1. _____ refers to an inability to retract the foreskin (prepuce). The condition is often caused by congenitally small foreskin; however, chronic inflammation at the glans penis and prepuce secondary to poor hygiene or infection also are etiologic factors. *(Phimosis, Paraphimosis, Torsion)*

2. Medical treatment for _____ consists of bed rest, scrotal elevation, analgesics, anti-inflammatory agents, and comfort measures such as local cold applications. Antibiotic therapy is initiated to eliminate the infectious agent. *(phimosis and paraphimosis, epididymitis and orchitis, hydrocele and spermatocele)*

3. _____ is a condition in which the penis becomes engorged and remains persistently erect. *(Phimosis, Paraphimosis, Priapism)*

4. When the number of nonmalignant cells in the prostate gland increases it is called _____. *(a spermatocele, benign prostatic hyperplasia, a hydrocele)*

5. Because residual urine is a good culture medium for bacteria, symptoms of _____ (inflammation of the bladder) may develop with benign prostatic hyperplasia. *(cystitis, epididymis, orchitis)*

6. _____ cancer is second to skin cancer in frequency among American men. It ranks second as the cause of deaths from cancer. About 1 American male in 6 will be diagnosed with this type of cancer, and 1 in 36 will die of the disease. *(Prostatic, Testicular, Penile)*

7. A _____ is a surgical attempt to reverse an elective sterilization by restoring patency and continuity to the vas deferens. It may take from 3 to 6 months after reversal procedures before sperm counts and motility are normal. Lack of success usually is the result of either scar formation or sperm leakage from the surgical connection. *(vasectomy, transurethral needle ablation, vasovasostomy)*

Activity B *Write the correct term for each description.*

1. Clients report a sudden, sharp testicular pain, with visible local swelling. The pain may be so severe that nausea, vomiting, chills, and fever occur. The condition may follow severe exercise, but it also may occur during sleep or after a simple maneuver such as crossing the legs. _____

2. A strangulation of the glans penis from an inability to replace the retracted foreskin. If the condition continues, severe edema and urinary retention may occur.

   _____

3. The underlying etiology of this disorder usually is a vascular problem, a medical condition that causes blood to thicken; it may also be a side effect of medications, including those prescribed to treat impotence.

   _____

4. The client notices that it takes more effort to void. Eventually, the urinary stream narrows and has decreased force. The bladder empties incompletely. As residual urine accumulates, the client has the urge to void more often and nocturia occurs. _____

5. In the early stage of benign prostatic hyperplasia, the progression of prostatic enlargement is monitored with this periodic examination. _____

6. This minor surgical procedure involves the ligation of the vas deferens and results in permanent sterilization by interrupting the pathway that transports sperm.

   _____

Activity C *Match the options for treating erectile dysfunction in Column A with their descriptions in Column B.*

Column A

_____ 1. Sildenafil (Viagra), a phosphodiesterase inhibitor

_____ 2. Apomorphine (Uprima), a dopamine agonist

_____ 3. Papaverine (Pavatine) with phentolamine (Regitine) or alprostadil (Caverject)

_____ 4. A vacuum device

_____ 5. Surgically implanted penile prosthesis

Column B

a. An injection site is selected on either of the lateral sides of the penis. The prescribed medication is injected into erectile tissue at a 90° angle.

b. One type contains a saline reservoir that is pumped to fill the implant when sexual activity is desired, and the other type maintains the penis in a semierect state at all times.

c. Administered as a nasal spray and acts within 15 to 25 minutes of administration. This medication is safer for men with coronary artery disease.

d. Facilitates penile erection by producing smooth muscle relaxation in the corpora cavernosa, facilitating an inflow of blood. This drug is typically taken on demand 15 minutes to 1 hour before sexual activity.

e. The device is used to engorge the penis with blood. A constricting attachment prohibits the outflow of blood to sustain the erection.

Activity D *Compare and contrast prostatic, testicular, and penile cancer based on the criteria listed in the table.*

Type of Cancer	Pathophysiology and Etiology	Signs and Symptoms	Treatment
Cancer of the prostate			
Cancer of the testes			
Cancer of the penis			

Activity E *Briefly answer the following questions.*

1. Describe the treatment for cryptorchidism.

_____

_____

_____

2. What are the recommendations for testicular self-examination?

_____

_____

_____

3. What information should the nurse provide clients with prostatitis?

_____

_____

_____

4. What are the signs and symptoms of epididymitis and orchitis?

_____

_____

_____

5. What conditions must be met for erectile dysfunction to be considered pathologic?

_____

_____

_____

6. How are physical origins of erectile dysfunction differentiated from psychological origins?

_____

_____

_____

7. Describe the action of the following medications used to treat benign prostatic hyperplasia: alpha-adrenergic blockers, androgen hormone inhibitors, and saw palmetto.

_____

_____

_____

SECTION 2: APPLYING YOUR KNOWLEDGE

Activity F *Give the rationale for the following questions.*

1. Why is cryptorchidism treated when the child is between 1 and 2 years of age?

_____

_____

_____

2. Why does the American Cancer Society not currently recommend regular testicular examinations, except in the case of those with specific testicular risk factors?

_____

_____

_____

3. Why is surgery immediately performed when torsion of the spermatic cord is present?

_____

_____

_____

4. Why does a varicocele usually require surgery, whereas a hydrocele and spermatocele usually do not?

_____

_____

_____

5. Why is it important to differentiate epididymitis from torsion of the spermatic cord within the testicle?

_____

_____

_____

6. Why does the nurse need to obtain a thorough medication record when evaluating a client with erectile dysfunction (ED)?

_____

_____

_____

7. Why is a client likely to be sterile after a transurethral resection of the prostate (TURP)?

_____

_____

_____

Activity G _Answer the following questions related to caring for clients with disorders of the male reproductive system._

1. Describe the pathophysiology, signs and symptoms, and treatment for prostatitis.

_____

_____

_____

2. Describe the etiology of epididymitis and orchitis.

_____

_____

_____

3. What are the processes necessary for an erection?

_____

_____

_____

4. What are possible complications that can occur following a penile implant?

_____

_____

_____

5. Describe the options for treating priapism.

_____

_____

_____

6. Identify the purpose and types of surgeries used to treat benign prostatic hyperplasia (BPH).

_____

_____

_____

7. Describe the use of PSA screening in prostatic cancer.

_____

_____

_____

Activity H *Think over the following questions. Discuss them with your instructor or peers.*

1. What home care instructions will you provide to the client following a vasectomy?

_____

_____

_____

2. What high-priority nursing diagnoses and interventions will you identify for a client following a transurethral resection of the prostate (TURP)?

_____

_____

_____

3. A client asks you what the signs and symptoms are for testicular cancer. What would you tell him?

_____

_____

_____

4. A client asks how to perform a testicular self-examination. How would you instruct him?

_____

_____

_____

5. What high-priority nursing diagnoses and interventions would you identify for the client following a radical prostatectomy with a bilateral orchiectomy?

_____

_____

_____

SECTION 3: GETTING READY FOR NCLEX

Activity I *Answer the following questions.*

1. Which of the following suggestions is best for the nurse to give a client with phimosis who is not a candidate for surgery?
 1. Apply a skin cream nightly and try retracting the tissue.
 2. Wash under the foreskin daily and seek care if retracting the tissue is unsuccessful.
 3. Apply warm soaks to the foreskin before having intercourse.
 4. Take sitz baths regularly until the tissue retracts.

2. Which of the following would a nurse suggest for a client with an inflammation of the prostate gland caused by an infectious pathogen? Select all that apply.
 1. Refer sexual partners for medical treatment.
 2. Avoid standing for long periods at a time.
 3. Eat fibrous foods daily to avoid constipation.
 4. Cease masturbation or intercourse until treated.
 5. Take mild analgesics for relieving pain.
 6. Utilize warm sitz baths to promote comfort.

3. Which of the following nursing interventions is most appropriate for a client undergoing treatment for epididymitis and orchitis?
 1. Use an alcohol rub to keep the scrotum dry.
 2. Apply skin cream to keep the scrotal skin supple.
 3. Elevate the scrotum to relieve the pain.
 4. Limit alcohol intake to two drinks per week.

4. Which of the following nursing interventions is advised for clients with prostate cancer to avoid a urinary tract infection during the home care of a Foley catheter?
 1. Boil the leg bag regularly in a solution of hot water and vinegar for 15 minutes during the cleaning.
 2. Before the insertion, disinfect several inches of the catheter with alcohol or any other antiseptic agent.
 3. Clean the leg bag by using soap and water and then rinse it with a 1:7 solution of vinegar and water.
 4. Separate the leg bag and the catheter only once a day to reduce microbial entry.

5. Which of the following suggestions from a nurse is best to give a client recovering from prostate surgery to deal with impotency?
   1. Substitute masturbation to provide sexual pleasure.
   2. Demonstrate sexual feelings in ways other than intercourse.
   3. Practice sexual intercourse at least two to three times daily until successful.
   4. Perform pelvic floor retraining exercises until erections occur.

6. Following a transurethral prostatectomy, a continuous bladder irrigation is used. The nurse anticipates which of the following electrolyte imbalances may occur?
   1. Hyperkalemia
   2. Hypocalcemia
   3. Hyponatremia
   4. Hypermagnesemia

7. A school nurse is called to the playground to assess an adolescent who experienced intense pain in his testicle after riding his bike. The nurse is correct in assuming that the trauma may most likely have caused which of the following?
   1. Torsion of the spermatic cord
   2. Acute epididymitis
   3. Paraphimosis
   4. Spermatocele

8. A client asks the nurse to explain the purpose of a continuous bladder irrigation (CBI) following a transurethral prostatectomy (TURP). Which of the following is the most accurate response?
   1. A CBI helps prevent urinary tract infections.
   2. A CBI helps remove blood clots and tissue.
   3. A CBI decreases postoperative discomfort.
   4. A CBI facilitates urinary continence after recovery.

9. Following a prostatectomy, which of the following is the best technique the nurse can teach a client to avoid urinary retention following catheter removal?
   1. Exhale against a closed airway like having a bowel movement.
   2. Perform several series of squats, push-ups and crunches each day.
   3. Contract abdominal muscles while breathing out through pursed lips.
   4. Apply even pressure from the umbilicus toward the lower abdomen.

10. What is the best nursing measure for ensuring continuous urinary drainage from a suprapubic catheter?
    1. Encourage a large fluid intake each day.
    2. Empty the urine collection bag frequently.
    3. Keep the drainage bag below the insertion site.
    4 Stabilize the catheter to the skin of the abdomen.

56 Caring for Clients With Sexually Transmitted Infections

LEARNING OBJECTIVES

1. Name five common sexually transmitted infections (STIs) and identify those that are curable.
2. List five STIs that by law must be reported.
3. Give two reasons why statistics on reportable STIs are not totally accurate.
4. Discuss several factors contributing to the transmission of STIs.
5. Give two reasons why women acquire STIs more often than men.
6. Name the most common and fastest-spreading STI.
7. Explain two ways STIs are spread.
8. Discuss methods that are helpful in preventing STIs.
9. Discuss information that is important to teach clients about using condoms.
10. Name the type of infectious microorganism that causes each of the common STIs.
11. Identify complications that are common among clients who acquire each of the most common STIs.
12. Name drugs used to treat common STIs.

SECTION 1: ASSESSING YOUR UNDERSTANDING

Activity A *Fill in the blanks by choosing the correct word from the options given in parentheses.*

1. Untreated _____ can cause sterility in infected women; infected pregnant women can transmit the microorganism to their infants during birth. *(chlamydia, herpes infection, genital warts)*

2. The incidence of _____ in the United States has been increasing among young black men having sex with men, a statistic that may correlate with the current incidence of HIV infection among this population. *(chlamydia, gonorrhea, syphilis)*

3. It is estimated that one in five Americans is infected with the virus that causes _____; at the current rate of infection, approximately 40% to 50% of the U.S. population may be infected by the year 2025. *(genital herpes, chancroid, genital warts)*

4. One in four Americans carry the _____ and are infectious but do not manifest symptoms. *(genital herpes virus, gonorrhea bacteria, human papilloma virus [HPV])*

5. _____ causes aortic regurgitation and insufficiency due to valvular changes. *(Syphilis, Chlamydia, Gonorrhea)*

Activity B *Write the correct term for each description.*

1. The study of the occurrence, distribution, and causes of human diseases. _____

2. The most common and fastest spreading bacterial STI in the United States. The number of new cases in 2010 totaled 1.3 million. _____

3. Tissue irritation, which may be permanent despite successful eradication of the bacteria, puts those with this type of infection at greater risk for acquiring other STIs, such as AIDS. _____

4. The second most frequently reported communicable disease in the United States. Its highest incidence occurs in the 15- to 24-year-old age group. _____

5. A highly contagious STI that is controllable but not curable. Presently, it affects 16.2% of people in the United States, with African American women being disproportionately affected. _____

6. Anyone can become infected, but people with AIDS as well as others with an immunodeficiency are particularly susceptible. _____

Activity C *Match the STIs in Column A with their usual treatments in Column B.*

Column A

_____ **1.** Chlamydia

_____ **2.** Gonorrhea

_____ **3.** Syphilis

_____ **4.** Herpes infection

_____ **5.** Genital warts (Human papilloma viral infection)

Column B

a. A single dose of parenterally administered penicillin G (Pfizerpen, Wycillin) is used to treat primary and secondary symptoms. Those with tertiary symptoms may require three doses of penicillin at 1-week intervals to prevent complications.

b. If treatment is necessary, either type responds to the antiviral drugs acyclovir (Zovirax), valacyclovir (Valtrex), and famciclovir (Famvir).

c. Antimicrobial drugs, such as a single oral dose of azithromycin (Zithromax) or a 7-day regimen of doxycycline (Vibramycin), erythromycin (E-Mycin), ofloxacin (Floxin), or levofloxacin (Levaquin) are used for treatment.

d. A single intramuscular dose of a broad-spectrum cephalosporin such as ceftriaxone (Rocephin), along with a second antibiotic such as azithromycin (Zithromax) in a single oral dose or oral doxycycline (Vibramycin); sexual partners in the preceding 60 days should also be treated.

e. The physician may prescribe podofilox (Condylox) solution or gel, or imiquimod (Aldara) cream for self-application. Physician-administered treatment involves surgical excision with scalpel or scissors, laser therapy, electrocautery (heat), cryotherapy (freezing) with liquid nitrogen, local applications of chemicals, or parenteral administration of natural or recombinant interferon.

Activity D *Identify the causative organisms, modes of transmission, and signs and symptoms for the following STIs.*

STI	Causative Organism and Mode of Transmission	Signs and Symptoms
Chlamydia		
Gonorrhea		
Syphilis		
Herpes infection		
Genital warts (HPV)		
Granuloma inguinale		
Chancroid		
Lymphogranuloma venereum		

Activity E   *Briefly answer the following questions.*

1. Identify the pathogens that cause STIs.

_____

_____

_____

2. Identify the possible reasons for the disproportionate reporting of higher incidences of STIs among racial and ethnic minorities.

_____

_____

_____

3. When testing for gonorrhea in women, why is the speculum moistened with water instead of lubricant?

_____

_____

_____

4. Besides AIDS, what are the five most common STIs?

_____

_____

_____

5. Out of the five most common STIs, which ones are curable?

_____

_____

_____

SECTION 2:   APPLYING YOUR KNOWLEDGE

Activity F   *Give rationale for the following questions.*

1. Why is the term *sexually transmitted infections* increasingly used rather than *sexually transmitted diseases?*

_____

_____

_____

2. Why is it difficult to determine the exact incidence of sexually transmitted infections (STIs)?

_____

_____

_____

3. Why do STIs occur more often in women?

_____

_____

_____

4. Why might an older adult be at risk for acquiring, or not receiving, treatment for an STI?

_____

_____

_____

5. Why does the Centers for Disease Control and Prevention (CDC) recommend annual screening for chlamydia in all sexually active women younger than 26 years of age and in women with new or multiple sexual partners?

_____

_____

_____

6. Why is it a common practice to test clients for chlamydia and gonorrhea as well as syphilis?

_____

_____

_____

Activity G *Answer the following questions related to caring for clients with sexually transmitted infections.*

1. Identify the factors that contribute to the high incidence of STIs.

_____

_____

_____

2. What complications may occur as a result of untreated gonorrhea?

_____

_____

_____

3. What questions will the nurse ask when obtaining a sexual history?

_____

_____

_____

4. How will the nurse instruct the client to reduce the risk of STIs?

_____

_____

_____

5. What information should the nurse provide the client with herpes simplex virus type 2 (HSV-2) infections?

_____

_____

_____

6. What information should the nurse provide to the client with genital warts?

_____

_____

_____

Activity H *Think over the following questions. Discuss them with your instructors or peers.*

1. A client requests information about the proper use of condoms. How will you instruct him or her?

_____

_____

_____

2. What high-priority nursing diagnoses and interventions will you identify for the client diagnosed with an STI?

_____

_____

_____

3. What information will you provide to the client diagnosed with an STI?

_____

_____

_____

SECTION 3: GETTING READY FOR NCLEX

Activity I   *Answer the following questions.*

1. Which nursing response is accurate when a client asks why a chlamydial infection creates a greater risk for acquiring AIDS?
   1. The tissue irritation may be permanent.
   2. The immune system is already compromised.
   3. The bacterium is genetically similar to the HIV virus.
   4. CD4 cells are damaged by the infecting bacterium.

2. Which of the following is a nurse most likely to detect when examining a client who acquired a chlamydial infection as a child while living in an undeveloped foreign country?
   1. Corneal scarring
   2. Anal ulceration
   3. Genital warts
   4. Urethral infection

3. When a school nurse discusses STIs, which of the following diseases is accurately identified as being curable with early treatment? Select all that apply.
   1. Gonorrhea
   2. Genital herpes
   3. Syphilis
   4. AIDS
   5. Chlamydia

4. When a client seeks treatment for a herpes simplex type 2 viral infection, which drug can the nurse anticipate the physician will prescribe?
   1. penicillin G (Bicillin)
   2. ciprofloxacin (Cipro)
   3. acyclovir (Zovirax)
   4. podofilox (Condylox)

5. Which of the following instructions would a nurse give a client undergoing treatment for an HSV-2 infection?
   1. Schedule an annual Papanicolaou smear.
   2. Have yearly mammograms.
   3. Perform breast self-examination monthly.
   4. Obtain a Western Blot test every 6 months.

6. What is the rationale for a nurse being unable to find statistics on STIs such as genital herpes, hepatitis B, and venereal warts?
   1. Clients don't seek treatment because of embarrassment.
   2. Healthcare providers are not required to report them.
   3. Healthcare providers are reluctant to report these statistics.
   4. Reporting is up to the client, not the provider.

7. A client reports having had a genital lesion that has spontaneously disappeared. Which of the following signs and symptoms will the nurse most likely elicit when assessing a client during the second stage of syphilis? Select all that apply.
   1. Ataxia
   2. Fever
   3. Rash
   4. Hyporeflexia
   5. Enlarged lymph nodes

8. A nurse is teaching a client in the doctor's office about genital warts. Which of the following is the best discharge instruction to give to a client with genital warts?
   1. Advise all sexual contacts to be examined and treated.
   2. Avoid intimate contact when warts are present.
   3. Use a condom when the warts are visible; otherwise, no condom is necessary.
   4. Suggest application of an antibiotic cream to sexual partner after intimate contact.

9. When a client who has gonorrhea is allergic to penicillin, which antibiotic can the nurse expect will be used as an alternative?
   1. erythromycin (E-mycin)
   2. amoxicillin (Amoxil)
   3. ceftriaxone (Rocephin)
   4. ampicillin (Omnipen)

10. A physician orders ceftriaxone 1 g IM in two equally divided doses for a client with gonorrhea. Calculate the volume the nurse should administer after reconstituting a 1 g vial of powdered ceftriaxone with 3.6 mL of diluent to yield 250 mg per mL.

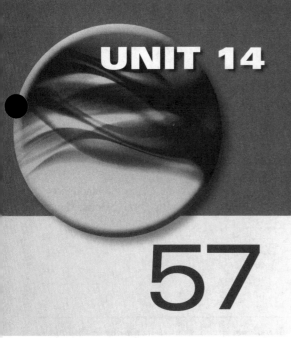

57 Introduction to the Urinary System

LEARNING OBJECTIVES

1. Name the parts of the urinary system.
2. Define the primary functions of the kidney and other structures in the urinary system.
3. List tests performed for the diagnosis of urologic and renal system diseases.
4. Identify laboratory tests performed to diagnose urologic and renal system diseases.
5. Discuss nursing management for a client undergoing diagnostic evaluation of the urinary tract.

SECTION 1:   ASSESSING YOUR UNDERSTANDING

Activity A   *Fill in the blanks by choosing the correct word from the options given in parentheses.*

1. The two _____ are paired, bean-shaped organs located in the upper abdomen on either side of the vertebral column. The blood supply to each consists of a renal artery and renal vein. The renal artery arises from the aorta and the renal vein empties into the vena cava. *(kidneys, ureters, bladders)*

2. The _____ contains calyces (pyramids), cone-shaped structures that open to the renal pelvis, a large funnel-like structure in the center of the kidney. The renal pelvis then empties into the ureter, which carries urine to the bladder for storage. *(medulla, bladder, urethra)*

3. _____ is a radiologic study used to evaluate the structure and function of the kidneys, ureters, and bladder. It locates the site of any urinary tract obstructions and is helpful in the investigation of the causes of flank pain, hematuria, or renal colic. It is based on the ability of the kidneys to excrete a radiopaque dye in the urine. *(A biopsy, Intravenous pyelography, Cystography)*

4. Severe pain in the back, shoulder, or abdomen following a biopsy can indicate _____. *(infection, bleeding, distention)*

5. _____ is performed to evaluate bladder and sphincter function. This noninvasive procedure measures the time and rate of voiding, the volume of urine voided, and the pattern of urination. Results are compared with normal flow rates and urinary patterns. Results vary by age and sex. *(Uroflowmetry, Postvoid residual, Cystometrography)*

6. _____ evaluates the bladder tone and capacity. *(Uroflowmetry, Cystometrography, Urinalysis)*

Activity B *Write the correct term for each description.*

1. These form a sling that supports the bladder and urethra, rectum, and some reproductive organs. _____

2. May result secondary to an overdistended bladder or other problems and may cause infections. _____

3. Clients receive this type of medication following a cystoscopy. _____

4. This is taken to diagnose cancer, assess prostatic enlargement, diagnose and monitor progression of renal disease, and assess and evaluate treatment of renal transplant rejection. _____

5. A diagnostic test similar to cystography except that the client is instructed to void (the urine contains the radiopaque dye), and a rapid series of x-rays are taken. _____

6. A measure of the amount of urine left in the bladder after voiding; provides information about bladder function. _____

Activity C *Match the diagnostic tests related to renal disorders listed in Column A with their descriptions in Column B*

Column A

_____ 1. Radiography

_____ 2. Ultrasonography

_____ 3. Computed tomography scan and magnetic resonance imaging

_____ 4. Angiography

_____ 5. Cystoscopy

Column B

a. Uses include identification of renal cysts or obstruction sites, assistance in needle placement for renal biopsy or nephrostomy tube placement, and drainage of a renal abscess.

b. Used to identify the cause of painless hematuria, urinary incontinence, or urinary retention. It is useful in the evaluation of structural and functional changes of the bladder.

c. Provides details of the arterial supply to the kidneys, specifically the location and number of renal arteries (multiple vessels to the kidney are not unusual) and the patency of each renal artery.

d. May be obtained to diagnose renal pathology, determine kidney size, and evaluate tissue densities with or without contrast material.

e. Performed to show the size and position of the kidneys, ureters, and bony pelvis as well as any radiopaque urinary calculi (stones), abnormal gas patterns (indicative of renal mass), and anatomic defects of the bony spinal column (indicative of neuropathic bladder dysfunction).

Activity D *Compare the following laboratory tests in terms of their purposes and how to perform them.*

Test	Purpose	How to Perform Test
Urinalysis		
Urine culture and sensitivity		
24-Hour urine collection		
Urine specific gravity		
Urine osmolality		
Urine protein test		
Creatinine clearance test		
Blood urea nitrogen (BUN)		

Activity E *Briefly answer the following questions.*

1. Describe the nephrons of the kidneys.

_____

_____

_____

2. What usually prevents the backflow of urine?

_____

_____

_____

3. What causes the urge to urinate?

_____

_____

_____

4. What can occur if the bladder muscles are impaired?

_____

_____

_____

5. During a physical examination, how does the nurse assess for kidney pain?

_____

_____

_____

6. If the client is being discharged the day after a biopsy, what instruction will the nurse provide?

_____

_____

_____

SECTION 2: APPLYING YOUR KNOWLEDGE

Activity F *Give rationale for the following questions.*

1. Why are periodic, small amounts of protein in the urine not considered a problem?

_____

_____

_____

2. Why would glucose be excreted in the urine?

_____

_____

_____

3. Why would older adults be at risk for drug toxicity?

_____

_____

_____

4. Why would older adults be at risk for dehydration?

_____

_____

_____

5. Why might the physician inject a minute amount of contrast and wait 5 to 10 minutes before proceeding?

_____

_____

_____

6. Why is intravenous pyelography scheduled prior to a barium test or gallbladder series using contrast material?

_____

_____

_____

Activity G *Answer the following questions related to the urinary system.*

1. Describe the structures and function of the urinary system.

_____

_____

_____

2. Explain the process of urine formation.

_____

_____

_____

3. How is intravenous pyelography performed?

_____

_____

_____

4. What postprocedure care will the nurse provide following intravenous pyelography?

_____

_____

_____

Activity H *Think over the following questions. Discuss them with your instructor or peers.*

1. Your client is scheduled for intravenous pyelography. What instructions would you provide?

_____

_____

_____

2. What high-priority nursing diagnoses and interventions would you identify for the client being evaluated for renal dysfunction?

_____

_____

_____

3. You need to obtain a clean-catch midstream urine specimen. How would you instruct the client?

_____

_____

_____

SECTION 3: GETTING READY FOR NCLEX

Activity I *Answer the following questions.*

1. For a client who is experiencing difficulty voiding, which method should the nurse use to assess the kidneys for tenderness and/or pain?
1. Auscultate the abdomen for bruits.
2. Lightly strike the fist at the costovertebral angle.
3. Palpate the suprapubic region.
4. Percuss the area over the bladder.

2. A client with a possible renal disorder, scheduled for a diagnostic test, is worried about the test and its results. Which of the following teaching strategies should the nurse use to alleviate the client's anxiety?
1. Use simple language with client or significant others.
2. Discuss medications that may be used to treat the renal disorder.
3. Explain in detail all the technicalities about the test.
4. Tell the client about the risk factors of the test.

3. Following an angiography procedure, why is it important for the nurse to frequently assess the client's pressure dressing in the femoral region?
   1. To note frank bleeding
   2. To assess for hypersensitivity responses
   3. To check for signs of arterial occlusion
   4. To assess peripheral pulses

4. When preparing a client for discharge following a renal biopsy, which of the following instructions needs to be included related to the prevention of bleeding?
   1. Increase fluid intake.
   2. Refrain from taking nephrotoxic drugs.
   3. Take sedative medications.
   4. Maintain limited physical activity.

5. A client who undergoes retrograde pyelography is transferred to postprocedure care. Which of the following measures should the nurse take when if there are signs of pyelonephritis?
   1. Report them to the physician.
   2. Advise the client to be bed rest.
   3. Observe further for signs of bleeding.
   4. Monitor pressure dressing to note any frank bleeding.

6. Before cystoscopy, the nurse checks for signs of fever and chills in the client because they may indicate which of the following?
   1. Bleeding
   2. A urinary infection
   3. An allergy to iodine
   4. A urinary tract disorder

7. Which of the following should the nurse closely monitor in older clients with renal dysfunction?
   1. Decreased urine output
   2. Urine discoloration
   3. Signs of ketonuria
   4. Signs of nephrotoxicity

8. A client, while collecting a 24-hour urine specimen, may have lost some urine during the night. What is the nurse's most appropriate action?
   1. Accept the sample and send it to laboratory for testing.
   2. Discard the test and ask the client to restart the urine collection.
   3. Send to the laboratory, informing the lab of the urine loss.
   4. Refrigerate the sample for 24 hours and then send it to the laboratory for the test.

9. When monitoring a client after an angiography, which of the following actions is most important?
   1. Palpate peripheral pulses in the lower extremities every hour.
   2. Monitor and document the intake and output every 8 hours.
   3. Assess the pressure dressing every 12 hours.
   4. Obtain a 24-hour urine specimen.

10. When reviewing a client's urinalysis report, which of the following values does the nurse report as abnormal?
    1. An absence of glucose
    2. A protein level of 0
    3. A specific gravity of 1.03
    4. A urine pH of 3.0

58

Caring for Clients With Disorders of the Kidneys and Ureters

LEARNING OBJECTIVES

1. Differentiate pyelonephritis and glomerulonephritis.
2. Name problems the nurse manages when caring for clients with glomerulonephritis.
3. Explain the pathophysiology and associated renal complications of polycystic disease.
4. Give examples of conditions that predispose to renal calculi.
5. Identify methods for eliminating small renal calculi and larger stones.
6. Discuss the nursing management of a client with a nephrostomy tube.
7. Describe conditions that cause a ureteral stricture.
8. Explain the classic triad of symptoms associated with renal cancer.
9. Discuss problems the nurse manages when caring for a client with a nephrectomy.
10. Differentiate acute and chronic renal failure.
11. Explain pathophysiologic problems associated with chronic renal failure.
12. Describe sources of organs for kidney transplantation.
13. Identify nursing methods for managing pruritus.
14. Explain the purposes and methods of dialysis.
15. Discuss nursing assessments performed when caring for clients undergoing dialysis.

SECTION 1: ASSESSING YOUR UNDERSTANDING

Activity A *Fill in the blanks by choosing the correct word from the options given in parentheses.*

1. Laboratory findings for _____ include urine findings of proteinuria, sediment, casts, and red and white blood cells. The urinary creatinine clearance is reduced. Serum electrolyte changes indicate nephron dysfunction. *(pyelonephritis, acute glomerulonephritis, chronic glomerulonephritis)*

2. _____ is performed by inserting a fine wire into the ureter by means of a cystoscope. A laser beam passes through it and repeated bursts of the laser reduce the stone to a fine powder, which is then passed in the urine. *(Laser lithotripsy, Extracorporeal shock wave lithotripsy, Ureteral stent placement)*

3. _____ disorders usually are obstructive problems in structures below the kidney(s) that have damaging repercussions for the nephrons above. *(Prerenal, Intrarenal, Postrenal)*

4. During the _____ phase of acute renal failure, fluid volume excess develops, which leads to edema, hypertension, and cardiopulmonary complications. *(initiation, oliguric, diuretic)*

5. Chronic renal failure is associated more often with _____ conditions or is a complication of systemic diseases such as diabetes mellitus and disseminated lupus erythematosus. *(prerenal, intrarenal, postrenal)*

6. In _____, the kidneys are so extensively damaged that they do not adequately remove protein by-products and electrolytes from the blood and do not maintain acid–base balance. *(acute renal failure, pyelonephritis, chronic renal failure)*

7. _____ is a neurologic condition believed to be caused by cerebral edema. The shift in cerebral fluid volume occurs when the concentrations of solutes in the blood are lowered rapidly during dialysis. Decreasing solute concentration lowers the plasma osmolality. Water then floods the brain tissue. *(Disequilibrium syndrome, Uremic frost, Azotemia)*

Activity B *Write the correct term for each description.*

1. The chief abnormality of pyelonephritis. _____

2. Laboratory findings include proteinuria and an elevated antistreptolysin O titer from the recent streptococcal infection. There is decreased hemoglobin, slightly elevated BUN and serum creatinine levels, and an elevated erythrocyte sedimentation rate. _____

3. An accumulation of nitrogen waste products in the blood; evidenced by elevated BUN, serum creatinine, and uric acid levels. _____

4. Distention of the renal pelvis, which may result from complete obstruction caused by renal calculi. _____

5. Refers to the death of cells in the collecting tubules of the nephrons, where reabsorption of water and electrolytes and excretion of protein wastes and excess metabolic substances occur. _____

6. A precipitate that may form on the skin in end-stage renal disease, when the skin becomes the excretory organ for the substances that the kidney usually clears from the body. _____

7. A procedure for cleaning and filtering the blood. It substitutes for kidney function when the kidneys cannot remove the nitrogenous waste products and maintain adequate fluid, electrolyte, and acid–base balances. _____

8. This syndrome is characterized by headache, disorientation, restlessness, blurred vision, confusion, and seizures. The symptoms are self-limiting and disappear within several hours after dialysis as fluid and solute concentrations equalize. The syndrome can be prevented by slowing the dialysis process to allow time for gradual equilibration of water. _____

Activity C *Match the congenital and obstructive disorders in Column A with the descriptions in Column B.*

Column A

_____ **1.** Adult polycystic kidney disease

_____ **2.** Urolithiasis

_____ **3.** Ureteral stricture

_____ **4.** Kidney tumor

Column B

a. Calculi traumatize the walls of the urinary tract and irritate the cellular lining, causing pain as violent contractions of the ureter develop to pass the stone along. If a stone totally or partially obstructs the passage of urine beyond its location, pressure increases in the area above the stone. The pressure contributes to pain, and urinary stasis promotes secondary infection.

b. The incidence is higher in older adults, which suggests chronic exposure to a carcinogen whose metabolites involve renal excretion. It is possible that the cause is exposure to an environmental toxin or volatile solvent.

c. The incidence is higher among those with chronic ureteral stone formation. Recurrent inflammation and infection cause scar tissue to accumulate in the ureter. This condition may also result from congenital anomalies or conditions that mechanically compress the ureter, such as pregnancy or tumors in the abdomen or upper urinary tract.

d. This is inherited as an autosomal dominant disorder. The disorder is characterized by the formation of multiple bilateral kidney cysts, which interfere with kidney function and eventually lead to renal failure. The fluid-filled cysts cause great enlargement of the kidneys, from their normal size of a fist to that of a football. As the cysts enlarge, they compress the renal blood vessels and cause chronic hypertension. Bleeding into cysts causes flank pain.

Activity D *Briefly answer the following questions.*

1. What is extracorporeal shock wave lithotripsy?

_____

_____

_____

2. What are the signs and symptoms of renal cancer?

_____

_____

_____

3. Identify the four phases of acute renal failure.

_____

_____

_____

4. Describe the diuretic phase of acute renal failure.

_____

_____

_____

_____

5. What signs and symptoms occur with chronic renal failure?

_____

_____

_____

6. Describe the process of hemodialysis.

_____

_____

_____

7. How does the nurse assess a vascular access?

_____

_____

_____

8. Compare the advantages and disadvantages of an arteriovenous fistula and an arteriovenous graft.

_____

_____

_____

SECTION 2: APPLYING YOUR KNOWLEDGE

Activity E *Give rationale for the following questions.*

1. Why does the nurse encourage an oral intake of 3000 to 4000 mL of fluid for the client with pyelonephritis?

_____

_____

_____

2. Why is it important that the client with glomerulonephritis receive adequate carbohydrates in his or her diet?

_____

_____

_____

3. Why is a low RBC volume detected through complete blood counts with chronic glomerulonephritis?

_____

_____

_____

4. Why can neurologic symptoms occur during the oliguric phase of acute renal failure?

_____

_____

_____

5. Why would a chest radiography and echocardiography be pertinent with a diagnosis of chronic glomerulonephritis?

_____

_____

_____

6. Why does urine have a very low specific gravity in clients with acute renal failure?

_____

_____

_____

7. Why are blood samples taken before and after dialysis?

_____

_____

_____

Activity F   _Answer the following questions related to caring for the client with disorders of the kidneys and ureters._

1. Describe the pathophysiology of pyelonephritis.

_____

_____

_____

2. What are the medical management goals for a client with chronic glomerulonephritis?

_____

_____

_____

3. What surgical treatment options are available for the treatment of calculi that are large or complicated by obstruction, ongoing UTI, kidney damage, or constant bleeding?

_____

_____

_____

4. Describe the treatment options for renal cancer.

_____

_____

_____

5. Describe the electrolyte and blood component changes that occur with chronic renal failure.

_____

_____

_____

6. How are acute and chronic renal failure medically and surgically managed?

_____

_____

_____

7. What are the options for vascular access with hemodialysis?

_____

_____

_____

8. Describe the process of peritoneal dialysis.

_____

_____

_____

Activity G *Think over the following questions. Discuss them with your instructor or peers.*

1. What high-priority nursing diagnoses and interventions would you identify for a client with chronic glomerulonephritis?

_____

_____

_____

2. What educational information related to diet would you provide to the client with renal calculi?

_____

_____

_____

3. What high-priority nursing diagnoses and interventions would you identify for a client with renal cancer?

_____

_____

_____

4. Your client is informed that he will need dialysis and asks you to explain the difference between hemodialysis and peritoneal dialysis as well as the process for each. What educational information will you provide?

_____

_____

_____

_____

Activity H *Read the following case study. Use critical thinking skills to discuss and answer the questions that follow it.*

A 30-year-old client is seen in his primary care physician's office by the nurse practitioner. The nurse begins by updating the client's current medications and family history. The client informs the nurse he has just discovered that his family history includes polycystic kidney disease (PKD). The client explains that his parents were killed in an auto accident when he was young. Both parents were unaffected carriers of the gene but did not have the disease. The client realizes that this can be a serious disease and has come for additional information and counseling about PKD. The nurse talks with the client about his concerns and discusses it with the physician. After examining the client, the physician orders some preliminary testing and refers the client for genetic counseling.

1. What information would the nurse give this client about the chances of developing PKD?

_____

_____

_____

2. When asked about signs and symptoms, which of these would the nurse anticipate a client with PKD to display?

_____

_____

_____

3. The client asks about prognosis and typical treatment options. What information would the nurse provide?

_____

_____

_____

SECTION 3: GETTING READY FOR NCLEX

Activity I   *Choose the best answer for each of the following questions.*

1. A client with pyelonephritis asks the nurse why it is necessary to drink 3000 to 4000 mL per day. What is the nurse's best response?
   1. "This assists us to evaluate your response to therapy."
   2. "Fluids flush the infectious microorganisms from the urinary tract."
   3. "Taking fluids determines the location of your discomfort."
   4. "Extra fluids helps to detect any evidence of changes."

2. A client is admitted with acute pyelonephritis. When assessing the client, the nurse expects to the client to report which of the following symptoms?
   1. Low urine output.
   2. Flank pain on the affected side.
   3. Periorbital edema.
   4. Intermittent headache.

3. A client with renal calculi complains of acute intense pain. Which of the following measures should the nurse include in the plan of care?
   1. Administer prescribed nephrotoxic drugs.
   2. Observe aseptic principles when changing dressings.
   3. Advise against protein restriction.
   4. Encourage ambulation and liberal fluid intake.

4. A 66-year-old client is admitted following a nephrolithotomy. One of the laboratory tests reveals a urinary tract infection. Which is the best nursing action?
   1. Administer IV fluids and blood transfusions.
   2. Administer narcotic analgesics as prescribed.
   3. Encourage fluid intake of 3000 mL/day.
   4. Suggest taking herbs or spices to increase food palatability.

5. A client is complaining of severe flank pain. A diagnosis of urolithiasis is made. Which of the following interventions is a priority?
   1. Encourage a low calcium diet.
   2. Inform client to remain on strict bed rest.
   3. Limit fluid intake to 50 mL per hour.
   4. Strain urine with each voiding.

6. A client is undergoing peritoneal dialysis. Which major complication should that the nurse should monitor for?
   1. Internal hemorrhage
   2. Ecchymosis
   3. Hydronephrosis
   4. Peritonitis

7. A client with chronic renal failure expresses frustration with managing all of the dietary restrictions. Which of the following would be the best nursing intervention to improve dietary compliance?
   1. Encourage the client to seek support from family members in managing the diet.
   2. Suggest that the client consume a specially formulated, high-protein food.
   3. Recommend that the client adjust calorie intake upward during dialysis.
   4. Recommend that the client increase intake of plant proteins.

8. A client is diagnosed with renal failure and is admitted for dialysis. Which of the following is the nurse's responsibility as the client undergoes dialysis?
   1. Keep dialysis supplies in a clean area.
   2. Inspect the catheter insertion site for signs of infection.
   3. Weigh the client before and after the procedure.
   4. Wash hands before and after handling the catheter.

9. A client is admitted for postoperative assessment and recovery after surgery for a kidney tumor. Knowing that a urinary tract infection is highly possible, which of the following nursing actions is a priority?
   1. Encourage the client to breathe deeply and cough every 2 hours.
   2. Monitor temperature every 4 hours.
   3. Measure intake and output every 8 hours.
   4. Irrigate tubes as ordered.

10. For a client in the oliguric phase of acute renal failure (ARF), which nursing intervention is most important?
    1. Maintain fluid restriction
    2. Encourage client to ambulate
    3. Promote a high carbohydrate diet
    4. Administer pain control medications

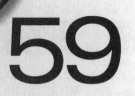

59 Caring for Clients With Disorders of the Bladder and Urethra

LEARNING OBJECTIVES

1. Explain urinary retention and appropriate nursing management.
2. Discuss urinary incontinence and appropriate nursing management.
3. Describe the pathophysiologic changes seen in cystitis, interstitial cystitis, and urethritis.
4. Explain the symptoms associated with bladder stones.
5. Discuss the cause and treatment of urethral strictures.
6. Identify the most common early symptom of a malignant tumor of the bladder, and outline treatment and nursing care.
7. Describe various types of urinary diversion procedures.
8. Identify components of a teaching plan for a client having a urinary diversion procedure.

SECTION 1: ASSESSING YOUR UNDERSTANDING

Activity A *Fill in the blanks by choosing the correct word from the options given in parentheses.*

1. _____ urinary retention requires immediate catheterization. *(Acute, Chronic, Delayed)*

2. Usually, clients with bladder stones are told to increase their _____ intake significantly, consume a moderate protein intake, and limit sodium. *(calcium, fluid, carbohydrate)*

3. Urethral strictures are treated by _____. *(urethroplasty, litholapaxy, dilatation)*

4. Small, superficial tumors may be removed by resection or _____ with a transurethral resectoscope. *(fulguration, dilatation, litholapaxy)*

5. _____ exercises increase muscle tone to assist bladder emptying and bladder training. *(Kegel, Credé, Valsalva)*

Activity B *Write the correct term for each description.*

1. This procedure uses a stone-crushing instrument and is suitable for small and soft stones. It is performed under general anesthesia. _____

2. Only clients who have *type II absorptive* hypercalciuria (approximately 50% of all clients with hypercalciuria) need to limit intake of this substance. _____

3. Often the first sign of bladder cancer and the reason clients seek medical attention. _____

4. The bladder and lower third of both ureters are removed in this procedure. _____

5. A method of bladder training that combines scheduled voiding with prompting and praising. _____

Activity C   *Match the terms related to voiding dysfunction in Column A to their descriptions in Column B.*

Column A

_____ **1.** Neurogenic bladder

_____ **2.** Residual urine

_____ **3.** Urinary retention

_____ **4.** Urinary incontinence

_____ **5.** Cystostomy

Column B

a. Urine retained in the bladder after the client voids.

b. Acute symptoms are the sudden inability to void, distended bladder, and severe lower abdominal pain and discomfort. A chronic condition may not produce symptoms because the bladder has stretched over time and accommodates large volumes without producing discomfort.

c. A bladder that does not receive adequate nerve stimulation.

d. A procedure in which a catheter is inserted through the abdominal wall directly into the bladder.

e. May result from either bladder or urethral dysfunction (or both); the bladder can contract without warning, fail to accommodate adequate volumes of urine, or fail to empty completely and become overstretched; the urethral sphincters may fail to hold urine in the bladder.

Activity D   *Compare the following infectious and inflammatory disorders of the bladder and urethra based on the following criteria.*

Disorder	Pathophysiology	Signs and Symptoms
Cystitis		
Interstitial cystitis (IC)		
Urethritis		

Activity E   *Briefly answer the following questions.*

1. Describe how the following medications can improve bladder retention, emptying, and control: anticholinergic drugs, tricyclic antidepressant medications, pseudoephedrine, and estrogen.

_____

_____

_____

2. What problems may interfere with the success of a bladder training program? What interventions would the nurse implement?

_____

_____

_____

3. What are the effects when incontinence cannot be avoided? What interventions would the nurse implement?

_____

_____

_____

4. What is involved in the nursing management of interstitial cystitis (IC)?

_____

_____

_____

5. Describe the nursing management implemented to prevent urethritis for the client with an indwelling urinary catheter.

_____

_____

_____

6. Describe the etiology of a urethral stricture.

_____

_____

_____

SECTION 2: APPLYING YOUR KNOWLEDGE

Activity F _Provide rationale for the following questions._

1. Why is permanent catheterization avoided?

_____

_____

_____

2. Why is it necessary to clamp the catheter if a large volume of urine is returned during catheterization?

_____

_____

_____

3. Why is it important to carefully assess the older client and the conditions that may contribute to incidents of incontinence?

_____

_____

_____

4. Why may cranberry juice or vitamin C be recommended for a client diagnosed with cystitis?

_____

_____

_____

5. Why would a client with bladder cancer exhibit symptoms of anemia?

_____

_____

_____

Activity G _Answer the following questions that relate to caring for clients with disorders of the bladder and urethra._

1. What options may be used to treat chronic urinary retention?

_____

_____

_____

2. A client with chronic urinary retention will be managed using intermittent catheterization. Describe the procedure that will be used.

_____

_____

_____

3. How is bladder training accomplished for a client with an indwelling catheter?

_____

_____

_____

4. What complications can result from a urethral stricture?

_____

_____

_____

5. Describe the medical treatment options for bladder cancer.

_____

_____

_____

6. Describe the two types of urinary diversions.

_____

_____

_____

Activity H　_Think over the following questions. Discuss them with your instructor or peers._

1. Your client has functional incontinence. What high-priority nursing diagnoses and interventions would you identify?

_____

_____

_____

2. How would you instruct the client to use Credé or Valsalva voiding?

_____

_____

_____

3. Which clients would you identify as being at risk for urinary incontinence?

_____

_____

_____

4. What high-priority diagnoses and interventions would you identify for the client with an infection of the bladder or urethra?

_____

_____

_____

5. What educational information would you provide to the client caring for a stoma and urinary ostomy?

_____

_____

_____

SECTION 3:　GETTING READY FOR NCLEX

Activity I　_Choose the best answer for the following questions._

1. What is a priority nursing intervention for a client having a ureterosigmoidoscopy procedure?
1. Inspect for bleeding or cyanosis
2. Assess the client's allergy to iodine
3. Inspect for symptoms of peritonitis
4. Check for signs of electrolyte losses

2. What is an important assessment on a client undergoing a urinary diversion?
1. The client's knowledge about effects of the surgery on sexual function
2. The client's medical history of allergy to iodine or seafood
3. The client's knowledge about the effects of the surgery on nervous control
4. The client's occupational and environmental health hazards

3. A client recently underwent a surgical procedure for malignant tumor. As a result of the surgery, The client's urine is diverted to a stomal pouch. What should the nurse suggest so that the client remains odor free?
1. Eating spicy foods
2. Eating eggs, asparagus, or cheese
3. Drinking cranberry juice
4. Drinking tea, coffee, and colas

4. While managing a client after a medical or surgical procedure for bladder stones, when should the nurse notify the physician?
1. When the temperature rises above 98° F
2. When the temperature rises above 99° F
3. When the temperature rises above 100° F
4. When the temperature rises above 101° F

5. A client who underwent litholapaxy surgery for removing bladder stones asks the nurse how long the urethral catheter needs to stay in place. Which of the following responses by the nurse is correct?
   1. The catheter should remain in place for 1 to 2 days.
   2. The catheter should remain in place for 2 to 3 days.
   3. The catheter should remain in place for 3 to 4 days.
   4. The catheter should remain in place for 7 days.

6. Which of the following is the most important factor in the nursing management of clients who undergo treatment for a malignant tumor following a urinary diversion procedure?
   1. Monitoring IV and central venous pressure lines
   2. Administering cleansing enemas as ordered
   3. Observing for leakage of urine or stool from the anastomosis
   4. Assessing the client's ability to manage self-catheterization

7. The nurse is instructed to perform preoperative preparation for the surgical management of a client with malignant tumors. Which of the following is the most important factor of the nursing management plan?
   1. Insertion of an ostomy pouch
   2. Maintaining the integrity of the urinary diversion procedure
   3. Assessing for symptoms of peritonitis
   4. Insertion of a nasogastric tube

8. A client experiences trauma to the urinary tract during an accident. Which of the following factors should the nurse consider while assessing the client?
   1. Sexual habits
   2. Abnormal findings
   3. Allergies to seafood
   4. Insurance coverage

9. A client diagnosed with urethritis is prescribed antibiotics and advised to drink at least eight large glasses of water daily. What is the nurse's best explanation for the increased water intake?
   1. "Increasing your fluid intake will assist in overcoming your incontinence."
   2. "Increasing your fluid intake will flush bacteria from the urinary tract."
   3. "Increasing your fluid intake will help eliminate urinary odors."
   4. "Increasing your fluid intake will alleviate pain and discomfort."

10. The nurse is reviewing procedures used to assist with urinary control with a client. As the nurse states that one procedure involves placing small amounts of collagen in the urethral walls to aid in closing pressure, what procedure is the nurse describing?
    1. Bladder augmentation
    2. Retropubic suspension
    3. Implantation of an artificial sphincter
    4. Periurethral bulking

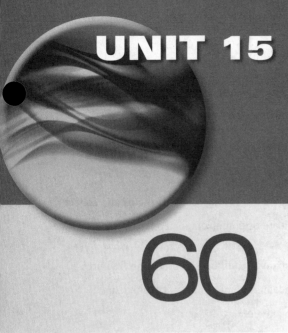

UNIT 15

CARING FOR CLIENTS WITH MUSCULOSKELETAL DISORDERS

60 Introduction to the Musculoskeletal System

LEARNING OBJECTIVES

1. Describe major structures and functions of the musculoskeletal system.
2. Discuss elements of the nursing assessment of the musculoskeletal system.
3. Identify common diagnostic and laboratory tests used in the evaluation of musculoskeletal disorders.
4. Discuss the nursing management of clients undergoing tests for musculoskeletal disorders.

SECTION 1:   ASSESSING YOUR UNDERSTANDING

Activity A   *Fill in the blanks by choosing the correct word from the options given in parentheses.*

1. The human body has _____ bones. *(206, 260, 620)*

2. _____ build bones; these cells secrete bone matrix (mostly collagen), in which inorganic minerals, such as calcium salts, are deposited. *(Osteocytes, Osteoblasts, Osteoclasts)*

3. A layer of tissue called _____ covers the bones (but not the joints). *(epiphyses, periosteum, diaphyses)*

4. A _____ is the junction between two or more bones. *(joint, ligament, tendon)*

5. _____ are cordlike structures that attach muscles to the periosteum of the bone. *(Joints, Bursae, Tendons)*

6. _____ are small sacs filled with synovial fluid. They reduce friction between areas (such as tendon and bone, and tendon and ligament). *(Cartilage, Bursae, Muscles)*

Activity B   *Write the correct term for each description.*

1. Bone cells involved in the destruction, resorption, and remodeling of bone. _____

2. These types of muscles are voluntary muscles; impulses that travel from efferent nerves of the brain and spinal cord control their function. They promote movement of the bones of the skeleton. _____

3. The lubricating fluid that is produced by the synovial membrane, which lines synovial joints. _____

4. A firm, dense type of connective tissue that consists of cells embedded in a substance called the matrix. The matrix is firm and compact, thus enabling it to withstand pressure and torsion. The primary functions are to reduce friction between articular surfaces, absorb shocks, and reduce stress on joint surfaces. _____

5. Lateral curvature of the spine. _____

6. Intake recommendations of this nutrient are set at 1000 mg/day for adults younger than age 50 years and 1200 mg/day for those over age 50 years. _____

Activity C *Match the blood test findings listed in Column A with the conditions they may indicate in Column B.*

Column A

_____ 1. Elevated alkaline phosphatase level and increased serum phosphorus level

_____ 2. Elevated acid phosphatase level

_____ 3. Decreased serum calcium level

_____ 4. Elevated serum uric acid level

_____ 5. Elevated antinuclear antibody level

Column B

a. May indicate Paget's disease and metastatic cancer.

b. May indicate osteomalacia, osteoporosis, and bone tumors.

c. May indicate bone tumors and healing fractures.

d. May indicate systemic lupus erythematosus.

e. May indicate gout.

Activity D *Compare the diagnostic tests of the musculoskeletal system based on the following criteria.*

Test	Purpose	How Test Is Performed
Imaging procedures		
Arthrogram		
Arthroscopy		
Arthrocentesis		
Synovial fluid analysis		
Bone densitometry		
Bone scan		
Electromyography		
Biopsy		

Activity E *Briefly answer the following questions.*

1. Describe the functions of the musculoskeletal system.

_____

_____

_____

2. Describe the types of involuntary muscles.

_____

_____

_____

3. Which results of a 24-hour urine test would be significant to the musculoskeletal system?

_____

_____

_____

4. How are the activities of smooth and cardiac muscles controlled?

_____

_____

_____

5. What is the purpose of hyaline cartilage, which covers diarthrodial joints?

_____

_____

_____

6. Identify nondairy sources of calcium.

_____

_____

_____

7. How are vitamin K, magnesium, and potassium related to bone health?

_____

_____

_____

SECTION 2: APPLYING YOUR KNOWLEDGE

Activity F   _Provide rationale for the following questions._

1. Why do older adults lose as much as 1 to 2 cm of height every two decades?

_____

_____

2. Why are older adults at higher risk for skeletal fractures?

_____

_____

_____

3. Why do older adults experience a greater amount of bone mass loss?

_____

_____

_____

4. Why should the nurse consult with the physician before applying a cold pack to a recent injury?

_____

_____

_____

5. Why is a swollen body part elevated above heart level?

_____

_____

_____

6. Why is vitamin D intake necessary for bone health?

_____

_____

_____

Activity G   _Answer the following questions related to the musculoskeletal system._

1. Identify the classification of bones and provide examples of each.

_____

_____

_____

2. Describe bone composition and the process of bone remodeling.

_____

_____

_____

3. Describe how skeletal muscles contract and relax.

_____

_____

_____

4. Describe the tendon attachments to a bone.

_____

_____

_____

5. What information is included in a general assessment of the musculoskeletal system?

_____

_____

_____

6. What information does the nurse gather if the client has experienced a traumatic injury to the musculoskeletal system?

_____

_____

_____

Activity H _Think over the following questions. Discuss them with your instructor or peers._

1. A client over age 50 years asks you how he can maintain his bone health and prevent loss of bone mass. What educational information would you provide?

_____

_____

_____

2. A client is brought in to the emergency department with a traumatic injury to the right ankle; there is no obvious deformity. What assessments and interventions would be appropriate for this client? What diagnostic tests would you anticipate?

_____

_____

_____

3. Your client is scheduled for an arthroscopy. What pre-procedure and postprocedure care would you provide?

_____

_____

_____

SECTION 3:   GETTING READY FOR NCLEX

Activity I   _Answer the following questions._

1. The nurse examines a client who fell while climbing stairs and now has swelling in the ankle and pain with movement. The nurse tells the client that there is ecchymosis. What is the best explanation for this term?
   1. "The area over the ankle is swollen."
   2. "The skin in the ankle area is very bruised."
   3. "There is mottling in the ankle region."
   4. "The skin on the ankle blanches when I apply pressure."

2. A client presents with a shoulder injury after falling from a stepladder. When the nurse examines the client, which finding most indicates that the shoulder is dislocated?
   1. The affected arm is longer than the other arm.
   2. The client complains of excruciating pain.
   3. There is obvious swelling above the joint.
   4. The client is afraid to move the affected arm.

3. Which of the following methods would best help the nurse determine the degree of a traumatic musculoskeletal injury?
   1. Palpating the injured area to assess the extent of pain experienced by the client
   2. Applying force to the client's extremity and asking the client to push back as much as possible
   3. Encouraging the client to move the injured area as much as possible
   4. Comparing structures and assessment findings on one side of the body with those on the opposite side

4. A client undergoes arthrography for an examination of the knee. What information should the nurse provide to the client?
   1. Expect crackling or clicking noises in the joint for up to 2 days.
   2. Expect fever, nausea, and vomiting for up to 2 days.
   3. Avoid dairy products for up to 2 days.
   4. Avoid potassium-rich foods for up to 2 days.

5. The nurse needs to detect the presence of ischemia in a client with tissue injury. Which of the following signs and symptoms may indicate the presence of ischemia?
   1. Signs of fatigue
   2. Signs of respiratory depression
   3. Absence of a peripheral pulse
   4. Heavy swelling in the injured area

6. Which of the following measures should be taken by the nurse to help relieve edema in a client with tissue injury?
   1. Massaging the swollen body part
   2. Taking a prescribed analgesic
   3. Applying a cold pack to the swollen body part
   4. Keeping the swollen body part above the level of the heart

7. Which of the following practices would delay the decline in muscle strength and bone mass in older adults?
   1. Maintaining an active lifestyle
   2. Maintaining a low-activity lifestyle
   3. Maintaining an adequate calcium intake after the age of 35 years
   4. Reducing the calcium intake after the age of 60 years

8. An elderly client has undergone electromyography tests to evaluate muscle weakness and deterioration. The client complains of slight pain after the tests. Which of the following nursing interventions would help relieve the client's discomfort?
   1. Administering topical analgesics to the area where the needle electrodes were inserted
   2. Massaging the area where the needle electrodes were inserted
   3. Applying a cold pack to the area where the needle electrodes were inserted
   4. Applying warm compresses to the area where the needle electrodes were inserted

9. A client recovering from a fractured knee wants to know if there are any nondairy sources of calcium that are absorbed well by the body. Which one of the following food items should the nurse suggest to enable the client to meet his daily calcium intake requirement?
   1. Green leafy vegetables
   2. Canned salmon with bones
   3. Broccoli
   4. Calcium-fortified orange juice

10. A nurse is assessing a client's musculoskeletal system and identifies symptoms of weak pulses, dusky color in the ankles, and +3 local edema. Which of the following does the nurse suspect to be an issue with this client?
    1. Problems with circulation
    2. Problems with sensation
    3. Problems with mobility
    4. Problems with pain

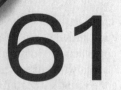

61 Caring for Clients Requiring Orthopedic Treatment

LEARNING OBJECTIVES

1. Differentiate types of casts.
2. Discuss the nursing management for a client with a cast.
3. State the reasons for using splints or braces.
4. Identify the principles for maintaining traction and describe nursing care for the client in traction.
5. Differentiate between closed reduction and open reduction and between internal fixation and external fixation.
6. Describe nursing care for the client with a fracture reduction.
7. Identify the reasons for performing orthopedic surgery.
8. Discuss the nursing management for a client undergoing orthopedic surgery.
9. Describe the positioning precautions after a conventional total hip replacement.
10. Explain the nursing needs of the client undergoing total knee replacement.
11. Discuss amputation, including reasons it may be performed and appropriate nursing management of the client.

SECTION 1: ASSESSING YOUR UNDERSTANDING

Activity A *Fill in the blanks by choosing the correct word from the options given in parentheses.*

1. _____ provides support, controls movement, and prevents additional injury. (*A reduction, A brace, Traction*)

2. In a(n) _____ reduction, the bone is restored to its normal position by external manipulation. (*closed, open, internal*)

3. In _____ fixation, the surgeon inserts metal pins into the bone or bones from outside the skin surface and then attaches a compression device to the pins. (*internal, closed, external*)

4. _____, death of bone tissue, occurs when there is diminished or absent blood supply. (*Subluxation, Avascular necrosis, Hemorrhage*)

5. Following an amputation, pain may result from a stump _____, which is formed when the cut ends of nerves become entangled in the healing scar. (*hematoma, neuroma, causalgia*)

6. A(n) _____ amputation is planned when a client has severe infection and gangrene. The guillotine method is first used, and then a few days later, after the infection is treated and the client is stable, a more definitive, closed amputation is done. (*open, closed, staged*)

Activity B *Write the correct term for each description.*

1. This type of cast surrounds one or both legs and the trunk. It may be strengthened by a bar that spans a casted area between the legs. _____

2. This is used to relieve muscle spasm, align bones, and maintain immobilization. The two most common types are skin and skeletal. _____

3. When this type of reduction is performed (in the operating room), the bone is surgically exposed and realigned. _____

4. Dislocation of the artificial joint. _____

5. A _____ machine promotes healing and flexibility in the knee and hip joint and increases circulation to the operative area.

6. In a _____ amputation (flap amputation), skin flaps cover the severed bone end.

Activity C *Match the methods to treat the fractures given in Column A with their correct descriptions in Column B.*

Column A

_____ **1.** Short leg cast

_____ **2.** Short arm cast

_____ **3.** Body cast

_____ **4.** Long arm cast

_____ **5.** Hip spica cast

_____ **6.** Long leg cast

_____ **7.** Shoulder spica cast

_____ **8.** Walking cast

Column B

a. Extends from below the elbow to the palmar crease and is secured around the base of the thumb. If the thumb is also casted, it is referred to as a thumb spica or gauntlet cast.

b. Extends from the upper level of the axillary fold to the proximal palmar crease. The elbow is usually immobilized at a right angle.

c. Extends from below the knee to the base of the toes. The foot is flexed at a right angle in a neutral position.

d. Extends from the junction of the upper and middle third of the thigh to the base of the toes. The knee may be slightly flexed.

e. A short or long leg cast reinforced for strength.

f. Encircles the trunk.

g. A body cast that encloses the trunk and the shoulder and elbow.

h. Encloses the trunk and a lower extremity. A double hip spica cast includes both legs.

Activity D *Briefly answer the following questions.*

1. Describe the purpose of a cast window.

_____

_____

_____

2. What is the purpose of a bivalve cast?

_____

_____

_____

3. Describe skin care once a cast is removed and describe limb care following cast removal from an extremity.

_____

_____

_____

4. What conditions must be met for the use of a splint?

_____

_____

_____

5. Describe the proper application of a splint.

_____

_____

_____

6. Describe reasons for orthopedic surgery.

_____

_____

_____

7. What interventions are used preoperatively to prevent excessive bleeding?

_____

_____

_____

8. What factors help the surgical team decide at which level to amputate the arm or leg?

_____

_____

_____

SECTION 2: APPLYING YOUR KNOWLEDGE

Activity E *Give rationale for the following questions.*

1. Why is a cast applied from the joint above the break to the one below it? Why is the joint slightly flexed?

2. Why do some fractures not require a cast?

3. Why are the palms of the hands used when repositioning a wet cast?

4. Why is Buck's traction or another form of skin traction applied if surgery for a fracture cannot be performed right away?

5. Why are porous-coated, cementless joint components used with an artificial joint (prosthesis)?

Activity F *Answer the following questions related to caring for clients requiring orthopedic treatment.*

1. Describe the advantages and disadvantages of plaster and fiberglass casts.

2. When is an open reduction required? When is internal fixation used?

3. What are general nursing measures following a reduction?

4. Explain precautions taken following a total hip replacement in order to prevent subluxation.

5. What are the discharge planning needs for the client following a joint replacement?

6. What conditions may necessitate an amputation?

7. What factors influence an amputee's rehabilitation?

Activity G *Think over the following questions. Discuss them with your instructor or peers.*

1. How will you manage care for the client in traction?

_____

_____

_____

2. What high-priority nursing diagnoses and interventions will you identify for the client following a total knee replacement?

_____

_____

_____

3. What steps will you take to provide pin care?

_____

_____

_____

4. What priority nursing diagnoses and interventions would you identify for the client following a traumatic amputation?

_____

_____

_____

Activity H *Read the following case study. Use critical thinking skills to discuss and answer the questions that follow it.*

A client is admitted to the local hospital for a left total knee arthroplasty. When the client returns from surgery, elastic stockings are placed on his lower extremities (TED hose). The client's left leg is placed in a CPM machine to provide passive range of motion to the extremity. The nurse checks peripheral pulses as part of the complete assessment and advances the CPM machine per protocol. The nurse completes a set of vital signs, inquires about the client's pain level, assesses the wound for any drainage, and hangs the last IV dose of an ordered prophylactic antibiotic. The nurse also explains to the client that he will be ambulating with a walker following weight bearing restrictions.

1. Why did the nurse assess peripheral pulses and apply elastic stockings to the client's lower extremities?

_____

_____

_____

2. To prevent postoperative infection, what prevention strategies would the nurse include in the plan of care for this client?

_____

_____

_____

3. What role does good nutrition play in this client's recovery process?

_____

_____

_____

SECTION 3: GETTING READY FOR NCLEX

Activity I *Answer the following questions.*

1. A cylinder cast needs to be applied to a client with a fracture. What is the role of the nurse during the procedure?
   1. Gently massage the arm or the leg.
   2. Hold the arm or the leg in place.
   3. Provide intense heat or a cast dryer to speed the evaporation.
   4. Compress the cast on a hard surface for better support.

2. Which of the following factors should the nurse emphasize while instructing a client with a cast about the lower extremities?
   1. The importance of following a regular diet
   2. The use of prescribed analgesics to manage the pain
   3. Instructions about ambulating with the crutches
   4. The importance of regular exercise

3. A client with a cast reports a throbbing pain. Which of the following actions should the nurse take to relieve the pain?
   1. Administer antibiotics.
   2. Elevate the extremity.
   3. Petal cast edges with waterproof tape.
   4. Massage the area of pain.

4. It is important for the nurse to maintain proper pin care for which of the following methods of treating a fracture?
   1. Closed reduction
   2. Open reduction
   3. External fixation
   4. Internal fixation

5. A client who has a musculoskeletal problem is being discharged after a few days of hospital care. Why should the nurse consider factors related to the home environment while determining a plan for the continued rehabilitation of the client?
   1. To include additional care for clients who lack the basic amenities at home
   2. To determine the client's access to the nearest drugstore
   3. To modify the client's living arrangements or make other accommodation changes
   4. To determine whether the client can continue with the self-care

6. A patient is being discharged following a leg amputation. Which of the following instructions should the nurse give the client regarding home care?
   1. Elevate the stump when sitting, as instructed by the physician.
   2. Apply a nonprescription ointment to the stump to relieve pain.
   3. Do not wash the bandages.
   4. Stretch the bandages when reapplying them.

7. Which of the following may reduce the risk of excessive bleeding in a client who is scheduled to undergo an orthopedic surgery?
   1. Withholding aspirin before the surgery
   2. Limiting antacids before the surgery
   3. Encouraging the intake of red meat before the surgery
   4. Avoiding excess fluid intake before the surgery

8. A client who underwent an amputation a week ago still feels an itching sensation or a dull pain in the missing limb. Which of the following nursing actions would help the client in getting relief?
   1. Seek an additional prescription for an analgesic from the physician.
   2. Advise the client to meet a psychiatrist.
   3. Discuss with the physician the possibility of a surgical removal of the nerve endings at the end of the stump.
   4. Discuss with the client the phenomenon of phantom pain.

9. A nurse is assisting a client who is scheduled for a leg amputation surgery. What are the presurgery nursing management strategies used to assist the client?
   1. Evaluate pain level and discomfort.
   2. Evaluate the client's mental acceptance.
   3. Evaluate bleeding and hemorrhage.
   4. Evaluate client for risk of infection.

10. A nurse evaluates a client for postoperative complications following joint replacement surgery. Upon discharge, the nurse teaches the client that the risk of infection is present for how long after surgery?
    1. Two weeks
    2. One month
    3. Three months
    4. Six months

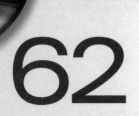

62 Caring for Clients With Traumatic Musculoskeletal Injuries

LEARNING OBJECTIVES

1. Differentiate strains, contusions, and sprains.
2. Define joint dislocations.
3. Discuss the nursing management of various types of sports or work-related injuries.
4. Identify the stages of bone healing after a fracture.
5. Describe the signs and symptoms of a fracture.
6. Explain the nursing management for clients with various types of fractures.
7. Discuss methods used to prevent complications associated with fractures.
8. Discuss potential complications associated with a fractured hip.

SECTION 1: ASSESSING YOUR UNDERSTANDING

Activity A *Fill in the blanks by choosing the correct word from the options given in parentheses.*

1. A _____ is confined to the soft tissues and does not affect the musculoskeletal structure. Many small blood vessels rupture, causing ecchymosis or a hematoma. *(strain, contusion, sprain)*

2. A test that elicits tingling, numbness, and pain, known as _____, may be used to diagnose carpal tunnel syndrome. *(Tinel's sign, Phalen's sign, Turner's sign)*

3. A _____ injury occurs with twisting of the knee or repeated squatting. *(tendon, ligament, meniscal)*

4. Rupture of the _____ occurs secondary to trauma. Because the client engages in an activity, the calf muscle contracts suddenly while the foot is grounded firmly in place. There is often a loud pop, and the client experiences severe pain and inability to plantar flex the affected foot. *(rotator cuff, Achilles tendon, collateral knee ligaments)*

5. Usually a hip fracture affects the _____ end of the femur. This type of fracture commonly results from a fall and occurs more frequently in older adults with osteoporosis. *(proximal, medial, distal)*

Activity B *Write the correct term for each description.*

1. Results from excessive stress, overuse, or overstretching. Small blood vessels in the muscle may rupture, and the muscle fibers sustain tiny tears. _____

2. A sprain of the cervical spine. _____

3. The client flexes the wrist for 30 seconds to determine if pain or numbness occurs, a positive sign for carpal tunnel syndrome. _____

4. Made up of four muscles and their tendons that connect the proximal humerus, clavicle, and scapula, which in turn connect with the sternum (clavicle) and ribs (scapula). _____

5. For torn menisci, the surgeon removes the damaged cartilage. _____

6. A break in the continuity of a bone. _____

Activity C *Match the terms in Column A with their correct descriptions in Column B.*

Column A

_____ **1.** Dislocation

_____ **2.** Subluxation

_____ **3.** Compartment syndrome

_____ **4.** Palsy

_____ **5.** Volkmann's contracture

Column B

a. A partial dislocation.

b. Decreased sensation and movement.

c. A clawlike deformity of the hand resulting from obstructed arterial blood flow to the forearm and hand.

d. When the articular surfaces of a joint are no longer in contact.

e. A condition in which a structure such as a tendon or nerve is constricted in a confined space.

Activity D *Describe these common complications of fractures and appropriate interventions based on the following criteria.*

Complication	Description	Intervention
Shock		
Fat embolism		
Pulmonary embolism		
Compartment syndrome		
Delayed bone healing		
Infection		
Avascular necrosis		

Activity E *Briefly answer the following questions.*

1. Describe the pathophysiology of a sprain and avulsion fracture.

_____

_____

_____

2. Describe the nursing care for a dislocation.

_____

_____

_____

3. Provide the names and locations of the common types of tendonitis that occur as a result of repeated sports and/or work activities.

_____

_____

_____

4. How do injuries to the ligaments of the knee occur? What are the signs and symptoms?

_____

_____

_____

5. How do rotator cuff injuries often occur? What are the signs and symptoms of a rotator cuff injury?

_____

_____

_____

SECTION 2: APPLYING YOUR KNOWLEDGE

Activity F *Give the rationale for the following questions.*

1. Why is a dislocation immobilized following a manipulation?

_____

_____

_____

2. Why are older adults more prone to skeletal fractures?

_____

_____

_____

3. Why do multiple injuries often accompany fractures of the femur?

_____

_____

_____

4. Why are fractures of the femur initially treated with some form of traction?

_____

_____

_____

5. Why are hip fractures a serious problem for older adults?

_____

_____

_____

_____

Activity G *Answer the following questions related to caring for clients with traumatic musculoskeletal injuries.*

1. Describe the medical management of a sprain.

_____

_____

_____

2. Describe the signs and symptoms of a dislocation.

_____

_____

_____

3. Describe the medical and surgical management of tendonitis.

_____

_____

_____

4. What are the signs and symptoms of a fracture?

_____

_____

_____

5. What is the nursing care for a client with a fracture?

_____

_____

_____

6. Describe the assessment findings with a femur fracture.

_____

_____

_____

7. What is the nursing management for a client with a femur fracture?

_____

_____

_____

Activity H *Think over the following questions. Discuss them with your instructor or peers.*

1. You are working at a community health fair. What information would you provide to clients for prevention of sports injuries or work-related injuries?

_____

_____

_____

2. Your client returns from surgery for treatment of a hip fracture. Which high-priority nursing diagnoses and interventions would you identify?

_____

_____

_____

3. You witness an individual take a fall; she complains of pain in her ankle. How would you assist the individual until additional assistance arrives?

_____

_____

_____

4. Your client is postoperative following musculoskeletal surgery. The client does not want to participate in any activities that involve movement. What educational information would you provide?

_____

_____

_____

_____

SECTION 3: GETTING READY FOR NCLEX

Activity I *Answer the following questions.*

1. The client tells the nurse that there was overstretching of the arm muscles when lifting a heavy suitcase. When examining the client the nurse expects which of the following signs and/or symptoms if the injury is a strain?
1. Ecchymosis and hematoma from ruptured blood vessels without loss of function.
2. Partial tearing of muscle and tendon without loss of function.
3. Loss of function following a over twisting of the joint.
4. Torn ligament with detachment of a bone fragment.

2. Which of the following measures should the nurse strongly recommend to a client recovering from a ruptured Achilles tendon to help regain mobility, strength, and the full range of motion?
1. Regular use of NSAIDs
2. Vigorous exercise
3. Physical therapy
4. Nonmedical interventions, such as yoga

3. A client, who spends hours working on the computer, complains of slight pain in the right hand, that is more prominent at night and early in the morning. Which of the following measures should the nurse suggest to help alleviate the pain?
1. Flexing the affected wrist
2. Shaking the affected hand
3. Using surgical intervention
4. Applying physical therapy

4. Which of the following symptoms should the nurse specifically monitor while assessing a client with a femoral neck fracture?
1. Severe pain at the site of the fracture
2. Bleeding from joint capsules
3. Muscle spasms
4. Crepitus at the site of the fracture

5. A nurse is working with an elderly client who is recovering from surgery for a fractured hip. For how long following surgery should the nurse leave the wound drain in place for this client?
1. 12 to 24 hours
2. 1 to 2 days
3. 3 to 4 days
4. 5 to 6 days

6. A client's leg was crushed when a steel girder fell on it at a construction site. The nurse recognizes that such an injury puts the client at risk for fat embolism. Which of the following interventions is needed to prevent this complication?
1. Provide early respiratory support.
2. Administer blood and fluid volume replacements as prescribed.
3. Elevate the extremity.
4. Apply ice to the extremity.

7. For which of the following symptoms should the nurse closely monitor in a client with a compartment syndrome in the upper arm?
   1. Epicondylitis
   2. Carpal tunnel syndrome
   3. Volkmann's contracture
   4. Ganglion cyst

8. A client has undergone surgery for a compound fracture that involved external fixation. Which of the following should the nurse do to prevent infection in this case?
   1. Position the client in line with the pull exerted by the traction.
   2. Administer an antibiotic.
   3. Clean the pin sites.
   4. Elevate the limb.

9. A fractured femur is found in a client with Paget's disease, but the client has been confined to the hospital bed for many days and has not suffered any kind of trauma of which the nurse is aware. Which type of fracture has this client experienced?
   1. Pathologic
   2. Compression
   3. Depressed
   4. Compound

10. A nurse receives word that a client is arriving with a compound fracture of the right tibia. What does the nurse expect to see in this client?
   1. No evidence of trauma to the right lower extremity.
   2. Client complains of pain when bearing weight.
   3. Signs of skin and mucus membrane trauma as well as bone protrusion.
   4. Areas of ecchymosis and swelling at site of injury.

63 Caring for Clients With Orthopedic and Connective Tissue Disorders

LEARNING OBJECTIVES

1. Explain the difference between rheumatoid arthritis and degenerative joint disease (osteoarthritis) and describe nursing management.
2. Describe the clinical manifestations of temporomandibular disorder (TMD).
3. Define the pathophysiology of gout, fibromyalgia, bursitis, and ankylosing spondylitis.
4. Delineate the nursing care required for clients with gout, fibromyalgia, bursitis, and ankylosing spondylitis.
5. Discuss the multisystem involvement associated with systemic lupus erythematosus.
6. Identify the causes of osteomyelitis.
7. Explain the inflammatory process associated with Lyme disease.
8. Identify risk factors for development of osteoporosis.
9. Distinguish the pathophysiology of osteomalacia and Paget's disease.
10. Differentiate between bunions and hammer toe.
11. Discuss characteristics of benign and malignant bone tumors.

SECTION 1: ASSESSING YOUR UNDERSTANDING

Activity A *Fill in the blanks by choosing the correct word from the options given in parentheses.*

1. A positive C-reactive protein (CRP) test, low red blood cell count and hemoglobin levels in later stages, and positive RF are laboratory findings that support the diagnosis of _____. *(rheumatoid arthritis, osteoarthritis, osteomyelitis)*

2. _____ is the most common form of arthritis. It also is known as the "wear and tear" disease and typically affects the weight-bearing joints. It is characterized by a slow and steady progression of destructive changes in weight-bearing joints and those that are repeatedly used for work. *(Rheumatoid arthritis, Osteoarthritis, Temporomandibular disorder)*

3. _____ is a painful metabolic disorder involving an inflammatory reaction in the joints. It usually affects the feet (especially the great toe), hands, elbows, ankles, and knees. *(Fibromyalgia, Gout, Ankylosing spondylitis)*

4. _____ is a chronic syndrome of musculoskeletal pain, fatigue, mood disorders, and sleep disturbances. The pain is widespread, affecting muscles, ligaments, and tendons. *(Fibromyalgia, Gout, Ankylosing spondylitis)*

5. The most common symptoms of _____ are low back pain and stiffness. As the disease progresses, the spine and hips become more immobile, thus restricting movement. The lumbar curve of the spine may flatten. The neck can be permanently flexed and the client appears to be in a perpetual stooped position. *(fibromyalgia, gout, ankylosing spondylitis)*

6. Approximately 60% to 70% of people with _____ have positive anti-dsDNA. *(systemic lupus erythematosus, osteomyelitis, Lyme disease)*

7. _____ is an infection of the bone, resulting in limited blood supply to the bone, inflammation of (and pressure on) the tissue, bone necrosis, and formation of new bone around devitalized bone tissue. This condition is difficult and challenging to treat. *(Systemic lupus erythematosus, Osteomyelitis, Lyme disease)*

8. _____ is a chronic bone disorder characterized by abnormal bone remodeling. It affects adults over the age of 60 years. The most common areas of involvement are the long bones, spine, pelvis, and skull. *(Osteomyelitis, Osteomalacia, Paget's disease)*

Activity B *Write the correct term for each description.*

1. In this disease, the synovial fluid usually appears cloudy, milky, or dark yellow and contains many inflammatory cells, including leukocytes and complement (a group of proteins in blood that affect the inflammatory process and influence antigen–antibody reactions).

_____

2. These products act as a lubricant, substituting for hyaluronic acid, the substance that provides joint fluid viscosity. Pain relief appears to last 6 to 13 months. Side effects include swelling, redness, or heat at the injection site. Clients allergic to eggs should not receive these injections. _____

3. An attack is characterized by a sudden onset of acute pain and tenderness in one joint. _____

4. Pregabalin (Lyrica) is the first drug approved by the Food and Drug Administration to treat this disorder. It is used to reduce pain and fatigue and improve sleep quality.

_____

5. Painful movement of a joint, such as the elbow or shoulder, is the most common symptom. A distinct lump may be felt. If there is a rupture, tissue in the area may become edematous, warm, and tender. _____

6. A chronic connective tissue disorder of the spine and surrounding cartilaginous joints, such as the sacroiliac joints and soft tissues around the vertebrae.

_____

7. Known as "the great imitator" because the clinical signs resemble many other conditions. _____

8. This type of bone tumor usually results from misplaced or overgrown clusters of normal bone or cartilage cells that cause the structure to enlarge and impair local function. They grow slowly and do not metastasize. Their growth can weaken the bone structure by compressing or displacing the normal tissue. _____

Activity C *Match the conditions given in Column A with their characteristics in Column B.*

Column A

_____ **1.** Gout

_____ **2.** Fibromyalgia

_____ **3.** Bursitis

_____ **4.** Ankylosing spondylitis

Column B

a. It is believed that repeated nerve stimulation results in abnormal levels of neurotransmitters that signal pain. The pain receptors in the brain develop a memory of the pain and are more sensitive to the signals. There are tender and painful points that can be identified on clients with this condition that other people without this condition do not have.

b. Usually begins in early adulthood and is more common in men than in women. Its etiology is unknown, although some theorize that an altered immune response occurs when T-cell lymphocytes mistake human cells for similar-appearing bacterial antigens. There also is a strong familial tendency for some affected individuals.

c. The disorder tends to be inherited and affects more men than women. It may occur secondary to other diseases marked by decreased renal excretion of uric acid. It also has been identified among clients who have received organ transplants and the antirejection drug cyclosporine.

d. Trauma is the most common cause. Other causes include overuse, stress, infection, and secondary effects of gout and rheumatoid arthritis (RA). Typical of any inflammation, pain and swelling occur with compromised function.

Activity D *Compare and contrast rheumatoid arthritis and osteoarthritis (degenerative joint disease) using the following criteria.*

Criteria	Rheumatoid Arthritis (RA)	Osteoarthritis (Degenerative Joint Disease)
Etiology		
Pathophysiology		
Signs and symptoms		
Medical management		

Activity E *Briefly answer the following questions.*

1. Describe the following proximal finger deformities associated with rheumatoid arthritis: swan neck deformity, Boutonnière deformity, and ulnar deviation.

_____

_____

_____

2. Temporomandibular disorder (TMD) is a cluster of symptoms localized near the jaw. Describe these symptoms.

_____

_____

_____

3. What are the two treatment approaches for gout?

_____

_____

_____

4. Describe the etiology of systemic lupus erythematosus (SLE).

_____

_____

_____

5. Describe how osteomyelitis may occur.

_____

_____

6. Describe the pathophysiology of osteoporosis.

_____

_____

_____

7. Where are malignant bone tumors usually found?

_____

_____

_____

SECTION 2: APPLYING YOUR KNOWLEDGE

Activity F *Give rationales for the following questions.*

1. Why does the nurse advise the client to take aspirin and NSAIDs with food?

_____

_____

_____

2. Why does the nurse place a cradle over the affected joint for the client with gout?

_____

_____

_____

3. Why does aging contribute to osteoporosis?

_____

_____

_____

4. Why is bone mass structurally weaker, and why do bone deformities occur with osteomalacia?

_____

_____

_____

5. Why would a client with systemic lupus erythematosus have coping issues? What assistance can the nurse provide?

_____

_____

_____

_____

6. Why would respiratory compromise be an issue for a client with ankylosing spondylitis?

_____

_____

_____

7. Why were some COX-2 inhibitors removed from the market?

_____

_____

_____

Activity G _Answer the following questions related to caring for clients with orthopedic and connective tissue disorders._

1. What are viscosupplements used for? Describe their effects and side effects.

_____

_____

_____

2. Describe the nursing management for the client with rheumatoid arthritis.

_____

_____

_____

3. Describe the nursing management for the client with osteoarthritis.

_____

_____

_____

4. What are the signs and symptoms of systemic lupus erythematosus?

_____

_____

_____

5. Describe the medical and surgical management of osteomyelitis.

_____

_____

_____

6. What are the three stages of Lyme disease?

_____

_____

_____

7. How is osteoporosis medically managed?

_____

_____

_____

8. Describe the pathophysiology of Paget's disease.

_____

_____

_____

Activity H *Think over the following questions. Discuss them with your instructor or peers.*

1. Your client does not understand the articular and extra-articular manifestations of rheumatoid arthritis. What educational information would you provide?

_____

_____

_____

2. Which high-priority nursing diagnoses and interventions would you identify for a client with rheumatoid arthritis?

_____

_____

_____

3. Your client has a family history of osteoarthritis. What educational information would you provide about the prevention of osteoarthritis?

_____

_____

_____

4. A client with systemic lupus erythematosus is distraught, related to her physical appearance and limitations. How would you support her and promote coping?

_____

_____

_____

5. Your client lives in an area where deer ticks are common. What educational information would you provide to promote prevention of Lyme disease?

_____

_____

_____

SECTION 3: GETTING READY FOR NCLEX

Activity I *Choose the correct response for the following questions.*

1. Which of the following should the nurse emphasize during the education of a client with degenerative joint disease?
   1. Sleep on a firm mattress.
   2. Maintain moderate activity.
   3. Take aspirin on an empty stomach.
   4. Avoid purine-rich foods.

2. When teaching a client about gout, the nurse is correct when stating which of the following increases the excretion of uric acid?
   1. A high fluid intake
   2. Use of salicylates
   3. A high intake of purine-rich foods
   4. A low intake of carbohydrates

3. When examining a client with ankylosing spondylitis, which symptom does the nurse expect to see?
   1. Painful movement of a joint
   2. Swelling and tenderness at a joint
   3. Low back pain and stiffness
   4. Partial paralysis of lower extremities

4. Which of the following should a nurse instruct a client with lupus erythematosus to use before performing ROM exercises?
   1. Prescribed analgesics
   2. Cold packs
   3. Moist heat
   4. Braces or splints

5. Which of the following symptoms would the nurse observe in a client who is in the midstage of Lyme disease?
   1. Joint erosion
   2. Fever, chills, and malaise
   3. Arthritis
   4. Facial palsy and meningitis

6. In providing care for clients with osteoporosis, the nurse emphasizes the need for a nutritious, well-balanced diet that is high in which of the following?
   1. Calcium
   2. Iron
   3. Zinc
   4. Carbohydrates

7. When reviewing lab results for a client with Paget's disease, a nurse is correct to expect which of the following results?
   1. Elevated serum alkaline phosphatase level
   2. Decreased urinary hydroxyproline excretion
   3. Elevated leukocyte count
   4. Elevated creatinine level

8. To reduce the risk of renal calculi, a complication of prolonged immobility and gout, the nurse should advise clients to drink at least _____ quarts of fluid daily.
   1. 1
   2. 2
   3. 3
   4. 4

9. A client with a disease of the bones is beginning to feel better. Which of the following critical instructions should a nurse provide this client at this stage?
   1. Advise the client to reduce the dosage of the prescribed drugs.
   2. Caution the client against discontinuing the prescribed drugs.
   3. Urge the client to resume heavy activity.
   4. Encourage the client to gain weight.

10. Which of the following teaching points does the nurse stress to the client with systemic lupus erythematosus (SLE)?
   1. Apply ice as instructed.
   2. Avoid sunlight and ultraviolet radiation.
   3. Use assistive devices appropriately.
   4. Change dressing as prescribed.

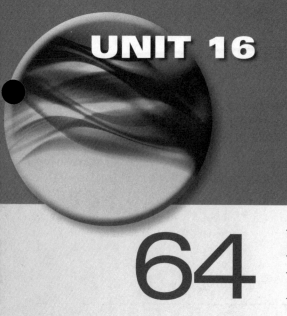
64 Introduction to the Integumentary System

LEARNING OBJECTIVES

1. Name the structures that form the integument.
2. List four functions of the integumentary system.
3. Identify the purpose of sebum and melanin.
4. Differentiate between eccrine and apocrine glands.
5. Name at least three facts about the integument that are pertinent to document when obtaining a health history.
6. Give the characteristics of normal skin.
7. Describe the criteria for staging pressure sores.
8. List characteristics of hair assessed during a physical examination.
9. Describe the characteristics of normal nails.
10. Name four diagnostic tests performed to determine the etiology of skin disorders.
11. Describe seven medical and surgical techniques for treating skin disorders.

SECTION 1: ASSESSING YOUR UNDERSTANDING

Activity A *Fill in the blanks by choosing the correct word from the options given in parentheses.*

1. The epidermis is constantly shed and replaced with epithelial cells from the dermis every day. The epidermis is totally replaced approximately every _____ days. *(25 to 35, 35 to 45, 45 to 55)*

2. The _____ is the layer of skin attached to muscle and bone. It is composed primarily of connective tissue and fat cells. *(dermis, subcutaneous tissue, epidermis)*

3. _____ are connected to each hair follicle and secrete an oily substance called sebum, which is a lubricant that prevents drying and cracking of the skin and hair. *(Sebaceous glands, Apocrine glands, Eccrine glands)*

4. A fungal culture requires incubation at room temperature for _____ weeks. *(1 to 2, 2 to 3, 3 to 4)*

5. _____ are prescribed when allergy is a factor in causing a skin disorder. They relieve itching and shorten the duration of the allergic reaction. *(Antihistamines, Antiseptics, Analgesics)*

6. Fingernails and toenails are layers of hard keratin that have a _____ function. *(sensory, protective, chemical synthesis)*

Activity B   *Write the correct term for each description.*

1. Consists of connective tissue and contains elastic fibers, blood vessels, sensory and motor nerves, sweat and sebaceous (oil) glands, and hair follicles (roots). _____

2. The color of the skin is determined by this pigment, which is manufactured by melanocytes located in the epidermis. _____

3. It covers all parts of the body except the palms, soles, dorsum of the fingers, lips, penis, labia, and nipples. _____

4. These commonly occur on the skin over the coccyx and sacrum in the lower spine, the hips, heels, elbows, shoulder blades, ears, and back of head. _____

5. A handheld device that can identify certain fungal infections that fluoresce under long-wave ultraviolet light. _____

6. Medications applied directly to the scalp or incorporated into shampooing products. They are used to control dandruff. _____

Activity C   *Match the stages of a pressure sore in Column A with their correct descriptions in Column B.*

Column A

_____ 1. Stage I

_____ 2. Stage II

_____ 3. Stage III

_____ 4. Stage IV

Column B

a. The most traumatic and life-threatening stage. The tissue is deeply ulcerated, exposing muscle and bone. The dead tissue produces a rank odor. Local infection, which is the rule rather than the exception, easily spreads throughout the body, causing a potentially fatal condition referred to as sepsis.

b. Characterized by redness of the skin; the reddened skin fails to resume its normal color, or blanch, when pressure is relieved.

c. A shallow crater extends to the subcutaneous tissue. These pressure sores may be accompanied by serous drainage from leaking plasma or purulent drainage (white or yellow-tinged fluid) caused by a wound infection. The area is relatively painless.

d. The area is reddened and accompanied by blistering or a shallow break in the skin, sometimes described as a skin tear. Impairment of the skin leads to microbial colonization and infection of the wound.

Activity D   *Provide the description and identify the purpose of the following medical and surgical treatments based on the given criteria.*

Treatment	Description	Purpose
Surgical excision		
Laser therapy		
Cryosurgery		
Electrodesiccation		
Photochemotherapy		

Activity E *Briefly answer the following questions.*

1. Describe the functions of the integumentary system.

_____

_____

_____

2. How does the skin facilitate the synthesis of vitamin D?

_____

_____

_____

3. How does a pressure sore occur?

_____

_____

_____

4. What causes an abnormal thickening of the nails?

_____

_____

5. What is the purpose of a skin biopsy?

_____

_____

_____

6. What medications are used to treat infectious skin disorders?

_____

_____

_____

7. Describe how keratolytics are used to treat warts, corns, and calluses.

_____

_____

_____

8. What is the purpose of a therapeutic bath?

_____

_____

_____

_____

SECTION 2: APPLYING YOUR KNOWLEDGE

Activity F *Give rationale for the following questions.*

1. Why is the skin considered protective?

_____

_____

_____

2. Why can exposure to warm temperatures and densely saturated moist air result in heat stroke?

_____

_____

_____

3. Why is thermoregulation altered in the older adult?

_____

_____

4. Why does odor occur with perspiration?

_____

_____

_____

5. Why are older adults more vulnerable to heat?

_____

_____

6. Why do nails have a pink semitransparent appearance?

_____

_____

7. Why would a physician order a potassium hydroxide test?

_____

_____

_____

8. Why are emollients, ointments, powders, and lotions used on the skin?

_____

_____

_____

Activity G *Answer the following questions related to the integumentary system.*

1. Describe the four methods of how heat is lost and provide an example of each.

_____

_____

_____

2. Describe the elements of a skin assessment and identify normal findings.

_____

_____

_____

3. Identify measures that reduce conditions under which pressure sores are likely to form.

_____

_____

_____

4. Describe the elements of a nail assessment.

_____

_____

_____

5. Describe the application and purpose of a wet dressing.

_____

_____

_____

6. Describe why lifestyle changes are important to some skin disorders.

_____

_____

_____

Activity H *Think over the following questions. Discuss them with your instructor or peers.*

1. Your client has a stage II pressure sore. What nutritional information would you provide to the client?

_____

_____

_____

2. Your older client requires assistance with moving and transferring. How would you educate the staff in the movement of this client to prevent a pressure sore?

_____

_____

_____

3. Your client requires the application of a topical medication. What is the nursing care required for this medication administration?

_____

_____

_____

SECTION 3: GETTING READY FOR NCLEX

Activity I *Answer the following questions.*

1. A nurse explains the purposes of the ridges and indentations on the ventral surface of the hands and feet. Which of the following are accurate? Select all that apply.
   1. They provide a unique means of identification.
   2. They facilitate the ability to grip and hold objects.
   3. They form a tough protective protein called keratin.
   4. They stretch with little damage after soft-tissue injury.

2. Which of the following actions helps the nurse assess the skin temperature?
   1. Palpating the skin lightly with the fingertips
   2. Using the palms of the hand on the skin surface
   3. Grasping the skin between the thumb and forefinger
   4. Placing the dorsum of the hand on the skin

3. What nursing advice is best when the nurse observes small, yellow or brown raised lesions on the face and trunk of an older adult?
   1. Limit the amount of time spent in direct sunlight.
   2. Consult a physician; these may be precancerous.
   3. Include a daily supplement of vitamin D.
   4. Apply an emollient such as lanolin liberally to the skin.

4. During the routine nail assessment of a client, the nurse notices that the angle between the nail base and the skin is greater than 160°. What does this finding indicate?
   1. Inadequate nutrition
   2. Iron-deficiency anemia
   3. Chronic cardiopulmonary disease
   4. Fungal infection

5. A nurse is caring for a client who has been bedridden for several years. Which of the following actions is most appropriate for the nurse to perform if reddened areas over bony prominences blanch with pressure relief?
   1. Massage bony red areas.
   2. Wash with soap and water.
   3. Increase time in a chair.
   4. Expose the skin to light.

6. Which of the following is the chief factor that predisposes a client in traction for a fractured femur to develop a pressure sore?
   1. Prolonged healing
   2. Physical immobility
   3. Reduced appetite
   4. Atrophy of muscle

7. A nurse identifies a skin lesion on a client noting that the lesion is elevated, round, and filled with serum. What is the correct term that describes the nurse's assessment finding?
   1. Macule
   2. Papule
   3. Wheal
   4. Vesicle

8. A nurse is taking care of a client and detects that the overall appearance of the skin is yellow. What is an explanation for the yellow skin color?
   1. Abnormal erythrocytes
   2. Liver or kidney disease
   3. Low tissue oxygenation
   4. Trauma to soft tissue

9. A client is concerned about the potential for side effects when a topical corticosteroid is prescribed for an inflammatory skin lesion? What information can the nurse provide this client?
   1. Side effects only occur after prolonged treatment.
   2. Side effects are temporary until the drug is discontinued.
   3. Side effects are unlikely with topical applications.
   4. Side effects can be minimized with fewer applications.

10. What is the best explanation a nurse can provide for leaving a wet dressing in place until it has dried?
   1. Allowing the dressing to dry prolongs cooling of the wound.
   2. A dry dressing results in less pain during its removal.
   3. Leaving the dressing until dry reduces the risk for infection.
   4. A dry dressing facilitates removing dead tissue and debris.

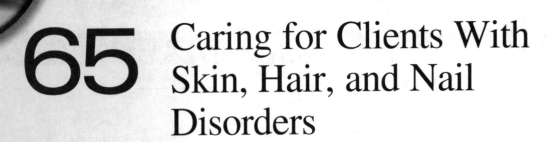

65 Caring for Clients With Skin, Hair, and Nail Disorders

LEARNING OBJECTIVES

1. Identify risks associated with tattooing and body piercing.
2. Describe general care following tattooing and body piercing.
3. Define and name two types of dermatitis.
4. Explain factors that lead to acne vulgaris.
5. Describe characteristics of rosacea.
6. Differentiate between a furuncle, furunculosis, and carbuncle.
7. Describe the appearance and cause of psoriasis.
8. Describe the process for eradicating a skin mite infection using a scabicidal medication.
9. Identify locations on the body where parasitic fungi known as dermatophytes are most likely to infect.
10. Describe the characteristics of an outbreak of shingles.
11. Discuss factors that promote skin cancer as well as measures that help prevent it.
12. Name two conditions characterized by hair loss and the etiology for each.
13. Describe the appearance of head lice and nits and explain how to remove them.
14. Discuss factors that promote fungal infections of the nails.
15. Name techniques for preventing onychocryptosis (ingrown toenails).

SECTION 1:   ASSESSING YOUR UNDERSTANDING

Activity A   *Fill in the blanks by choosing the correct word from the options given in parentheses.*

1. With _____, the skin response is characterized by dilation of the blood vessels, causing redness and swelling, and sometimes by vesiculation and oozing. Itching is a prominent symptom. *(dermatitis, psoriasis, rosacea)*

2. _____ is a method of removing surface layers of scarred skin. It is useful in lessening scars such as the pitting from severe acne. The outermost layers of the skin are removed by sandpaper, a rotating wire brush, chemicals (chemical face peeling), or a diamond wheel. *(Scarification, Salabrasion, Dermabrasion)*

3. _____ is a chronic, noninfectious inflammatory disorder of the skin that affects both men and women. Its onset is in young and middle adulthood. Periods of emotional stress, hormonal cycles, infection, and seasonal changes appear to aggravate the condition. *(Dermatitis, Psoriasis, Rosacea)*

4. _____ is a dermatologic condition associated with excessive production of secretions from the sebaceous glands. Although it is not always confined to the scalp, it is one of the primary sites. *(Alopecia, Seborrhea, Lice)*

5. _____ is a fungal dermatophyte infection of the fingernails or toenails. *(Onychomycosis, Seborrhea, Onychocryptosis)*

Activity B *Write the correct term for each description.*

1. The insertion of a metal ring or barbell, which is a straight or curved rod, into a body part. Common locations include lips, ear cartilage, cheeks, nose, tongue, eyebrows, navel, nipples, or genital area. _____

2. Mild cases improve with gentle facial cleansing and nonprescription drying agents containing benzoyl peroxide. _____

3. Factors that contribute to vasodilation or irritation of the skin may trigger blushing; examples include consuming hot beverages, spicy food, or alcohol; exposure to sun, wind, or cold; bathing with hot water; stress; or use of skin care products. _____

4. A combination of UV light therapy and a photosensitizing psoralen drug such as methoxsalen (Oxsoralen-Ultra). It also has been used for severe, disabling psoriasis that does not respond to other methods of treatment. _____

5. The medical term for an ingrown toenail. _____

6. A person trained to care for feet. _____

Activity C *Describe the pathophysiology and signs and symptoms of the skin disorders that follow.*

Disorder	Pathophysiology	Signs and Symptoms
Scabies		
Dermatophytoses		
Shingles		

Activity D *Briefly answer the following questions.*

1. Describe the medical management of dermatitis.

_____

_____

_____

2. Describe the medical management of a furuncle, furunculosis, or carbuncle.

_____

_____

_____

3. Describe the etiology of psoriasis.

_____

_____

_____

4. Describe the medical management of scabies.

_____

_____

_____

5. Describe the appearance and treatment for lice.

_____

_____

_____

SECTION 2: APPLYING YOUR KNOWLEDGE

Activity E *Give rationale for the following questions.*

1. Why does the American Association of Blood Banks reject potential blood donors who have received a tattoo within 1 year?

_____

_____

_____

2. Why is furunculosis associated with diabetes?

_____

_____

_____

3. Why should pediculicides not be used on pets?

_____

_____

_____

4. Why does the nurse instruct the client or family not to rinse with a conditioner after shampooing the hair before applying a pediculicide?

_____

_____

_____

5. Why are sutures not required for the surgical treatment of onychocryptosis?

_____

_____

_____

Activity F *Answer the following questions related to caring for clients with skin, hair, and nail disorders.*

1. What are the risks associated with body tattooing?

_____

_____

_____

2. What are the risks associated with body piercing?

_____

_____

_____

3. What treatment options are available for clients with severe acne vulgaris?

_____

_____

_____

4. Describe the nursing management of a client with a furuncle, furunculosis, or carbuncle.

_____

_____

_____

5. Describe the pathophysiology and signs and symptoms of psoriasis.

_____

_____

_____

6. What factors predispose a client to malignant changes in the skin?

_____

_____

_____

Activity G   *Think over the following questions. Discuss them with your instructor or peers.*

1. A neighbor has received a tattoo and asks you how to care for the affected area of the skin. What educational information would you provide?

_____

_____

_____

2. A coworker is considering a body piercing but is unfamiliar with the risks and care following a piercing. What educational information would you provide?

_____

_____

_____

3. You volunteer to provide educational information about skin cancer prevention at a health promotion fair. What information will you provide?

_____

_____

_____

4. A friend calls and states that her child has been sent home from school due to head lice. The friend asks you what to do. How would you advise her on the treatment and procedure for removing lice?

_____

_____

_____

Activity H   *Read the following case study. Use critical thinking skills to discuss and answer the questions that follow it.*

A client is referred by a primary healthcare provider to the dermatologist's office to have a suspicious new skin lesion examined. The client is seen initially by the nurse who examines and measures the skin lesion, which is located on the client's right lower forearm. The skin lesion appears small and shiny with gray plaque. The nurse inquires regarding when the lesion was first noticed and about any changes that may have occurred since then. The nurse notes in the chart that the client is light skinned and works outside several hours of the day as part of employment. The nurse educates the client on how to prevent further skin damage and skin cancer and then updates the physician.

1. Based on the appearance of the skin lesion, location, and the client's information, what type of skin lesion does this client most likely have?

_____

_____

_____

2. Which treatment options are available for this client?

_____

_____

_____

3. If this client continues to fail to protect skin from exposure to UV radiation, for what other potential health problems is this client at risk?

_____

_____

_____

SECTION 3: GETTING READY FOR NCLEX

Activity I *Answer the following questions.*

1. What is the best nursing suggestion for an elderly client who experiences itching from dry skin in the winter time?
   1. Take hot baths with antibacterial soap daily.
   2. Apply lotion or cream to the skin.
   3. Take an antipruritic to control the itching.
   4. Wear clothing that exposes the skin to the air.

2. Following the diagnosis of dermatophytosis, a client asks the nurse to identify its cause. What is the most accurate answer?
   1. The skin disorder is caused by an itch mite.
   2. The skin disorder is caused by a parasitic fungi.
   3. The skin disorder is caused by a reactivated virus.
   4. The skin disorder is caused by a lice infestation.

3. A client will undergo surgical treatment of a persistent ingrown toenail. Which of the following nursing statements indicates correct information?
   1. Fast overnight to avoid vomiting from general anesthesia.
   2. Bleeding will be minimal as the physician will clamp blood vessels.
   3. The entire nail will be removed from the affected toe.
   4. The procedure will not require suturing the site.

4. What nursing instruction is best regarding self-care for a client with onychomycosis of the foot?
   1. Take antifungal medication for 10 days.
   2. Change from leather shoes to tennis shoes.
   3. Avoid walking barefoot.
   4. Keep the feet moist.

5. What is the most important measure the nurse can teach a diabetic client with a carbuncle on the foot to prevent the spread of infection?
   1. Soak the foot in warm epsom salt solution.
   2. Dispose of soiled dressings in a paper bag.
   3. Wash hands before and after touching the area.
   4. Use hydrogen peroxide to clean the infected area.

6. A client is using acne preparations containing benzoyl peroxide. What instruction should the nurse give to the client to prevent fabric discoloration?
   1. Thoroughly wash hands after each application.
   2. Wash clothing in a strong detergent and bleach.
   3. Use an atomizer to spray the benzoyl peroxide.
   4. Don disposable vinyl gloves for drug applications.

7. Which of the following actions from the nurse is best for helping a client with psoriasis who is distressed by the fact that the condition is incurable?
   1. Suggest joining a psoriasis support group.
   2. Recommend dermabrasion.
   3. Suggest applications of anthralin.
   4. Refer the client for a skin graft.

8. What information is important to provide a female client with acne who will be treated with isotretinoin (Accutane)? Select all that apply.
   1. Take the drug only when acne is at its worst.
   2. Have a pregnancy test before treatment.
   3. Consult the physician if breastfeeding an infant.
   4. Use a reliable contraceptive during drug use.

9. Which of the following is the most important measure for preventing skin cancer when a nurse instructs a client who frequents a swimming pool?
   1. Wear a hat with a wide brim and cover the back of the neck.
   2. Use a sunscreen with an SPF of at least 15 and reapply every 2 hours.
   3. Use a lip balm with sunscreen and apply frequently.
   4. Stay in the shade when outdoors and only swim after 2:00 p.m.

10. A client is frustrated because of her hair loss. Which of the following is most appropriate for the nurse to recommend?
    1. Use a narrow-toothed comb
    2. Style hair in a ponytail or braids
    3. Use of a conditioner or detangler after shampooing
    4. Ask the physician to prescribe finasteride (Propecia).

66 Caring for Clients With Burns

LEARNING OBJECTIVES

1. Explain how the depth and percentage of burns are determined.

2. Name three life-threatening complications of serious burns.

3. Differentiate between open and closed methods of wound care for burns.

4. Name three sources of skin grafts.

5. Describe nursing management for the client with a burn injury.

SECTION 1: ASSESSING YOUR UNDERSTANDING

Activity A *Fill in the blanks by choosing the correct word from the options given in parentheses.*

1. A burn is a _____ injury to the skin and underlying tissues. Heat, chemicals, or electricity cause burn injuries. *(superficial, traumatic, deep)*

2. _____ is a quick assessment technique to estimate how much of the client's skin surface is involved. *(Comparing the client's foot with the size of the burn wound, Comparing the client's palm with the size of the burn wound, Rule of tens)*

3. _____ is the removal of necrotic tissue. *(Autograft, Debridement, Allograft)*

4. A disadvantage of surgical debridement is _____. *(infection, bleeding, pain)*

5. Skin grafting is necessary for _____ burns because the skin layers responsible for regeneration have been destroyed. *(superficial and superficial partial-thickness, superficial partial-thickness and deep partial-thickness, deep partial-thickness and full-thickness)*

6. _____ or homograft is human skin obtained from a cadaver. *(An autograft, An allograft, A heterograft)*

7. _____ is a temporary covering that promotes wound healing by interacting directly with body tissues. It can be applied all over the burn wound as soon as the skin is cleaned and debrided instead of having to wait until enough skin is available for grafting purposes. *(Skin substitutes, Cultured skins, Autografts)*

Activity B *Write the correct term for each description.*

1. Generally, the drug of choice to manage severe pain for a burn victim. _____

2. If the eschar constricts the area and impairs circulation, this procedure, which involves an incision into the eschar, is done to relieve pressure on the affected area. _____

3. The regrowth of skin. _____

4. Only skin transplanted from one identical twin to another, or this type of graft, can become a permanent part of the client's own skin. _____

5. The epidermis and a thin layer of dermis are harvested from the client's skin. This type of autograft is usually obtained from the buttocks or thighs. _____

6. This type of autograft includes epidermis, dermis, and some subcutaneous tissue. It is used when the burned area is fairly small or involves the hands, face, or neck. _____

7. A wound-closure product that is developed by growing the client's own skin cells in a laboratory culture medium. From a piece of postage stamp–sized skin, a sheet of epithelial cells may be grown, which is then transferred to the burned areas. _____

Activity C *Match the zones of burn injury in Column A with their correct descriptions in Column B.*

Column A

_____ **1.** Zone of coagulation

_____ **2.** Zone of stasis

_____ **3.** Zone of hyperemia

Column B

a. The area of least injury, where the epidermis and dermis are only minimally damaged.

b. The area of intermediate burn injury, it is here that blood vessels are damaged, but the tissue has the potential to survive.

c. The area at the center of the injury, where the injury is most severe and usually deepest.

Activity D *Differentiate between the various depths of burn injury based on the given criteria.*

Burn Injury	Depth and Characteristics
Superficial burn	
Superficial partial-thickness burn	
Deep partial-thickness burn	
Full-thickness burn	

Activity E *Briefly answer the following questions.*

1. Describe the difference between the pathophysiologic changes in thermal, chemical, and electrical burns.

_____

_____

_____

2. What neuroendocrine changes occur with serious burns?

_____

_____

_____

3. What factors increase the mortality rate from burn injuries?

_____

_____

_____

4. Name three potential complications of burns that can be life threatening.

_____

_____

_____

5. What are the goals of fluid resuscitation?

_____

_____

_____

6. What three microorganisms most commonly cause infection in burned tissue?

_____

_____

_____

7. Name the three major antimicrobial agents used for the treatment of burn victims.

_____

_____

_____

SECTION 2: APPLYING YOUR KNOWLEDGE

Activity F   *Give rationale for the following questions.*

1. Why are burns caused by electricity characteristically the most severe?

_____

_____

_____

2. Why can burns result in serious complications for the older adult?

_____

_____

_____

3. Why may the estimate of burn depth be revised in the first 24 to 72 hours?

_____

_____

_____

4. Why is impaired ventilation associated with a burn involving the upper airway?

_____

_____

_____

5. Why do healthcare providers wear powder-free sterile gloves when caring for a burn victim?

_____

_____

_____

6. Why is the body hair around the perimeter of the burn shaved?

_____

_____

_____

7. Why is skin grafting performed?

_____

_____

_____

Activity G   *Answer the following questions that relate to caring for clients with burns.*

1. Describe the pathophysiology of a burn.

_____

_____

2. Describe the initial first aid for a burn victim.

_____

_____

_____

3. Describe the acute care for a burn victim.

_____

_____

_____

4. Describe the closed method of wound management.

_____

_____

_____

5. What are the disadvantages of harvesting the client's own tissue for a graft?

_____

_____

_____

6. Describe the care for a client following a skin graft.

_____

_____

_____

Activity H *Think over the following questions. Discuss them with your instructor or peers.*

1. Your client with full-thickness burns is upset because everyone entering the room is in sterile attire. The client feels detached from people. How would you explain the importance of sterile attire to the client?

_____

_____

_____

2. Your client needs nutritional support via a nasogastric tube. However, the client is refusing to have the tube inserted. How would you explain the importance of nutritional support to the client?

_____

_____

_____

3. A burn victim is brought in to the emergency department. How would you assess the client to determine whether there are signs of heat injury or smoke inhalation injury?

_____

_____

_____

4. Your client has carbon monoxide poisoning and is going for hyperbaric oxygen treatment. How would you explain this treatment to the client?

_____

_____

_____

SECTION 3: GETTING READY FOR NCLEX

Activity I *Answer the following questions.*

1. Which of the following are correctly identified by a nurse as goals of fluid resuscitation following a burn injury? Select all that apply.
  1. Restoration of nutrition
  2. Replacing vascular volume
  3. Reducing blood loss
  4. Preventing cellular ischemia
  5. Maintaining organ functions

2. The nurse observes that some burned areas appear black and leathery. What is the most accurate nursing identification of this burned area?
  1. Superficial burn
  2. Superficial partial thickness burn
  3. Deep partial thickness burn
  4. Full thickness burn

3. Which of the following nursing assessment findings suggest that a burn victim is experiencing hypovolemic shock? Select all that apply.
  1. Hypotension
  2. Dilated pupils
  3. Capillary refill <3 seconds
  4. Tachycardia
  5. Anuria
  6. Respiratory stridor

4. When a client asks a nurse about the advantages in using cultured skin to cover a burn wound, what is the most accurate answer? Select all that apply.
   1. Healing occurs rapidly.
   2. Culturing skin is a speedy process.
   3. A large burn area can be covered.
   4. Tissue rejection is unlikely.

5. Which of the following nursing instructions is best for preventing permanent pigment changes where a client has undergone skin grafting?
   1. Wear several layers of clothing.
   2. Use a high SPF sunscreen outdoors.
   3. Slowly expose the graft to sunlight.
   4. Rub the skin graft with vitamin D.

6. Which of the following nursing interventions is essential for minimizing the risk of mortality when caring for a client with extensive burns?
   1. Administering prescribed analgesics.
   2. Relieving the client's depression.
   3. Maintaining bowel elimination.
   4. Providing adequate nutrition.

7. Which of the following assessment findings suggest to the nurse that a client may have experience smoke inhalation? Select all that apply.
   1. Burn involving the chest
   2. Oxygen saturation <90 mmHg
   3. Singed nasal hair
   4. Carbon particles in sputum
   5. Dry oral mucous membranes

8. What is the best reason the nurse can provide for performing an escharotomy on a burned client?
   1. This procedure promotes epithelialization.
   2. This procedure reduces the potential for infection.
   3. This procedure relieves tissue constriction.
   4. This procedure decreases pain intensity.

9. The nurse applies mafenide acetate (Sulfamylon) to a burn wound. The nurse is correct in identifying which advantage for its use?
   1. It is relatively painless when applied.
   2. It effectively penetrates eschar.
   3. It is a low-cost antimicrobial.
   4. It avoids acid-base imbalances.

10. Calculate the volume of Lactated Ringers intravenous solution a client should receive for fluid resuscitation when the physican orders 4 mL/kg/% of burn. The client weighs 186 lbs. and has a 50% total body surface burned area. Round the client's weight to the nearest whole number.

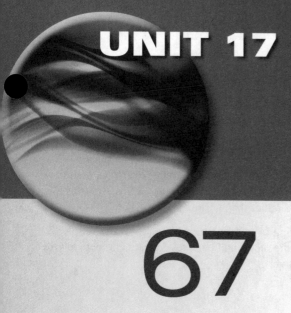

UNIT 17

CARING FOR CLIENTS WITH PSYCHOBIOLOGIC DISORDERS

67 Interaction of Body and Mind

LEARNING OBJECTIVES

1. Discuss new areas of neuroscience being studied to learn more about mind-body connections and their effect on health.
2. Name chemical substances transmitted between neurons, giving examples of each.
3. Explain why mental illnesses are now considered psychobiologic disorders.
4. Name biologic and psychologic components that contribute to disorders affecting the body and mind.
5. List examples of techniques used to assess clients with psychobiologic disorders.
6. Describe treatment and nursing care for psychobiologic disorders.
7. Distinguish between stress, eustress, and distress.
8. Describe the general adaptation syndrome, naming its three stages.
9. Explain the purpose of coping mechanisms and the outcomes that may result from their use.
10. List the defining features of hardiness.
11. Discuss techniques that the nurse can suggest for helping clients cope with stressors.
12. Discuss the rationale for a mind–immune system connection.
13. Discuss four explanations for the development of psychosomatic disorders.
14. Describe treatment and nursing care for psychosomatic disorders.
15. Explain the placebo effect.

SECTION 1: ASSESSING YOUR UNDERSTANDING

Activity A *Fill in the blanks by choosing the correct word from the options given in parentheses.*

1. _____ are conditions in which evidence affirms a connection between abnormalities in the brain and altered cognition, perception, emotion, behavior, and socialization. *(Psychological disorders, Psychosocial disorders, Psychobiologic disorders)*

2. _____ aims at correcting the underlying biochemical abnormality. *(Drug therapy, Psychotherapy, Cognitive therapy)*

3. According to Selye's theory (1956), _____ is a physiologic response to biologic stressors such as surgical trauma or infection, psychological stressors such as worry and fear, or sociologic stressors, including a new job or increased family responsibilities. *(fear, stress, emotion)*

4. _____ are the unconscious tactics humans use to protect the self from feeling inadequate or threatened. *(Physiological responses, Coping mechanisms, General adaptation syndromes)*

5. Psychosomatic disorders are also known as _____ -related disorders. *(stress, mood, anxiety)*

6. The effect of chronically suppressing _____ and the neurochemical changes that accompany it, however, may be the triggering mechanism for a dysfunctional immune response. *(anger, dependence, ambivalence)*

Activity B *Write the correct term for each description.*

1. It is the structure in the brain for sensory perception, voluntary movement, personality, intelligence, language, thoughts, judgment, emotions, memory, creativity, and motivation. _____

2. A technique that compares a client's brain activity patterns (from an EEG or other electronic image) with a computerized database of electrophysiologic abnormalities. _____

3. Implicated in the development or exacerbation of autoimmune diseases, anorexia nervosa, obsessive-compulsive disorder, panic attacks, thyroid conditions, heart disease, functional and inflammatory disorders of the gastrointestinal tract, chronic pain conditions, and diabetes. _____

4. A nonspecific physiologic response to a stressor. _____

5. Characteristics include a commitment to something meaningful versus a sense of alienation, a sense of having control over sources of stress versus a feeling of helplessness, and the perception of life events as a challenge rather than a threat. _____

6. The healing or improvement that takes place simply because the individual believes a treatment method will be effective. _____

Activity C *Match the theorists in Column A with their proposed theory in Column B.*

Column A

_____ 1. Sigmund Freud

_____ 2. Erik Erikson and Harry Stack Sullivan

_____ 3. B. F. Skinner

Column B

a. Proposed the theory that adaptive and maladaptive behaviors are learned and repeated because of rewarding reinforcement.

b. Proposed that mental health or illness is a consequence of social relationships and interpersonal interactions.

c. Proposed that disordered behavior is the result of intra-personal (within oneself) conflicts that arise during particular stages of development that occur between infancy and adolescence.

Activity D *Identify some of the functions of the following neurotransmitters.*

Neurotransmitter	Functions
Serotonin	
Dopamine	
Norepinephrine	
Acetylcholine	
Gamma-aminobutyric acid	
Glutamate	

Activity E   *Briefly answer the following questions.*

1. Describe the structures in the brain that play the greatest role in connecting the mind with physiologic functions.

_____

_____

_____

2. Identify three types of neuropeptides.

_____

_____

_____

3. What suggests that the brain, endocrine system, and immune system communicate with each other?

_____

_____

_____

4. Which components of an extensive mental status examination elicit information about a person's cognitive and mental state?

_____

_____

_____

5. Describe the advantages and disadvantages of coping mechanisms.

_____

_____

_____

6. How can stress affect the immune system?

_____

_____

_____

SECTION 2:   APPLYING YOUR KNOWLEDGE

Activity F   *Give rationale for the following questions.*

1. Why might an older adult be more vulnerable to stressors?

_____

_____

2. Why are clients with psychosomatic illnesses given anti-inflammatory and corticosteroid drugs?

_____

_____

3. Why might an excessive expression of hostility be related to increased incidents of heart disease?

_____

_____

4. Why is it important to conduct tests before assuming that a disorder is stress induced?

_____

_____

5. Why do clients taking placebos experience improvement?

_____

_____

Activity G *Answer the following questions related to caring for clients with psychobiologic disorders.*

1. Describe the relationship between receptors and neurotransmitters.

_____

_____

_____

2. Describe the physiologic stress response.

_____

_____

_____

3. How can a nurse foster effective coping skills?

_____

_____

_____

Activity H *Think over the following questions. Discuss them with your instructor or peers.*

1. A client with irritable bowel syndrome asks you how his symptoms are related to stress. How would you explain this relationship to him?

_____

_____

_____

2. A client is diagnosed with a mood disorder and does not understand how neurotransmitters play a part in her diagnosis. What would you tell her?

_____

_____

_____

3. Describe how the effects of psychobiology, intrapersonal conflicts, learned behavior, and social relationships/interpersonal interactions play a role in mental illness.

_____

_____

_____

SECTION 3:   GETTING READY FOR NCLEX

Activity I *Answer the following questions.*

1. Which of the following nutritional instructions should a nurse give to stress-prone clients?
   1. Eat at regular intervals.
   2. Eat only when hungry.
   3. Eat only one meal a day.
   4. Avoid products containing lactose.

2. When a nurse assesses a client, which of the following findings are most suggestive a stress response? Select all that apply.
   1. Tachycardia
   2. Hypertension
   3. Hyperperistalsis
   4. Hypoglycemia

3. When a client asks the nurse to describe the Minnesota Multiphasic Personality Inventory (MMPI), which response is most correct?
   1. You will be asked what you see when shown various inkblots.
   2. You will self-rate your mood by answering written questions.
   3. You will need to respond to many questions as true or false.
   4. You will need to tell a story about pictures you are shown.

4. When a nurse is asked to explain what a placebo is, which of the following is the best response?
   1. It is the equivalent of a biologically active substance.
   2. It is an inactive substance that can alter physiology.
   3. It is a healing technique used traditionally in folk medicine.
   4. It is an inert substance that becomes biologically active.

5. What techniques can the nurse suggest to increase a client's assertiveness? Select all that apply.
   1. Recommend keeping a diary
   2. Stating feelings clearly
   3. Delegating unwanted tasks
   4. Encourage setting priorities
   5. Saying "no" to requests

6. The nurse is correct in explaining that medications that mimic which of the following neurotransmitters help to relieve stress?
   1. Glutamate
   2. Norepinephrine
   3. Acetylcholine
   4. Gamm-aminoabutyric acid

7. Which of the following measures is most important for the nurse to recommend for promoting a client's ability to cope with stressors?
   1. Cultivate supportive relationships
   2. Drink alcohol in moderation
   3. Eliminate sources of caffeine
   4. Performing daily exercise

8. Which theorist is the nurse correct in identifying as one who proposed that adaptive and maladaptive behaviors are learned and repeated because of rewarding reinforcement?
   1. B.F. Skinner
   2. Harry Stack Sullivan
   3. Erik Erikson
   4. Sigmund Freud

9. A nurse is attending an in-service program on common mental disorders. Which of the following is a diagnostic category of mental disorders within the psychiatric illness domain?
   1. Uncontrolled anger
   2. Sleep deprivation
   3. Failed relationships
   4. Generalized anxiety

10. Which of the following are nursing responsibilities when caring for clients with psychobiologic disorders? Select all that apply.
    1. Administering prescribed psychotropic medications
    2. Implementing behavior modification protocols
    3. Promoting healthy coping strategies 4. Participating in group therapy meetings
    5. Measuring neurotransmitter blood levels
    6. Reviewing the results of brain mapping

68 Caring for Clients With Anxiety Disorders

LEARNING OBJECTIVES

1. Differentiate anxiety from fear.
2. Name four levels of anxiety, explaining the differences among the various levels.
3. Give six areas of nursing management that apply to the care of anxious clients.
4. Name examples of anxiety disorders.
5. List categories of drugs used to treat anxiety disorders.
6. Name and discuss two types of psychotherapy used to treat anxiety disorders.
7. List six nursing interventions that are helpful for reducing anxiety.
8. Discuss areas of teaching for clients with anxiety disorders.

SECTION 1: ASSESSING YOUR UNDERSTANDING

Activity A *Fill in the blanks by choosing the correct word from the options given in parentheses.*

1. _____ is a vague, uneasy feeling, the cause of which is not readily identifiable. It is evoked when a person anticipates nonspecific danger. *(Anxiety, Fear, Apprehension)*

2. _____ is manifested by the performance of an anxiety-relieving ritual to terminate a disturbing, persistent thought. *(A phobic disorder, A post-traumatic stress disorder, An obsessive-compulsive disorder)*

3. _____ are drugs that relieve the symptoms of anxiety. These medications include benzodiazepines and nonbenzodiazepines. *(Anxiolytics, Beta-adrenergic blockers, Central-acting sympatholytics)*

4. _____ are prescribed more often to control primary hypertension; however, they potentially have beneficial effects in anxious people with elevated blood pressure. *(Anxiolytics, Central-acting sympatholytics, Antidepressants)*

5. _____ involves talking with a psychiatrist, psychologist, clinical nurse specialist, or mental health counselor. *(Psychotherapy, Cognitive therapy, Behavioral therapy)*

Activity B *Write the correct term for each description.*

1. A feeling of terror in response to someone or something specific that a person perceives as dangerous or threatening. _____

2. A group of psychobiologic illnesses that result from activation of the autonomic nervous system, chiefly the sympathetic division. _____

3. A condition that involves a delayed anxiety response 3 or more months after an emotionally traumatic experience. _____

4. Following an emotionally traumatic event, the affected person avoids dealing with the tragedy and detaches himself or herself from others by using this technique. _____

5. Antidepressants prescribed for obsessive-compulsive disorder and post-traumatic stress disorder that sustain levels of serotonin. _____

6. A type of psychotherapy in which the therapist helps clients alter their irrational thinking, correct their faulty belief systems, and replace negative self-statements with positive ones. _____

Activity C *Match the levels of anxiety in Column A with the associated behavioral manifestations listed in Column B.*

Column A

_____ **1.** Mild

_____ **2.** Moderate

_____ **3.** Severe

_____ **4.** Panic

Column B

a. The client is more easily distracted and concentration is slightly impaired, but attention can be redirected. Learning takes more effort, perception narrows, problem solving becomes difficult, and the client is irritable and feels inadequate.

b. The client exaggerates details, perception is distorted, and learning is disabled. Thoughts are fragmented. The client cannot control emotions and feels helpless.

c. Attention is heightened, and sensory perception is expanded. The focus is on the stimuli, and reality is intact. Information processing is accurate, and the client feels in control.

d. The attention span decreases; the person cannot concentrate or remain focused, and perception is reduced. The ability to learn is impaired, and information processing is inaccurate or incomplete. The client is aware of extreme discomfort, and effort is needed to control emotions. The client feels incompetent.

Activity D *Briefly answer the following questions.*

1. Describe the changes that occur as anxiety escalates.

_____

_____

_____

2. What are the manifestations of a phobic disorder?

_____

_____

_____

3. What situations may trigger a flashback for a client with post-traumatic stress disorder?

_____

_____

_____

4. Describe the medical management of clients with anxiety disorders.

_____

_____

_____

5. Describe the process of desensitization.

_____

_____

_____

SECTION 2: APPLYING YOUR KNOWLEDGE

Activity E *Give rationale for the following questions.*

1. Why do some clients with post-traumatic stress disorder abuse substances?

_____

_____

_____

2. Why is long-term treatment with benzodiazepines not recommended?

_____

_____

_____

3. Why is it important to decrease external stimuli for the client with an anxiety disorder?

_____

_____

_____

4. Why is the client with an anxiety disorder advised to avoid caffeine, nicotine, or stimulating drugs such as non-prescription diet pills and cold and allergy medications?

_____

_____

_____

Activity F *Answer the following questions related to caring for clients with anxiety disorders.*

1. What are the manifestations of panic disorder?

_____

_____

_____

2. What are the manifestations of an obsessive-compulsive disorder?

_____

_____

_____

3. Describe the purpose and side effects of beta-adrenergic blocking agents.

_____

_____

_____

4. What assessments will the nurse include when caring for the client with an anxiety disorder?

_____

_____

_____

5. What interventions can the nurse use to decrease the client's anxiety?

_____

_____

_____

Activity G *Think over the following questions. Discuss them with your instructor or peers.*

1. What physical manifestations would cue you that your client is experiencing an escalating level of anxiety?

_____

_____

_____

2. Your client's chart reveals that a T3, T4, blood chemistry panel, and drug screen were performed prior to admission. Why would these laboratory tests be performed?

_____

_____

_____

3. What high-priority nursing diagnoses and interventions would you identify for a client diagnosed with an anxiety disorder?

_____

_____

_____

4. What educational information related to nutrition would you provide to your client with an anxiety disorder?

_____

_____

_____

Activity H *Read the following case study. Use critical thinking skills to discuss and answer the questions that follow it.*

A daughter accompanies her 72-year-old mother to her primary care physician's office. The daughter explains to the nurse that she has been worried about her mother since her father's death over 8 months ago. The client has become withdrawn, forgetful, and is not sleeping. The nurse begins by obtaining the client's vital signs and asks the client how she is feeling. The nurse notes that the client's blood pressure and heart rate are elevated from normal. The client verbalizes her fears over financial concerns, the loss of her spouse, the burden of care placed on her children, and her perceived deteriorating health. The client continues fidgeting while informing the nurse about her worries, fears, and anxieties. The nurse asks the client how long she has been experiencing this anxiety and to rate it on a scale of 0 to 10. The client rates it a 4 out of 10 and states that it has existed for 7 or 8 months. The nurse asks how the client is currently coping with her anxiety at home. The client admits to drinking alcohol daily to deal with her anxiety. The nurse completes the interview with a medication history and passes the information on to the physician. Once the physician examines the client, a diagnosis of generalized anxiety disorder is made and the client is prescribed buspirone (Buspar).

1. Why is the medication buspirone (Buspar) a good choice for this client?

_____

_____

_____

2. What precautions might the nurse provide the client when taking this medication?

_____

_____

_____

3. What level of anxiety is this client currently experiencing?

_____

_____

_____

4. In addition to medication treatment, what other treatment options are available to this client?

_____

_____

_____

SECTION 3: GETTING READY FOR NCLEX

Activity I   *Answer the following questions.*

1. Before administering a benzodiazepine to an older client with anxiety, which of the following are important for the nurse to assess? Select all that apply.
   1. Sleep problems
   2. Memory impairment
   3. Fall potential
   4. Renal function
   5. Digestive disturbances

2. What should the nurse teach a client who is recommended antianxiety drugs?
   1. Take the medication with food.
   2. Avoid antiinflammatory agents.
   3. Use caution when driving.
   4. Stop when you feel better.

3. Which of the following nursing actions are appropriate when teaching a client who is highly anxious? Select all that apply.
   1. Use a group setting.
   2. Talk in a loud voice.
   3. Use short sentences.
   4. Give brief instructions.
   5. Reduce area noise.
   6. Repeat information.

4. When the nurse assists a client with problem-solving, what action is most appropriate after the client identifies possible solutions?
   1. Select the best option for the client.
   2. Suggest the client consult the physician.
   3. Have the client examine the pros and cons of each option.
   4. Discourage the client from making an unwise decision.

5. When interacting with a client who is experiencing panic level anxiety, which nursing action is best?
   1. Avoid the client's personal space.
   2. Touch the client to show concern.
   3. Sit or stand close to the client.
   4. Seek help from additional staff.

6. When a nurse gathers information about a client's current health problems, which one of the following is a condition that can mimic signs and symptoms of anxiety?
   1. Type 2 Diabetes
   2. Hyperthyroidism
   3. Seizure disorder
   4. Crohn's disease

7. When interviewing a client with recurring panic attacks, which of the following is a common coping strategy?
   1. Alcohol abuse
   2. Social isolation
   3. Psychic numbing
   4. Compulsive rituals

8. What is the best nursing action when caring for a client with obsessive compulsive disorder who washes his hands for up to a half hour several times a day?
   1. Interrupt each hand washing ritual after 3 minutes.
   2. Allow the client to complete the hand washing ritual.
   3. Substitute hand sanitizer for the soap.
   4. Offer the client a moisturizer to soothe skin.

9. Which of the following nursing actions are most appropriate for reducing a client's anxiety? Select all that apply.
   1. Maintain a calm manner.
   2. Be available to the client.
   3. Vary the daily schedule.
   4. Engage the client in large-muscle activity.
   5. Help the client visualize a pleasant experience.

10. When caring for a client with post-traumatic stress disorder, which of the following nursing actions is appropriate?
    1. Correct the client's faulty belief system.
    2. Encourage the client to repeat positive self-statements.
    3. Avoid waking the client suddenly from sleep.
    4. Engage the client in some form of distraction.

69 Caring for Clients With Mood Disorders

LEARNING OBJECTIVES

1. Discuss common signs and symptoms of mood disorders.
2. Name three neurotransmitters that, when imbalanced, affect mood.
3. Identify the types of drugs that are used to treat depression and nursing considerations related to their administration.
4. Discuss the causes, manifestations, and management of serotonin syndrome.
5. Identify the reasons electroconvulsive therapy is used in the management of depression.
6. Name three interventions that are alternatives to electroconvulsive therapy for recurrent depression.
7. Give three criteria that indicate a high risk for suicide.
8. Discuss nursing measures that are useful in preventing suicide.
9. Discuss the nursing management of clients with depression.
10. Describe seasonal affective disorder, its treatment, and nursing management.
11. Explain bipolar disorder and describe its treatment and nursing management.

SECTION 1:   ASSESSING YOUR UNDERSTANDING

Activity A   *Fill in the blanks by choosing the correct word from the options given in parentheses.*

1. Brain function, and consequently mood, depends on the dynamic interplay of neurotransmitters. Moods are most likely generated by the _____ system, which is the center for emotions. *(limbic, ventricle, reticular activating)*

2. _____ block the reuptake of serotonin and norepinephrine. *(MAOIs, TCAs, Atypical antidepressants)*

3. The lag time before the client experiences a therapeutic effect is approximately _____ weeks after beginning MAOI therapy. *(1 to 2, 3 to 6, 6 to 8)*

4. _____ uses the application of an electric stimulus to one or both temporal regions of the head to produce a brief, generalized seizure. *(Electroconvulsive therapy, Vagus nerve stimulation, Deep brain stimulation)*

5. Treatment for seasonal affective disorder may include _____. *(electroconvulsive therapy, phototherapy, vagus nerve stimulation)*

6. _____, a chemical element, usually is the initial drug of choice for bipolar disorder. It controls depressive as well as manic symptoms in clients. *(SNRIs, Atypical antidepressants, Lithium)*

7. _____ may be prescribed for a brief period for clients with bipolar disorder in order to induce sedation and control hallucinations and delusions. *(Atypical antidepressants, Lithium, Antipsychotics)*

8. Providers must stress the importance of maintaining an adequate ingestion of _____ to all clients who rely on lithium to control their disorder. *(potassium, salt, calcium)*

Activity B   *Write the correct term for each description.*

1. A potentially life-threatening condition that results from elevated levels of serotonin in the blood secondary to drug therapy. _____

2. Consequence of combining an MAOI and substances containing tyramine. _____

3. Clinical evidence has shown that children and adolescents experience increased risk of suicidal thoughts and behavior with the use of these drugs. _____

4. This type of multiple reuptake inhibitor provides rapid relief of symptoms with fewer sexual side effects, as compared to SSRIs. _____

5. Treatment involves implanting an electrode in the brain through a small opening in the skull eventually connecting to a neurostimulator implanted under the skin near the clavicle, chest, or abdomen. _____

6. A mood disorder that has its onset during darker winter months and spontaneously disappears in the spring. _____

Activity C *Psychotherapy is a treatment for major depression. Match the types of psychotherapy given in Column A with their corresponding benefits given in Column B.*

Column A

_____ **1.** Psychodynamic psychotherapy

_____ **2.** Interpersonal psychotherapy

_____ **3.** Supportive psychotherapy

_____ **4.** Cognitive therapy

_____ **5.** Behavioral therapy

Column B

a. Facilitated by a bond that develops between the therapist and client; the empathy and trust help clients gain an understanding of their condition and the courage and support to overcome it.

b. Helps clients replace negative, and often illogical, ways of thinking with more positive outlooks.

c. Endeavors to change unhealthy ways of behaving; clients are rewarded verbally (or in some other way) when they alter their behavior positively.

d. Clients discuss their early life experiences to raise repressed feelings to a conscious level.

e. Helps clients learn about their disorder and treatment techniques, improve or develop new social skills, obtain positive reinforcement for progress, and gain encouragement to persevere.

Activity D *Describe the following moods and mood disorders.*

Mood or Mood Disorder	Description
Euthymia	
Dysthymia	
Cyclothymia	
Reactive (secondary) depression	
Unipolar depression (major depression)	
Psychotic depression	
Bipolar disorder (manic-depressive syndrome)	
Mania	
Seasonal affective disorder	

Activity E *Briefly answer the following questions.*

1. Describe the relationship between mood disorders and genetics.

_____

_____

_____

2. Describe the role of a neuroendocrine imbalance on mood.

_____

_____

_____

3. What are the signs and symptoms of serotonin syndrome?

_____

_____

_____

4. How do MAOIs work?

_____

_____

_____

5. What is a leading cause of noncompliance with SSRIs?

_____

_____

_____

6. How is transcranial magnetic stimulation utilized?

_____

_____

_____

7. Describe the etiology and pathophysiology of bipolar disorder.

_____

_____

_____

8. How are anticonvulsants used in the treatment of bipolar disorder?

_____

_____

_____

SECTION 2: APPLYING YOUR KNOWLEDGE

Activity F *Give rationale for the following questions.*

1. Why should alternative reasons for clinical findings be considered when a tentative diagnosis of depression is thought to be the cause for alterations in mood?

_____

_____

_____

2. Why might older adults be reluctant to admit depressive feelings?

_____

_____

_____

3. Why is closer observation of the depressed client essential once antidepressant therapy is initiated?

_____

_____

_____

4. Why are the MAOIs tranylcypromine (Parnate) and phenelzine (Nardil) the least prescribed category of antidepressants?

_____

_____

_____

5. Why are SSRIs currently the most prescribed group of drugs used to treat depression?

_____

_____

_____

6. Why is it essential that clients taking antidepressants consult with their physicians before taking herbal remedies or dietary supplements?

_____

_____

_____

7. Why is a history of substance abuse significant when assessing a client who has bipolar disorder?

_____

_____

_____

8. Why are clients who take anticonvulsants at risk for infection?

_____

_____

_____

Activity G *Answer the following questions related to caring for clients with disorders.*

1. Describe the hypothesis of neurotransmitter dysregulation in relation to major depressive disorder.

_____

_____

_____

2. What are the disadvantages of TCAs?

_____

_____

_____

3. Describe the differences in action of the following multiple reuptake inhibitors: SSRIs, SNRIs, and atypical antidepressants.

_____

_____

_____

4. Describe the nursing assessment of a suicidal client.

_____

_____

_____

5. Differentiate between the various types of bipolar disorders.

_____

_____

_____

6. Describe the signs and symptoms of bipolar disorder.

_____

_____

_____

Activity H *Think over the following questions. Discuss them with your instructor or peers.*

1. Antidepressant therapy has been initiated for your client diagnosed with major depression. You are concerned about the risk for suicide. What behavioral clues will you watch for to identify an increased risk for suicide?

_____

_____

_____

2. Your client is currently in a manic phase of a bipolar disorder. What high-priority nursing diagnoses and interventions will you implement to keep the client safe and healthy?

_____

_____

_____

3. The family members of a client diagnosed with bipolar disorder are feeling the strain of dealing with the disorder. What interventions and educational information can you provide to support the family members?

_____

_____

_____

4. A friend tells you he has been experiencing depression since his divorce 3 months ago. The friend is having difficulty adjusting to the changes in the family dynamics. What educational information would you provide?

_____

_____

_____

SECTION 3: GETTING READY FOR NCLEX

Activity I _Answer the following questions._

1. The nurse is correct in consulting the physician when which of the following could result in serotonin syndrome?
1. Coprescription of antidepressants from different classes
2. Abnormal blood levels of cortisol in the body
3. Weaning from one antidepressant before initiating another
4. Substances containing tyramine have been consumed

2. Which of the following will the nurse most likely detect when assessing a client immediately after electroconvulsive therapy? Select all that apply.
1. Headache
2. Seizures
3. Myalgia
4. Confusion
5. Impaired memory
6. Reddened scalp

3. When reviewing the trend and a client's current lithium level, which results indicate to the nurse that it is safe to administer the medication? Select all that apply.
1. 0.8 mEq
2. 1.2 mEq
3. 1.5 mEq
4. 1.8 mEq
5. 2.0 mEq

4. Which of the following statements reported to the nurse is an indication that a client with bipolar disorder may be experiencing an adverse effect from anticonvulsant drug therapy?
1. "I have a terribly sore throat."
2. "I have been having nightmares."
3. "I have lost my appetite for food."
4. "I have developed blurred vision."

5. Which health teaching is most appropriate for the nurse to provide to a client who has been prescribed lithium carbonate (Eskalith)?
1. Consume fluids liberally.
2. Restrict the use of salt.
3. Include fresh fruits daily.
4. Avoid hard, aged cheese.

6. When client with bipolar disorder shows signs of aggression and is at risk for violence, which nursing interventions is most appropriate for ensuring the safety of others?
1. Orient the client to events.
2. Suggest relaxation exercises.
3. Take the client to a secluded area.
4. Increase distracting stimuli.

7. When a nurse assesses a client who takes lithium carbonate (Eskalith), which of the following are side effects of the medication? Select all that apply.
1. Hand tremors
2. Ataxia
3. Polyuria
4. Skin rash

8. A nurse is teaching a client who takes an MAOI inhibitor that tyramine in some foods can cause a fatal side effect. What are examples the nurse should tell the client to avoid? Select all that apply.
1. Overripe bananas
2. Aged, hard cheese
3. Grapefruit
4. White bread
5. Red wine

9. Which of the following should the nurse consider as an indication of suicidal ideation when caring for a client with major depression?
   1. The client says, "Things are just not going my way."
   2. The client says, "I only have one friend in the world."
   3. The client gives away valued possessions.
   4. The client creates a living will.

10. Which of the following is most appropriate for the nurse to tell a client with seasonal affective disorder who will use phototherapy at home?
    1. Glance briefly at the artificial light throughout use.
    2. Stare at the artificial light for 30 minutes.
    3. Insert a standard fluorescent bulb in the device.
    4. Use the artificial light for no more than 15 minutes.

70 Caring for Clients With Eating Disorders

LEARNING OBJECTIVES

1. Differentiate normal eating from an eating disorder.
2. Name four types of eating disorders.
3. Describe two forms of anorexia nervosa.
4. Name the neurotransmitters, neurohormones, and other chemicals that affect the appetite and satiety center in the brain.
5. Discuss two reasons why most people with anorexia nervosa induce self-starvation.
6. Identify the tool used to evaluate a person's size in relation to norms within the adult population.
7. Give the healthy range for body mass index.
8. List four components of treatment for clients with anorexia nervosa.
9. Discuss the nurse's role in managing the care of a client with anorexia nervosa.
10. Give two examples of how people with bulimia nervosa compensate for binging.
11. Name two problems, besides nutrition, that are the nursing focus when caring for clients with bulimia nervosa.
12. Differentiate between binge eating disorder and compulsive overeating.
13. Discuss at least three psychosocial problems that may accompany overeating syndromes.
14. Describe nursing care for a client with binge eating disorder or compulsive overeating.

SECTION 1: ASSESSING YOUR UNDERSTANDING

Activity A *Fill in the blanks by choosing the correct word from the options given in parentheses.*

1. Eating disorders are most prevalent in young women between _____ years of age. *(10 and 17, 12 and 25, 15 and 30)*

2. _____ is characterized by an obsession with thinness that is achieved through self-starvation. *(Anorexia nervosa, Bulimia nervosa, Binge eating)*

3. A healthy body mass index is between _____. *(16 and 18.5, 18.5 and 24.9, 25 and 29.9)*

4. _____ is a technique in which clients with anorexia attempt to demonstrate weight gain by consuming a large volume of water and avoiding urination before being weighed. *(Water intoxication, Water loading, Water dumping)*

5. A nursing intervention for the anorexic client is to remove the eating tray after _____ minutes without commenting on uncomsumed food to avoid a power struggle. *(30, 45, 60)*

Activity B *Write the correct term for each descriptions.*

1. Almost universally, people with this disorder consider themselves obese despite appearing emaciated. _____

2. The body mass index in people with anorexia nervosa. _____

3. Characterized by a minimum of two episodes of secret food binges per week, followed by behaviors intended to prevent weight gain. The abnormal eating pattern must have persisted for at least 6 months. _____

4. Natural chemicals with marijuana-like properties that activate the appetite center. _____

5. Acts as a major anorexic signal that limits the consumption of calories, increases energy expenditure, and promotes sustained weight loss. _____

Activity C

Compare and contrast the physical, emotional, and behavioral manifestations of the eating disorders in the table based on the given criteria.

Eating Disorder	Physical	Emotional	Behavioral
Anorexia nervosa			
Bulimia nervosa			
Binge eating and compulsive overeating			

Activity D

Briefly answer the following questions.

1. Name the four types of eating disorders.

_____

_____

_____

2. Describe the two types of anorexia.

_____

_____

_____

3. What complications can result from anorexia?

_____

_____

_____

4. How is a body mass index calculated?

_____

_____

_____

5. Describe the two different types of bulimia.

_____

_____

_____

6. What complications can result from bulimia?

_____

_____

_____

SECTION 2: APPLYING YOUR KNOWLEDGE

Activity E

Provide rationale for the following questions.

1. Why are family and friends often not aware an eating disorder exists?

_____

_____

_____

2. Why might as few as 1500 calories/day be prescribed initially for the treatment of anorexia nervosa?

_____

_____

_____

3. When caring for an anorexic client, why does the nurse work with the dietitian to provide at least six to eight meals each day, beginning with a low caloric value and then gradually increasing the total calories?

_____

_____

_____

4. Why does the nurse formulate a contract with the bulimic client to seek out the nurse or another support person when the client feels the urge to purge?

_____

_____

_____

5. Why does the nurse advise the client with an overeating disorder to follow a sensible weight loss regimen prescribed by a dietitian in conjunction with nutritional counseling?

_____

_____

_____

6. Why do some clients with overeating disorders consider suicide or perform self-mutilation, such as cutting and burning themselves, pulling their hair, and interfering with wound healing?

_____

_____

_____

Activity F   _Answer the following questions related to caring for clients with eating disorders._

1. Discuss the etiology of anorexia.

_____

_____

_____

2. What are the assessment findings with anorexia?

_____

_____

_____

3. How is anorexia medically managed?

_____

_____

_____

4. Discuss the etiology of bulimia.

_____

_____

_____

5. What are the signs and symptoms of bulimia?

_____

_____

_____

6. What are complications of overeating syndromes?

_____

_____

_____

Activity G   _Think over the following questions. Discuss them with your instructor or peers._

1. What high-priority nursing diagnoses and interventions would you identify for the anorexic client?

_____

_____

_____

2. What nursing assessments would you perform to identify complications of anorexia?

_____

_____

_____

3. What high-priority nursing diagnoses and interventions would you identify for the client with bulimia?

_____

_____

_____

4. How would you provide support to the client diagnosed with an overeating disorder?

_____

_____

_____

SECTION 3: GETTING READY FOR NCLEX

Activity H *Answer the following questions.*

1. When caring for an emaciated client, which nursing assessment finding is most suggestive that the client has anorexia nervosa?
   1. There is the presence of lanugo.
   2. The enamel on the teeth is eroded.
   3. The voice is unusually hoarse.
   4. There are conjunctival hemorrhages.

2. Which of the following laboratory findings is the nurse correct in identifying as those that most often accompany anorexia nervosa? Select all that apply.
   1. Hypokalemia
   2. Hyperlipidemia
   3. Anemia
   4. Hypoalbuminemia
   5. Hyperglycemia

3. Upon assessing the psychosocial history of a client with anorexia nervosa, which characteristic is the nurse most likely to detect?
   1. Extreme vanity
   2. Negative attitude
   3. Drive for perfection
   4. Intense introversion

4. When reviewing the health history of a client with chronic anorexia nervosa, which of the following is the most likely complication the client may have experienced?
   1. Enlarged heart
   2. Gastric ulcer
   3. Degenerative joints
   4. Stress fractures

5. Which of the following nursing interventions is most appropriate to add to the nursing care plan of a client with anorexia nervosa?
   1. Restrict eating to a specific time and place.
   2. Allow the client unlimited time for eating.
   3. Weigh the client regularly, but randomly.
   4. Assign care to multiple different nurses.

6. When discussing a bulimic client's eating patterns, which of the following is most common?
   1. Eating when not hungry
   2. Overeating without guilt
   3. Binging in private
   4. Eating when bored

7. To which of the following organizations is it most appropriate for the nurse to refer a client with bulimia?
   1. American Dietetic Association
   2. Overeaters Anonymous
   3. National Institute of Mental Health
   4. Recovery International

8. Which of the following are measures the nurse should recommend to clients whose dentition may be damaged by chronic vomiting? Select all that apply.
   1. Rinse with water after vomiting.
   2. Drink water throughout the day.
   3. Brush with a fluoride toothpaste.
   4. Choose energy drinks when thirsty.
   5. Eat dried fruit when snacking.
   6. Take a calcium supplement.

9. Which instruction is best for the nurse to recommend to clients who are compulsive overeaters?
   1. Avoid strict dieting or fasting.
   2. Select foods labeled "sugar free."
   3. Supplement with OTC diet pills.
   4. Enroll in a weight loss center.

10. Which nursing suggestion is most likely to help a compulsive overeater comply with their food plan?
    1. Stock large amounts of low calorie items at home.
    2. Use a scale and measuring utensils for portion sizes.
    3. Eat alone to avoid being tempted by non-dieters.
    4. Consume 3 meals, but avoid snacking in between.

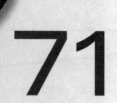

71 Caring for Clients With Chemical Dependence

LEARNING OBJECTIVES

1. Discuss the health and social consequences of substance abuse.
2. Name four commonly abused addictive substances and at least three other categories of abused drugs.
3. Discuss the meaning of withdrawal.
4. Explain tolerance and give two mechanisms by which it occurs.
5. List four steps in the progression toward chemical dependence.
6. List two physiologic explanations and two psychosocial factors for the development of chemical dependence.
7. Explain two ways abused drugs produce their effects.
8. Define alcoholism and list three accompanying symptoms.
9. Describe treatment and nursing management for clients with alcoholism.
10. List five potential health consequences of tobacco use.
11. Discuss the components of a successful smoking cessation program.
12. Discuss elements of recovery programs.
13. Describe signs and symptoms of cocaine and methamphetamine abuse as they relate to the manner of use.
14. Describe treatment and nursing management for clients addicted to cocaine and methamphetamine.
15. Discuss methods for managing opiate dependence.

SECTION 1: ASSESSING YOUR UNDERSTANDING

Activity A *Fill in the blanks by choosing the correct word from the options given in parentheses.*

1. _____ refers to the reduction in a drug's effect that follows persistent use. *(Withdrawal, Chemical dependence, Tolerance)*

2. _____ involves stabilizing the client with a sedative drug while alcohol is eventually metabolized. Withdrawal symptoms are controlled until they subside. *(Cross-tolerance, Detoxification, Psychotherapy)*

3. Alcoholism may result in _____ deficiency, which can lead to dementia. *(riboflavin, thiamine, niacin)*

4. _____ therapy prevents neurologic complications, known as Wernicke's encephalopathy and Korsakoff's psychosis, which affect memory and cognitive functions among alcoholic clients. *(Hydration, Sedation, Vitamin)*

5. _____ is the most heavily used addictive, mood-altering substance in the United States. *(Alcohol, Nicotine, Cocaine)*

Activity B *Write the correct term for each description.*

1. The use of a drug for a purpose that is different from its intended use. _____

2. A chronic, progressive, multisystem disease characterized by an inability to control the consumption of alcohol. _____

3. Therapy that deters drinking by causing unpleasant physical reactions when alcohol is consumed or absorbed through the skin. _____

4. Triad of elevated vital signs manifested during alcohol withdrawal that suggests the need for sedative medication. _____

5. Refers to the smoke given off by the burning end of a cigarette, pipe, or cigar and the exhaled smoke from the lungs of a smoker, which is potentially injurious to others. _____

6. Abuse of more than one substance. _____

Activity C   *Match the chemicals in Column A with their descriptions in Column B.*

Column A

_____ **1.** Cocaine

_____ **2.** Crack

_____ **3.** Methamphetamine

_____ **4.** Opiate

_____ **5.** Opioid

Column B

a. Causes sedation after initial euphoria.

b. A purified form of cocaine with a crystalline or rocklike appearance.

c. A term for synthetic narcotics.

d. An addicting stimulant that is made by combining over-the-counter medications containing ephedrine and pseudoephedrine with other chemicals such as ammonia, acetone, and lye.

e. A CNS stimulant obtained from the leaves of the coca plant.

Activity D   *Compare and contrast the commonly abused substances based on the given criteria.*

Substance Abuse	Signs and Symptoms	Complications
Cocaine and methamphetamine dependence		
Opiate dependence		

Activity E   *Briefly answer the following.*

1. Identify commonly abused drugs.

_____

_____

_____

2. Describe the etiology of alcoholism.

_____

_____

_____

3. How does dopamine contribute to addictive behavior?

_____

_____

_____

4. What complications may result from alcoholism?

_____

_____

_____

5. What is the purpose of psychotherapy for alcoholism?

_____

_____

_____

6. How can Alcoholics Anonymous benefit a client with alcoholism?

_____

_____

_____

7. What are the complications of smoking?

_____

_____

_____

SECTION 2: APPLYING YOUR KNOWLEDGE

Activity F *Give rationale for the following questions.*

1. Why is tobacco considered one of the most harmful substances?

_____

_____

_____

2. Why does tolerance occur?

_____

_____

_____

3. Why is initiating treatment one of the most difficult hurdles in treating chemical dependence?

_____

_____

_____

4. Why must glucose solutions be avoided until thiamine is administered to clients withdrawing from chronic alcoholism?

_____

_____

_____

5. Why must cocaine toxicity be treated immediately?

_____

_____

_____

Activity G *Answer the following questions related to caring for chemically dependent clients.*

1. What factors contribute to the development of substance abuse?

_____

_____

2. Describe the signs and symptoms of alcoholism.

_____

_____

_____

3. Describe the addictive quality of tobacco.

_____

_____

_____

4. What are the risks associated with environmental tobacco smoke?

_____

_____

5. Explain the purpose and advantages of methadone maintenance therapy.

_____

_____

_____

Activity H *Think over the following questions. Discuss them with your instructor or peers.*

1. Your client is admitted for an opiate overdose. What nursing care would you provide?

_____

_____

_____

2. The parents of a young adult who abuses substances are hopeless about their child's recovery. What educational assistance would you provide?

_____

_____

_____

3. Your client is chemically dependent. What high-priority nursing diagnoses and interventions would you identify?

_____

_____

_____

4. A client seeks information about smoking cessation. What educational information would you provide?

_____

_____

_____

SECTION 3: GETTING READY FOR NCLEX

Activity I *Answer the following questions.*

1. Which of the following indicates to the nurse that a client is an alcoholic?
  1. The client drinks at various social gatherings.
  2. The client drinks despite negative consequences.
  3. The client limits the number of drinks consumed.
  4. The client experiences a hangover after drinking.

2. Which of the following is an indicator of escalating withdrawal used by a nurse when assessing a client with alcohol dependence?
  1. Systolic blood pressure <100 mm Hg
  2. Temperature <100° F
  3. Heart rate >100 bpm
  4. Pain intensity rated >100

3. When providing postoperative nursing care, which of the following is most suggestive that a client suffers from alcoholism?
  1. The rating for pain is less than expected.
  2. Narcotic analgesics provide little pain relief.
  3. Arousal is difficult after receiving a narcotic.
  4. Vital signs escalate after administering a narcotic.

4. Which of the following must a nurse ensure before administering prescribed naltrexone (ReVia) to a client with a history of opiate dependence?
  1. Client has consumed adequate fluid.
  2. Client's pulse rate is at least 100 beats/minute.
  3. Client has been opiate free for at least 7 days.
  4. Client's diastolic blood pressure is at least 100 mm Hg.

5. Which of the following instructions should a nurse provide to a client with alcohol dependence after discontinuing disulfiram?
  1. Be compliant with periodic checks every week.
  2. Consume small amounts of alcohol in the interim.
  3. Continue rehabilitation by joining a support group.
  4. Avoid all forms of alcohol for at least 2 weeks.

6. Which of the following is the most serious complication that the nurse may detect when a client is withdrawing from alcohol?
  1. Hypotension
  2. Hand tremors
  3. Seizures
  4. Ataxia

7. When a nurse cares for a client with a history of chronic alcoholism, which of the following assessments is most suggestive that the client has portal hypertension?
  1. The client vomits bloody emesis.
  2. The client complains of constipation.
  3. The client has abdominal pain.
  4. The client's skin is jaundiced.

8. A physician orders naloxone (Narcan) 0.6 mg IV stat for a client with suspected opioid overdose. The nurse asks the LPN to co-check the dosage calculation. If the naloxone is supplied in a 10 mL multidose vial labeled 0.4 mg/mL, calculate the volume the nurse should administer.

9. Upon assessing a client who abuses methamphetamine, which of the following is the nurse most likely to find?
1. Needle track marks on the arms
2. Singed eyebrows and facial burns
3. Blackened and stained teeth
4. Ulceration of the nasal mucosa

10. The nurse advises a pregnant client to cease smoking cigarettes based on the fact that if continued, smoking can cause which of the following problems in the newborn infant?
1. Mucus accumulation in the airway
2. Acute respiratory failure
3. Sudden infant death syndrome
4. Periods of apnea at birth

72 Caring for Clients With Dementia and Thought Disorders

LEARNING OBJECTIVES

1. Differentiate between delirium and dementia, and give an example of a condition that causes each.
2. List five etiologic factors linked to Alzheimer's disease.
3. Discuss the pathophysiologic changes associated with Alzheimer's disease.
4. Name the first symptom of Alzheimer's disease.
5. Identify two methods for diagnosing Alzheimer's disease.
6. Explain the mechanism of drug therapy in Alzheimer's disease.
7. Describe nursing management for clients with Alzheimer's disease.
8. Name three characteristics of schizophrenia.
9. Describe two psychobiologic explanations for schizophrenia.
10. Differentiate between positive and negative symptoms of schizophrenia, and give two examples of each.
11. Discuss the medical management of most people with schizophrenia.
12. Name three examples of antipsychotic drugs and their mechanisms of action.
13. Explain the term *extrapyramidal symptoms*, and list four examples.
14. Describe a technique used to prevent non-compliance with drug therapy in clients with schizophrenia.
15. Describe the nursing management of clients with schizophrenia.

SECTION 1: ASSESSING YOUR UNDERSTANDING

Activity A Fill in the blanks by choosing the correct word from the options given in parentheses.

1. _____ is a sudden, transient state of confusion. (*Delirium, Dementia, Alzheimer's disease*)

2. _____ is a progressive, deteriorating brain disorder. (*Delirium, Alzheimer's disease, Schizophrenia*)

3. _____ is a thought disorder characterized by deterioration in mental functioning, disturbances in sensory perception, and changes in affect. (*Alzheimer's disease, Dementia, Schizophrenia*)

4. _____ produce their effects with reduced incidence of extrapyramidal symptoms. (*Traditional antipsychotics, Atypical antipsychotics, Typical antipsychotics*)

Activity B Write the correct term for each description.

1. Conditions in which decline in memory, thinking, and reasoning is severe enough to affect the daily life of an alert person. This condition is manifested by a gradual, irreversible loss of intellectual abilities. _____

2. These drugs, used to treat Alzheimer's disease, increase acetylcholine by inhibiting cholinesterase, the enzyme that degrades it. _____

3. These drugs are also called major tranquilizers or neuroleptics. _____

4. This antipsychotic medication has the potential adverse effect of dangerously depressing bone marrow function, and clients who take this drug must have a blood count done weekly or biweekly. _____

Activity C
Match the extrapyramidal side effects (EPS) given in Column A with their correct descriptions given in Column B.

Column A

_____ **1**. Akinesia

_____ **2**. Akathisia

_____ **3**. Dystonia

_____ **4**. Tardive dyskinesia

Column B

a. The client cannot sit or stand still.

b. The client appears to have symptoms of Parkinson's disease, such as hand tremors, stooped posture, and stiff shuffling gait.

c. The client makes involuntary muscle movements, usually in the face, such as tongue thrusting, continuous chewing, grimacing, lip smacking, or blinking; irreversible once manifested.

d. Sudden severe muscle spasm occurs, usually in the neck, tongue, or eyes.

Activity D
Compare and contrast the positive and negative signs of schizophrenia.

Positive Symptoms of Schizophrenia	Negative Symptoms of Schizophrenia

Activity E
Briefly answer the following questions.

1. What conditions can result in delirium? How is mentation restored?

_____

_____

_____

2. What is the etiology of early-onset and late-onset Alzheimer's disease?

_____

_____

_____

3. What is the action of *N*-methyl-D-aspartate (NMDA) antagonists? How effective are they?

_____

_____

_____

4. How is schizophrenia medically managed?

_____

_____

_____

SECTION 2: APPLYING YOUR KNOWLEDGE

Activity F *Give rationale for the following questions.*

1. Why are older adults at high risk for loss of identity?

_____

_____

_____

2. Why would institutionalization be necessary for a schizophrenic client?

_____

_____

_____

3. Why are anticholinergic drugs given to clients with schizophrenia?

_____

_____

_____

4. Why are depot injections used for the nonhospitalized schizophrenic client?

_____

_____

_____

_____

Activity G *Answer the following questions related to caring for clients with dementia and thought disorders.*

1. Describe the pathophysiology of Alzheimer's disease.

_____

_____

_____

2. What are the signs and symptoms of Alzheimer's disease?

_____

_____

_____

_____

3. Describe the pathophysiology of schizophrenia.

_____

_____

_____

4. What are the classic symptoms of schizophrenia?

_____

_____

_____

_____

Activity H *Think over the following questions. Discuss them with your instructor or peers.*

1. What high-priority nursing diagnoses and interventions would you identify for a client with Alzheimer's disease?

_____

_____

_____

2. What educational information would you provide to a client starting on a traditional antipsychotic medication?

_____

_____

_____

3. What high-priority nursing diagnoses and interventions would you identify for a client with schizophrenia?

_____

_____

_____

4. What educational information would you provide to family members caring for a client living at home with dementia?

_____

_____

_____

Activity I

Read the following case study. Use critical thinking skills to discuss and answer the questions that follow it.

A client presents to the emergency room (ER) with symptoms of confusion, dyspnea, tachycardia, severe muscle stiffness, and high fever. The client's family is extremely concerned and informs the nurse that the client was discovered exhibiting these symptoms while in bed at their apartment. The family also explains that the client has a mental illness called schizophrenia and takes risperidone (Risperdal) to treat it. They stated that the client's primary healthcare provider had just increased the client's dosage a week ago to better manage symptoms. The nurse obtains a complete history along with information about the client's current medications and the client's primary healthcare provider is notified.

1. Given the client's history, symptoms, and current medication, what is the likely cause of the client's sudden illness?

_____

_____

_____

2. Upon admission, what type of nursing care would you provide for this client?

_____

_____

_____

3. What precautions must the nurse keep in mind when caring for older clients who require antipsychotic medication?

_____

_____

_____

SECTION 3: GETTING READY FOR NCLEX

Activity J

Answer the following questions.

1. When a nurse assesses a client, which of the following suggest the client is experiencing delerium rather than dementia? Select all that apply.
   1. Symptoms occurred gradually.
   2. The client is awake and alert.
   3. The client has a high fever.
   4. The client is middle-aged.

2. When relatives of a client with Alzheimer's disease ask the nurse to identify a test that can indicate if they will develop the same disease, which test is most accurately identified?
   1. Computed tomography (CT scan)
   2. Magnetic resonance imaging (MRI)
   3. Electroencephalogram (EEG)
   4. Genetic chromosomal testing

3. The family of a client with Alzheimer's disease asks the nurse to explain the term apraxia that the physician used during a conference with them. What is the best nursing explanation?
   1. Apraxia means difficulty speaking.
   2. Apraxia means problems reading.
   3. Apraxia means difficulty walking.
   4. Apraxia means unable to perform activities of daily living.

4. Which of the following nursing care problems is the most difficult to manage due to the impaired ability to communicate experienced by client's with Alzheimer's disease?
   1. Adequate nutrition
   2. Bowel elimination
   3. Pain management
   4. Sleep requirement

5. Which of the following nursing interventions are most appropriate when caring for a client with impaired memory? Select all that apply.
   1. Ask family to participate in care.
   2. Reorient the client frequently.
   3. Keep a consistent daily routine.
   4. Assign consistent caregivers.
   5. Keep the environment well-lighted.

6. Which of the following is an appropriate nursing intervention when a client with schizophrenia expresses a delusional belief or experiences a hallucination?
   1. Leave the client alone throughout the hallucination.
   2. Inform the physician about the client's hallucination.
   3. Question the validity of the client's hallucination.
   4. Stay with the client throughout the hallucination.

7. What is the best nursing response when a client with schizophrenia says, "I need help with the aptronometer"?
   1. "I'll help you in a few minutes".
   2. "Can you bring the device to me?"
   3. "I don't understand your request."
   4. "Is there someone more qualified?"

8. Which of the following indicates to the nurse that a client who has been prescribed clozapine (Clozaril) should have the medication temporarily withheld?
   1. The client's leukocyte count is very low.
   2. The client's blood pressure is elevated.
   3. The client is experiencing polyuria.
   4. The client has a weight gain of 10 lbs.

9. A physician orders fluphenazine (Prolixin) decanoate 12.5 mg IM now and q 2weeks. Calculate the volume to administer when the medication is supplied in a 5 mL multidose vial labeled 25 mg/mL.

10. Which of the following is an indication to the nurse that a client receiving a typical antipsychotic medication is experiencing an extrapyramidal side effect?
    1. The client is unusually drowsy.
    2. The client has urinary retention.
    3. The client has a pounding headache.
    4. The client has a severe neck spasm.